Meg Blandford
(606) 223-2530

# CLINICAL MANAGEMENT OF COMMUNICATION DISORDERS IN CULTURALLY DIVERSE CHILDREN

**Thalia J. Coleman**
*Appalachian State University*

**Allyn and Bacon**
Boston • London • Toronto • Sydney • Tokyo • Singapore

*This work is presented with deep appreciation to my professional mentors
and friends: Dr. Thomas B. Abbott, Dr. Ronald E. Brown,
Ms. Quenie L. Crawford, Dr. Linda J. Lombardino, Dr. Michael Marlowe,
Dr. Harold Powell, Dr. Ida Stockman
And to the townsfolk of Lake View, South Carolina who collectively
sent me to college.
And in loving memory of my mother Mrs. Lily Mae Ford Coleman.*

*Executive Editor:* Stephen D. Dragin
*Editorial Assistant:* Bridget McSweeney
*Senior Editorial-Production Administrator:* Joe Sweeney
*Editorial-Production Service:* Walsh & Associates, Inc.
*Composition Buyer:* Linda Cox
*Manufacturing Buyer:* Dave Repetto
*Cover Administrator:* Jenny Hart

Copyright © 2000 by Allyn & Bacon
A Pearson Education Company
160 Gould Street
Needham Heights, MA 02494

*Library of Congress Cataloging-in-Publication Data*

Clinical management of communication disorders in culturally diverse
    children / [edited by] Thalia J. Coleman.
        p.      cm.
    Includes bibliographical references and index.
    ISBN 0-205-26724-6
    1. Communicative disorders in children.    2. Communicative
disorders in children Miscellanea.    I. Coleman, Thalia J., 1948– .
    [DNLM: 1. Communication Disorders—therapy—Child—United States.
2. Cultural Diversity—United States.    3. Early Intervention
(Education)—United States.    WL 340.2 C6408 1999]
RJ496.C67C556    1999
618.92'855—dc21
DNLM/DLC
for Library of Congress                                          99-34179
                                                                     CIP

Printed in the United States of America

10   9   8   7   6   5   4   3   2   1        03   02   01   00   99

# CONTENTS

# FOREWORD

In terms of the information available to persons who provide therapeutic services to a diverse population, this book takes a road less frequently traveled. The authors are professionals who have had extensive clinical experiences with individuals from the groups to which these chapters are devoted. Many of those persons have been underserved; others may have been misserved. The information in this book can do much to improve both of those situations.

This book will be valuable to the extent that it helps to (1) remove stereotypical perceptions of persons from formerly "unfamiliar" groups and (2) replace them with a genuine appreciation of the differences among us. Even though the authors have written about clinical intervention with persons who may be off the beaten path of our usual clients, they are not writing about a monolithic group. Rather, these potential clients are subgroups of subgroups, which makes them unique individuals. They should be served by professionals who at least appreciate and accept their differences. The professionals need, most of all, an open mind. This comes from information and understanding.

The very competent authors of the chapters in this book do not have all of the answers; however, they do present some provocative ideas that can initiate dialogues among service providers. A number of positives can result from these dialogues that can affect clients, clinicians, and the environment in which they interact.

In regard to the environment, information from this book, if used properly, can help to disprove some myths, objectify some perceptions, and remove some stereotypes. All of these changes can reduce possible sources of tensions and produce more open communication. For the professional, the information that follows can remove apprehensions, thereby freeing the individual to function with more confidence. For the clients, the results could mean an increase in the quantity and an improvement in the quality of services received. The overall consequence: more benefits for the client and more professional satisfaction for the clinician, that is, a more effective intervention process for all concerned.

## ESTABLISHING EFFECTIVE PROFESSIONAL RELATIONSHIPS WITH INDIVIDUALS FROM NONMAINSTREAM POPULATIONS

Nonmainstream populations are those whose members, for one or more reasons, are not included in the American "middle class." The reasons are neither age nor gender specific. The exclusion of individuals or groups from the American middle class may be completely or partially a function of their income, education, ethnicity, religion, history, occupation, place of residence, or tradition. The critical criterion is that they have been isolated sufficiently, be it over time or distance, for there to have developed a real lack of understanding between the groups in some important aspects of their lives.

In the past, these inaccurate or incomplete understandings may have led to "official" interpretations that were misleading and, subsequently, to actions that were inappropriate, counterproductive, and even insulting. As a result, there may now be some mistrust of and negative suspicions about any interactions with professionals who are perceived as representing the middle class. To be effective, one must move beyond unfortunate preconceptions to an atmosphere of mutual trust and understanding—to the extent possible. There may always be some uneasiness, but there should not be enough to prevent a frank exchange of the essential information.

Developing positive interpersonal relationships is seldom easy and never simple. The process becomes more challenging when the persons involved are interacting with each other only on a professional level, and the interaction is limited to a single activity, event, or concern. In such instances, the participants may not have the benefit of other shared experiences from which they may derive information and reach mutual understandings. This chasm widens if, as is most likely, the participants are from different cultural, ethnic, socioeconomic, or age groups.

Each of the groups above has values that are unique in some way. The variations among these groups increase with the presence of subdivisions. Each client represents an infinite variety. That is not always the case with the professional. The backgrounds of the individual professionals may not have the same range of differences from the norms. Actually, professional training obliterates some of the individual differences.

The aforementioned factors create an absolute necessity for the professional to develop an information base about the community in which he or she will work or the one from which his or her clients will come. Among the areas about which information will be sought are: demographics, economy, history, housing patterns, politics and religion, and speech patterns. Even though the group data gathered about the community will not tell specifically how to react to an individual client, they will provide a foundation on which intervention strategies can be developed. Such data enable the speech-language pathologist to approach the client with more confidence.

There must be trust and understanding between client and clinician if they are to work effectively toward resolution of any issue or the accomplishment of any objective. The clinician needs valid information about the client's concerns. The most direct, and ultimately most fruitful, method is to ask the client forthrightly for the needed information.

Because the clinician will probably be a stranger to the client, there is some information that will not be obtainable early in the relationship. It is preferable to be patient and work to develop trust so that the information can be obtained from the primary source. To seek alternative sources could be counterproductive. If the client learns that he or she is being discussed with someone else, the flow of information could be cut off completely.

Rapport must be established without showing undue familiarity too quickly. A must to avoid is addressing adult or elderly clients by their first names. This can be especially grating if the client is a senior citizen and the clinician is a peer of his or her grandchildren.

The clinician should never patronize the client. A possible lack of education does not necessarily indicate a lack of common sense or a diminution of the person's ability to "read" a new acquaintance and ascertain his or her motives. The clinician should be clear about the information that he or she hopes to obtain and the reasons for wanting it. Be truthful. There should be no reason for a hidden agenda.

## SOME COMMENTS ON RELATING TO CLIENTS FROM DIFFERENT CULTURES

Avoid patronizing the client. The use of a seeming unnatural speech pattern suggests that you are talking down to a listener. Characteristics of an unnatural speech pattern include switching from a mainstream to a non-mainstream dialect when talking with the client and using "slang" words

viii   *Foreword*

that are really foreign and inappropriate in that particular situation. These acts detract from the building of trust because they brand the speaker as a fake.

There are some facts of life that you must face.

1. Experiences are not universal. The fact that something is true for you (the clinician) does not make it true for everyone else.
2. The ability to communicate well with speech and language is not of equal importance to everyone. That ability does not make a significant difference in the lives of everyone; consequently, it is not always valued.
3. When the resources available to a given family are paired with the needs, the necessary prioritization may not make the needs of the children, no matter how special, the paramount ones.
4. Everyone does not discuss feelings, life, or perceptions in great detail. Sometimes a statement such as, "I don't like that," is the extent of the description. Pressing for more details before the clinician knows the client can be counterproductive.
5. You do not have to like all patients, but you must accept and respect them. The patients do not have to meet your approval.
6. The fact that a particular opinion, statement, or observation from the client does not seem meaningful to you does not reduce its meaningfulness to the client. Listen to what the client is saying.
7. Comparing the client's performance negatively with that of someone else from the same environment as a motivating device may not be motivating at all.
8. Be observant during the interview. Get cues from the client's responses to your questions and actions. Factors to observe:

    a. Variations in speed of responses
    b. Changes in directions of responses
    c. Certainty or uncertainty in responses
    d. Signs of tension, or the lack thereof
    e. Tone of voice
    f. Receptiveness or resistance to questions

*Harold Powell, Ph.D.*
*ASHA Fellow*
*Retired Chairperson, Department of Speech-Language Pathology*
*and Audiology, South Carolina State University*

# ABOUT THE AUTHORS

**Rhoda L. Agin**, Ph.D., is Professor of Communicative Sciences and Disorders at California State University-Hayward and Owner-Director of Communication Associates in Berkeley, California. Dr. Agin specializes in voice disorders and therapeutics. She received the Post-Doctoral Fellowship in Communicative Diversity in Multicultural Populations at Howard University in Washington, DC and served as the voice specialist at ASHA conferences on "Teaching Cultural Diversity Within the Professional Education Curriculum." She is co-author of *Guide to the Pronunciation of Asian Names*. Dr. Agin was Visiting Professor of Voice at the Department of Communicative Disorders of the Sackler School of Medicine at Tel Aviv University, Visiting Professor of Speech at the Department of Orthodontics of the School of Dental Medicine at Tel Aviv University, and Director of the International Students Program of the California State University System at Hebrew University in Jerusalem, Israel. Her current interests include vocal dynamics and disorders in culturally and linguistically diverse populations.

**Sheila J. Bridges**, Ph.D., is an assistant professor in the Department of Counseling and Communication Disorders at North Carolina Central University in Durham, North Carolina. She specializes in augmentative and alternative communication and cultural diversity. Her clinical work, teaching, and research experiences have focused on service delivery to culturally and linguistically diverse families, ethnographic assessment, and family-centered services. During her eighteen years of professional practice, Dr. Bridges has provided numerous presentations on AAC and cultural diversity at national and state conferences and conventions and serves on professional boards and committees. She is an executive staff member of the National Black Association for Speech-Language and Hearing and editor of ECHO, the professional publication of the association. Sheila received a B.S. degree from the University of Massachusetts-Amherst, an M.A. from Bowling Green State University, and her Ph.D. from Michigan State University.

**Thalia J. Coleman**, Ph.D., is Professor of Communication Disorders and Assistant to the Provost for Women's Concerns at Appalachian State University in Boone, North Carolina. Dr. Coleman was the principal investigator for a research project to study language performance of preschool children in remote/rural areas of South Carolina. She has presented numerous seminars, workshops, and short courses at state, regional, and national conferences and conventions. Dr. Coleman's current areas of interest include culturally appropriate service provision to families with preschool children who have special needs. She is a multicultural consultant for several state/regional boards and task forces. During her 27-year career in higher education, she has supervised students in Head Start centers and public schools, served as administrator of a university clinic, and been a consultant to SLPs in public schools and private practice.

**Thomas Crowe**, Ph.D., is chair and professor in the Department of Communicative Disorders and Director of the Center for Speech and Hearing Research at The University of Mississippi. He is also Director of Speech and Hearing Services at Baptist Memorial Hospital-North Mississippi. Dr. Crowe is president of a private practice and is a Fellow of ASHA. He established and formerly directed both the Center for Enhancement of Rural Life at The University of Mississippi and the Communication Disorders Laboratory in the Mississippi Department of Corrections.

**Linda McCabe-Smith**, Ph.D., is an assistant professor and clinical supervisor at Southern Illinois University at Carbondale. Dr. McCabe-Smith's doctoral focus was on communication disorders in multicultural populations. She has published in the area of language development among African American children. Her research emphasis relates to Head Start and public school programs.

**Lemmietta McNeilly**, Ph.D., is an Assistant Professor in the Department of Communicative Disorders, College of Health Professions at the University of Florida. Since 1992, she has served as the Multicultural Issues Consultant to the National Speech Language Hearing Association Executive Council. She has conducted numerous national-level presentations regarding working with families of children with language delays from culturally diverse groups and has authored several articles in that area. She also has served as Director of Speech and Hearing in hospitals and as director of an early intervention program. Dr. McNeilly received her doctoral degree from Howard University, which integrates information on cultural and linguistic diversity throughout its curriculum. Dr. McNeilly's research areas include language disorders in young children from culturally and linguistically diverse populations.

**Thomas E. Midgette**, Ph.D., is an Associate Professor of Education in the Department of Counseling and Communication Disorders at North Carolina Central University. Dr. Midgette has taught/counseled at the University of Arkansas, University of Akron, Michigan State University, Pitt Community College, and schools in North Carolina, Michigan, and Ohio. Dr. Midgette has published over forty articles and reviews in the areas of multicultural education, counseling, psychology, and human development. He serves on the Journal Advisory Committee for *The Journal of Intergroup Relations*. He is an ad hoc reviewer for the *Research Association for Minority Professors Journal*.

**Corine Myers-Jennings**, Ph.D., is an Associate Professor in the Department of Special Education and Communication Disorders at Valdosta State University. She has taught in the area of speech-language pathology for twenty-one years. For seventeen of those years she has worked with clients and taught students from culturally diverse and underserved populations. Dr. Myers-Jennings' research, teaching, and clinical interests are in the area of child language and phonological development and disorders. She is particularly interested in issues concerning child language/phonology with culturally diverse and underserved populations and has done extensive research and clinical work in rural areas.

**Barbara Pullen-Smith**, M.P.H., is Executive Director of the North Carolina Office of Minority Health. She provides leadership and develops initiatives to improve the public health system's ability to respond to the specific needs of racial and ethnic minorities. She works closely with the seven DEHNR health divisions, offices, local health departments, and other public and private agencies and organizations, including minority community-based organizations, in a collaborative and advocacy role to insure that minority health issues are addressed. She has made numerous presentations to community groups, administrators, policymakers, and students on challenges and opportunities regarding the health status of minorities.

**Tommie L. Robinson**, Jr., Ph.D., is Director of the Scottish Rite Center for Childhood Language Disorders in the Department of Hearing and Speech at the Children's National Medical Center in Washington, DC and an assistant professor of pediatrics at The George Washington University School of Medicine and Health Sciences. He specializes in the assessment and treatment of children with speech fluency disorders. Dr. Robinson has served on various boards and committees of ASHA and is a legislative councilor. He is an ASHA Fellow and presently serves on the board of directors for the National Black Association for Speech, Language, and Hearing. Dr. Robinson received his B.A. and M.S. degrees from The University of Mississippi and his Ph.D. degree from Howard University.

**Diane M. Scott**, Ph.D. served as the Director of the Office of Multicultural Affairs at the American Speech-Language-Hearing Association from 1993 until early 1997. She has published articles and made presentations on issues concerning sickle cell disease and hearing impairment, aging and hearing loss, hearing science and cultural diversity, and cultural competence. Dr. Scott has recorded a videotape entitled "Managing Diversity." Presently she is a visiting associate professor in the Department of Communication Disorders at North Carolina Central University, where she also serves as the campus coordinator for the North Carolina Consortium for Distance Education in Communication Sciences and Disorders.

**Lori Stewart-Gonzalez**, Ph.D., is an associate professor at the University of Kentucky in Lexington. Dr. Gonzalez was born in a small town in eastern Kentucky and worked in rural areas for a number of years in a variety of settings. Her research interests include communication issues in rural populations and phonological development and disorders in young children. She is currently investigating characteristics of Appalachian dialect.

**Wanda Woods**, M.P.H., is Assistant Director of the North Carolina Office of Minority Health. She also functions as resource development/conference planner/training liaison for the Office of Minority Health. She has an extensive history as a health educator, project coordinator, trainer, and author. In her current position Woods provides consultation and technical assistance to a variety of state, regional, and local public health agencies; colleges/universities; community-based organizations; and public/private health agencies in the design and implementation of minority health programs/initiatives.

**Johnny R. Wilson**, Ph.D., Director of Upstate Telecommunication Services with the Spartanburg Regional Healthcare System, is a communication technology specialist with both technological and literary expertise. He is a scientist, former university professor, and writer with over twenty years of university teaching and international healthcare management experience. Dr. Wilson received his B.A. in English and his M.S. in Speech and Hearing Sciences from the University of North Carolina at Durham, NC. He earned his Ph.D. in Speech Science and Speech Communication from Florida State University. Dr. Wilson has written several articles and made presentations on vocal and speech differences that are associated with cultural, ethnic, linguistic, and sociological factors in both children and adults.

**W. Freda Wilson**, Ph.D., CCC-SLP, is the Director of Rehabilitation and Sports Medicine at Spartanburg Regional Rehabilitation Center. She has over twenty years of national and international university teaching and healthcare management experience. Dr. Wilson is a Fellow of the American Speech-Language-Hearing Association. She lectures, writes, and researches in the areas of multicultural communication, international affairs, neurogenics, language development and disorders, and healthcare management. Dr. Wilson received a B.A. in Speech-Language Pathology and Audiology from South Carolina State University and her A.M. and Ph.D. from the University of Illinois.

# INTRODUCTION

Demographic data shows that the United States is increasingly becoming a pluralistic society. Furthermore, the "minority" population in the United States is projected to increase. According to the 1990 Census, more than 60 million people fall into one minority group or another, reflecting dozens of different cultures (ASHA, 1994). Simultaneously, the majority white population will increase at a slower rate and will thus become a smaller proportion of the entire U.S. population. Currently in the United States approximately one in four Americans identifies with a minority group. In at least 14 percent of homes in our nation, a language other than English is spoken (Owens, 1992). Washington, DC demographer Martha Farnsworth Riche was quoted as saying, "'Normal' is no longer everyone being White, everyone being a family. The old community—the middle class, Leave-it-to-Beaver community—simply isn't going to be there, and the rhetoric associated with it isn't going to bring it back" (What is a real American? 1992, p. 2A). Cole (1989) reported that minorities represent more than 50 percent of the population in at least one state, twenty-five U.S. cities, and numerous U.S. counties. She further commented that although there are many unknowns that may impact upon these projections, we know that our nation will become less and less European and increasingly more pluralistic.

The American Speech-Language-Hearing Association (ASHA) estimates at least 3.5 million speakers of various "minority languages" have speech, language, or hearing disorders that are related to the use of a minority language (1994). While the demographic characteristics of our nation are changing rapidly, those of ASHA members have remained relatively constant; individuals from diverse backgrounds comprise only 4 to 5 percent of the membership of ASHA. Consequently, middle-class white speech-language pathologists will be called upon to serve increasing numbers of individuals with communication disorders from diverse backgrounds (Campbell, Brennan, & Steckol, 1992; Keough, 1990). Although it is possible for white speech-language pathologists to be sensitive to the needs of clients from diverse backgrounds, cultural differences between speech-language pathologists and their clients may create barriers to appropriate and effective clinical practice (Cary, 1992).

## PREPARATION TO SERVE A DIVERSE SOCIETY

Several researchers have studied the preparedness of ASHA-certified speech-language pathologists and audiologists to provide clinical services to individuals from diverse backgrounds (Campbell, 1986; Cary, 1992; Coleman & Lieberman, 1995; Keough, 1990; Taylor, 1989). According to the 1988 ASHA Omnibus Survey, only 17 percent of ASHA members reported that they had specific graduate course work pertaining to communication disorders in multicultural populations. The combined results of the above studies found that 83 to 91 percent of the ASHA-certified respondents, working in a variety of settings across the United States, did not feel competent to evaluate persons with limited English proficiency; 68 percent did not feel competent to evaluate speakers of nonstandard English; and 83 percent had no professional education about the assessment and management of communication disorders in diverse populations. These data clearly indicate that the majority of ASHA-certified speech-language pathologists may not be qualified to provide services to almost one-fourth of our nation's population (Coleman & Lieberman, 1995; Taylor, 1989).

To address this deficiency in the sensitivity to and the knowledge of cultural and linguistic diversity in the academic preparation of speech-language pathologists, the Executive Board of ASHA approved the Multicultural Action Agenda 2000 in 1991. That agenda consisted of strategies for addressing the changing needs of a pluralistic society. The task force that drafted the plan pointed out that most course content in speech-language pathology and audiology pertains to the dominant middle-class, standard-English-speaking population. Among the action steps recommended were the inclusion of coursework on and clinical practice with individuals from diverse backgrounds as well as increased emphasis on research on the communication disorders of the populations (ASHA, 1990; Coleman & Lieberman, 1995). Since 1993, educational programs in communication sciences and disorders have been required to include coursework about the communication disorders of individuals from diverse backgrounds in the program of study leading to ASHA certification.

Results of a survey conducted by Coleman and Lieberman (1995) suggest that training programs in communication disorders may not be doing an adequate job of ensuring that students who graduate from those programs are sensitive to and knowledgeable of cultural and linguistic diversity. Some university programs have begun to introduce awareness of cultural and linguistic diversity to student clinicians. However, research findings support the conclusion of Taylor (1989) that clinical training in academic programs is woefully inadequate.

Only 49 percent of survey respondents reported that their programs required students to observe assessment of and intervention practices with clients from culturally diverse populations. Only 30 percent required students to obtain clinical clock hours with clients from diverse populations.

The volume of calls for help I receive from speech-language pathologists and other special-service providers further supports the conclusion that not enough is being done to prepare students to work with an increasingly diverse clientele. One recent graduate of an ASHA-accredited university program reported that she felt "robbed." She commented on the changing demographics of our nation and on projections that may mean that soon one-third or more of our caseloads will consist of individuals from minority populations. She also expressed her concerns about what will happen to the credibility of our profession if we continue to provide services to culturally diverse populations knowing that we do not have the necessary preparation (Hunter, 1989).

Federal mandates, including The Education for All Children Act of 1975 (PL 94-142), make it illegal to use assessment instruments and strategies that unfairly penalize people who are from culturally or linguistically different backgrounds. Several individuals have discussed the importance of using culturally appropriate intervention strategies as we employ current best practices in the professions of speech-language pathology (Adler, 1993; Anderson, 1991, Battle, 1998, Taylor, 1990, Taylor & Payne, 1991). Clearly there is a need for more information that will help clinicians and educators be more qualified to help those they serve.

## PREVIOUS CONTRIBUTIONS OF SCHOLARS

Those of us who work in the helping professions are deeply indebted to several scholars who have published books, chapters, and journal articles providing excellent insight into general characteristics of racial, ethnic, and cultural groups (e.g., Adler, 1990; Anderson, 1992, 1994; Battle, 1998; Campbell, 1994; Cheng, 1991; Cole, 1989; Damico & Damico, 1993; Ellis, 1994; Iglesias & Anderson, 1993; Taylor, 1986a). Others have provided extremely valuable information about the nature of linguistic differences among certain culturally diverse groups and the implications for speech-language pathologists (Butler, 1994; Friedlander, 1993; Seymour & Bland, 1991; Stockman, 1993; Westby, 1994; Wilkerson, 1994; Wolfram, 1993). These scholars agree that we are just beginning to amass a body of knowledge regarding normal development of speech and language skills in people from "different" backgrounds. All issue an urgent call for more research and the development of local norms.

## STATEMENT OF THE PROBLEM

It is an awesome, and perhaps impossible, task for any one book to include all of the information needed in order to achieve cultural competence. Some of the books now being used serve as rich resources of information about professional ethics and characteristics of certain minority groups (Adler, 1992; Battle, 1998; Hanson & Lynch, 1990; Screen & Anderson, 1994; Taylor, 1986a, 1986b). They are available and being used as textbooks and references for courses now being taught by professors in some communication disorders programs. As has been discussed above, there remains a large proportion of speech-language pathologists who are not being exposed to that information. Furthermore, even those who benefit from that kind of exposure are seeking more knowledge about how they can apply that information in their everyday interactions with others.

Suggestions have been offered for modifications of traditional assessment and intervention strategies. Some of these suggestions are quite specific. Most, however, are more general in nature and often appear in lists of "culturally sensitive" behavior. Often the listed suggestions are presented with no explanation or elaboration. For example, one commonly offered suggestion is "use culturally appropriate materials." An individual who has had very little training on cultural diversity and little or no interactions with individuals who are "different" may need help deciding what is culturally appropriate. Without elaboration and explanation, the suggestions may be subject to misuse or misinterpretation. The lists contain only facts. Those facts are interpreted from the perspective of the person reading them. If readers interpret the information based on an ethnocentric perspective, the appropriate strategies be ignored, misused, or misapplied.

## NATURE AND SCOPE OF THIS BOOK

This text focuses on clinical application of research findings on communication differences and disorders in culturally diverse children (preschool and school-age).

People with a little background knowledge about cultural diversity will find this book to contain a wealth of information that will help them as they engage in clinical activities. Individuals who already have considerable knowledge about cultural diversity will benefit by having so much information about clinical strategies and procedures in a single source. In addition to a rich review of strategies previously published by other scholars, readers will find innovative suggestions for assessment and intervention of communication disorders in culturally diverse children. Unique aspects of this book include chapters on rural service delivery, interagency collaboration, culturally different learning styles, and strategies for working with families.

Case studies and vignettes are included with the chapters to provide opportunities for students to practice applying the principles discussed. Study questions and activities are provided at the end of chapters to help students focus on key issues and important concepts discussed in the chapters. The case studies, vignettes, and study questions may also be used to stimulate discussions and facilitate group learning opportunities within class settings.

Some information about characteristics, beliefs, and values of various racial, cultural, and ethnic groups is provided in chapter 14 of this text. However, issues directly related to clinical or educational practices will be the primary focus of the other chapters. The writers have chosen to focus on discussing values and belief systems of culturally and linguistically diverse groups primarily as they would have a direct impact upon appropriate clinical interactions, assessment procedures, interpretation of test results, goal setting, and teaching strategies and activities. This book was written specifically for early interventionists and speech-language pathologists. However, it would be a valuable reference tool for all special-service providers who work with children from culturally diverse backgrounds.

In a work of this nature, with many scholars collaborating on a single project, the finished work itself becomes a lesson in diversity. The authors live and work in different parts of the country; represent different racial, ethnic, and cultural backgrounds; and have engaged in an array of scholarly and clinical activities related to issues of cultural diversity. They may sometimes use slightly different terms to refer to similar concepts, and, even though they generally agree regarding service delivery to culturally different individuals, their own unique experiences are reflected in their approaches to dealing with the various subjects about which they have written. We view this diversity of writing styles and approaches as an asset rather than a liability to this project. It is our belief that this provides an additional opportunity for students to experience first-hand the richness of diversity that exists even among scholars who share a strong commitment to culturally appropriate service delivery.

Readers may find some redundancy of information across chapters. We have attempted to keep this to a minimum. However, we did not try to eliminate all redundancy for at least two reasons:

**1.** We believe that some repetition of information, presented by different writers in slightly different ways, can serve as a tool to enhance learning, especially for individuals who are being exposed to that information for the first time. One strategy that is often suggested for facilitating generalization or transfer of newly acquired skills and information is the use of redundancy; to teach the same thing in a variety of different ways employing different people in different settings. Students should benefit from having repeated exposure to the same or similar information from slightly different perspectives.

**2.** It is important to address certain issues in any discussion of culturally appropriate service delivery. In some instances, total elimination of redundant information may have fostered confusion as some readers would have been forced to "dive right in" to the discussion at hand with no review of or elaboration on key terms, concepts, and issues pertinent to the chapter. Not all readers of an individual chapter would have read all of the previous chapters where there was discussion of those key terms, concepts, and issues.

Several terms and concepts with which one should be familiar in order to provide appropriate services to individuals from backgrounds that are not white or middle-class are discussed in chapter 1. As discussed above, writers sometimes use slightly different terminology to refer to similar concepts. Chapter 1 is an attempt to address this issue. Key terms and concepts used throughout this textbook are defined as they are used by its contributors. Chapter 2 deals with issues and considerations regarding work with individuals who are "different." There is considerable discussion of assumptions we make about people whose race or culture differs from ours and how those assumptions affect our attitudes as we interact with them. Suggestions are offered for making adjustments in the previously held assumptions so that our attitudes may change. This should result in a change in our professional behavior.

There are volumes of research studies documenting that learning styles are culturally based. A discussion of how we can and should apply this information as we work with children from "different" backgrounds is presented in chapter 3.

Many special services are provided for children by members of teams. Team members may represent several agencies and may themselves be from different backgrounds. Culturally based professional practices will influence service delivery systems within and across agencies. In order for the services provided to be the most effective, there must be coordination of those services among the various agencies involved. Issues regarding interagency service provision are discussed in chapter 4. The author discusses possible barriers to culturally appropriate service delivery and provides several suggestions for fostering better relations across agencies.

Most states are now requiring services to be provided to families with very young children who are at risk for or have developmental disabilities. Chapter 5 deals with current best practices in early intervention when working with families from culturally and/or linguistically diverse populations. Valid assessment is not only good, as well as ethical, clinical educational practice, it is required by federal law. Chapter 6 examines the appropriateness of some of the most popular methods of assessments in schools and clinical facilities. Suggestions for culturally sensitive and culturally fair assessment strategies are offered. The suggestions include all aspects of assessment from evaluating caregiver–child interactions and family strengths and needs to determining intervention goals.

Service-delivery options for individuals who live in remote rural areas are presented in chapter 7. The author briefly reviews some of the problems unique to rural service delivery. Most of her discussion focuses on possible solutions. She presents examples of models that have been used successfully. These models may be adjusted and adapted to the needs of specific rural areas in various states.

Chapters 8 through 13 provide information concerning intervention decisions and practices for specific communication disorders. Clinical strategies are suggested for working with culturally diverse preschool and school-age children who have language, phonological, voice, fluency, and hearing disorders. The phonology chapter includes some discussion of how to make distinctions between dialectal variations and speech sound disorders. An extensive discussion of dialects is not presented in this book. We have chosen to focus on discussions about treating *communication disorders*. A reading list that begins on page xxii identifies excellent resources for professionals who want to read more on the subject of dialects. Chapter 14 relates to working with culturally diverse children who use augmentative/assistive technology for communicative purposes.

## CONCLUDING STATEMENT

The American Speech-Language-Hearing Association issued a Position Paper on Social Dialects in 1983. That report declared that:

1. No dialectal variety of English is a disorder or pathological form of speech or language.

2. The traditional role of the speech-language pathologist has been to provide services to those who have communication disabilities.
3. In order for speech-language pathologists to conduct accurate assessments of communicative disorders, they must have certain competencies that allow them to distinguish between those aspects of linguistic variation that represent communication differences and those that represent communication disorders.
4. The speech-language pathologist who has the necessary competencies may provide *elective* services to speakers of nonstandard English who do not have a communication disorder.
5. The speech-language pathologist who has the necessary competencies may serve in a consultative role to educators who work with speakers of social dialects (ASHA, 1983).

ASHA published its Position Paper on Clinical Management of Communicatively Handicapped in Minority Language Populations in 1985. In addition to reinforcing guidelines presented in the 1983 position paper, this document presented several guidelines for providing clinical services to individuals from minority language populations.

According to the two position papers, cultural variables may influence how speech-language pathology and audiology services are accepted by people with culturally/linguistically diverse backgrounds. Furthermore, the assessment of many aspects of speech, language, and hearing of these individuals requires specific background and skills (ASHA, 1983, 1985). The collective focus of the authors of this book has been to discuss many of the variables that may have an impact on the nature of service delivery and on how these services are received by people from diverse cultural backgrounds. In addition, we have provided specific information about what to do and how to do it in order to facilitate culturally competent service delivery.

## REFERENCES

Adler, S. (1990). Multicultural clients: Implications for the SLP. *Language, Speech and Hearing Services in Schools, 21*, 135–139.

Adler, S. (1992). *Multicultural communication skills in the classroom.* Old Tappan, NJ: Longwood Division, Allyn & Bacon.

Adler, S. (1993). Nonstandard language: Its assessment. In S. Adler, *Multicultural communication skills in the classroom.* Boston: Allyn & Bacon.

American Speech-Language-Hearing Association. (1983). Social dialects: A position paper. *Asha, 25* (9), 23–24.

American Speech-Language-Hearing Association. (1985). Clinical management of communicatively handicapped minority language populations. *Asha, 27* (6), 29–32.

American Speech-Language-Hearing Association. (1990). Multicultural professional education in communication disorders: Curriculum approaches. In L. Cole (Ed.), *Multicultural literacy in communication disorders: A manual for teaching cultural diversity within the professional education curriculum*. Rockville, MD: Author.

American Speech-Language-Hearing Association. (1994). LET'S TALK: I know the answer, I just didn't recognize the question! *Asha, 61*, 51–52.

Anderson, N. B. (1991). Understanding cultural diversity. *American Journal of Speech-Language Pathology, 1*, 9–10.

Anderson, N. B. (1992). Understanding cultural diversity. *American Journal of Speech-Language Pathology, 1*, 11–12.

Anderson, R. T. (1994). Cultural and linguistic diversity and language impairment in preschool children. *Seminars in Speech and Language, 15*, 115–124.

Battle, D. E. (1998). *Communication disorders in multicultural populations* (2nd ed.). Boston: Butterworth-Heinemann.

Butler, K. (1994). *Cross-cultural perspectives in language assessment and intervention*. Gaithersburg, MD: Aspen Publishers.

Campbell, L. R. (1986). *A study of the comparability of master's level training and certification needs of SLPs*. Doctoral dissertation, Howard University, Washington, DC. Dissertation Abstracts International, 46, 10B. (University Microfilms # 85-28, 727).

Campbell, L. R. (1994). Learning about culturally diverse populations. *Asha, 36*, 40–41.

Campbell, L. R., Brennan, D. G., & Steckol, K. F. (1992). Preservice training to meet the needs of people from diverse cultural backgrounds. *Asha, 34*, 27–32.

Cary, A. L. (1992). Get involved: Multiculturally. *Asha, 34*, 3–4.

Cheng, L. L. (1991). *Assessing Asian language performance: Guidelines for evaluating limited English proficient students* (2nd ed.). Oceanside, CA: Academic Communication Associates.

Cole, L. (1989). E Pluribus Pluribus: Multicultural imperatives for the 1990s and beyond. *Asha, 31*, 65–70.

Coleman, T. J., & Lieberman, R. J. (1995). *Preparing speech-language pathologists for work with diverse populations: A survey*. Paper presented at the Annual Convention of the American Speech-Language-Hearing Association. Anaheim, CA.

Damico, J. S., & Damico, S. K. (1993). Language and social skills from a diversity perspective: Considerations for the speech-language pathologist. *Language, Speech and Hearing Services in Schools, 24* (4), 236–243.

Ellis, D. M. (1994). *Trends, projections and practices for developing cultural sensitivity*. Paper presented at the Multicultural Institute: Challenges in the expansion of cultural diversity in communication sciences and disorders. American Speech-Language and Hearing Association, Sea Island, GA.

Friedlander, R. (1993). BHSM comes to the Flathead Indian Reservation. *Asha, 35*, 29–30.

Hanson, M. J., & Lynch, E. W. (1990). Honoring cultural diversity of families when gathering data. *Topics in Childhood Special Education, 10*, 112–131.

Hunter, S. L. (1989). Multicultural professional educational education: Student perspectives. *Asha, 31*, 76–77.

Iglesias, A., & Anderson, N. (1993). Dialectal variations. In J. E. Berthal & N. W. Bankson (Eds.), *Articulation and phonological disorders* (3rd ed.; pp. 147–161). Englewood Cliffs, NJ: Prentice Hall.

Keough, K. (1990). Emerging issues for the professions in the 1990s. *Asha, 32*, 55–58.

Owens, R. (1992). Language differences: Bidialectism and bilingualism. In *Language development: An introduction* (3rd ed.). Boston: Allyn & Bacon.

Screen, R., & Anderson, N. B. (1994). *Multicultural perspectives in communication disorders*. San Diego, CA: Singular Publishing Company.

Seymour, H. N., & Bland, L. (1991). A minority perspective in the diagnosis of child language disorders. *Clinical Communication Disorders, 1*, 39–50.

Stockman, I. J. (1993). Variable word initial and medial consonant relationships in children's speech and articulation. *Perceptual Motor Skills, 76*, 675–689.

Taylor, O. L. (1986a). Historical perspectives and conceptual framework. In *Nature of communication disorders in culturally diverse populations*. San Diego: College Hill Press.

Taylor, O. L. (1986b). Treatment of communication disorders in culturally diverse populations. Austin, TX: Pro-Ed.

Taylor, O. L. (1989). Old wine and new bottles: Some things change yet remain the same. *Asha, 31*, 72–73.

Taylor, O. L. (1990). Language and communication differences. In G. H. Shames & E. H. Wiig (Eds.), *Human communication disorders* (3rd ed., pp. 126–158). Columbus, OH: Merrill.

Taylor, O. L., & Payne, K. T. (1991). *Language and communication disorders: An introduction* (4th ed.). Boston: Allyn & Bacon.

Westby, C. E. (1994). The effects of culture on genre, structure, and style of oral and written texts. In G. P. Wallach & K. G. Butler (Eds.), *Language learning disabilities in school-age children and adolescents: Some principles and applications* (pp. 180–218). New York: Macmillan College Publishing.

What is a real American? (1992, May 29). *USA Today*.

Wilkerson, D. (1994). *Differences in learning styles*. Multicultural Institute: Challenge in the expansion of cultural diversity in communication sciences and disorders. American Speech-Language-Hearing Association, Sea Island, GA.

Wolfram, W. (1993). A proactive role for speech-language pathologists in sociolinguistic education. *Language, Speech, and Hearing Services in Schools, 24*, 181–185.

## APPENDIX: RECOMMENDED READINGS ON DIALECTS/LINGUISTIC VARIATION

Adler, S. (1987). Bidialectalism? Mandatory or elective? *Asha, 29*, 41–44.

Adler, S. (1989). *An annotated bibliography relevant to nonstandard and non-native speakers of English*. Knoxville: University of Tennessee-Knoxville.

American Speech-Language-Hearing Association. (1985). Clinical management of communicatively handicapped minority language populations. *Asha, 26*, 55–57.

American Speech-Language-Hearing Association Committee on the Status of Racial Minorities. (1987). Social dialects position paper. *Asha, 29,* 45.

Battle, D. E. (1983). Social dialects. *Asha, 25,* 23–24.

Baugh, J. (1983). *Black street speech.* Austin: University of Texas Press.

Beile, K. M., & Wallace, H. (1992). A sociolinguistic investigation of the speech of African American preschoolers. *American Journal of Speech-Language Pathology, 1,* 54–62.

Campbell, L. (1993). Maintaining the integrity of home linguistic varieties: Black English vernacular. *American Journal of Speech-Language Pathology, 2,* 11–12.

Carver, C. (1987). *American regional dialects: A word geography.* Ann Arbor: University of Michigan Press.

Cheng, L. L. (1987). Cross-cultural and linguistic considerations in working with Asian populations. *Asha, 29,* 33–38.

Cheng, L. L. (1990). The identification of communication disorders in Asian Pacific students. *Journal of Child Communication Disorders, 13,* 113–119.

Cheng, L. L. (1991). *Assessing Asian language performance: Guidelines for evaluating LEP students* (2nd ed.). Oceanside, CA: Academic Communication Associates.

Cole, L. (1980). *Developmental analysis of social dialect features in the spontaneous language of preschool black children.* Ph.D. dissertation, Northwestern University.

Cole, L. (1983). Implications of the position of social dialects. *Asha, 25,* 25–27.

Cole, P. A., & Taylor, O. L. (1990). The performance of working class African American children on three tests of articulation. *Language, Speech, and Hearing Services in Schools, 21,* 171–176.

Craig, H. K., & Washington, J. A. (1994). The complex syntax skills of poor, urban, African American preschoolers at school entry. *Language, Speech, and Hearing Services in Schools, 25,* 181–190.

Fang, X., & Ping-an, H. (1992). Articulation disorders among speakers of Mandarin Chinese. *American Journal of Speech-Language Pathology, 1,* 15–16.

Fields, C. (1997). Ebonics 101: What we have learned. *Black Issues in Higher Education, 13,* 18–28.

Fletcher, J. D. (1983). What problems do American Indians have with English? *Journal of American Indian Education, 23,* 1–14.

Hamayan, E. V., & Damico, J. (1991). *Limiting bias in the assessment of bilingual students.* Austin, TX: Pro-ed.

Harris, G. A. (1985). Considerations in assessing English language performance of Native American children. *Topics in Language Disorders, 5,* 42–52.

Haynes, W., & Moran, M. (1989). A cross-sectional developmental study of final consonant production in Southern Black children from preschool through third grade. *Language, Speech, and Hearing Services in Schools, 20,* 400–406.

Iglesias, A., & Anderson, N. (1993). Dialectal variations. In J. E. Berthal & N. W. Bankson (Eds.), *Articulation and phonological disorders* (3rd ed., pp. 147–161). Upper Saddle River, NJ: Prentice Hall.

Jimenez, B. C. (1987). Acquisition of Spanish consonants in children. *Language, Speech, and Hearing Services in Schools, 18,* 357–363.

Kayser, H. G. (1989). Speech and language assessment of Spanish-English speaking children. *Language, Speech, and Hearing Services in Schools, 20,* 226–244.

Kayser, H. G. (1995). *Bilingual speech-language pathology: An Hispanic focus.* San Diego, CA: Singular.

Kayser, H. (1996). Cultural/linguistic variations in the United States and its implications for assessment and intervention in speech-language pathology: An epilogue. *Language, Speech, and Hearing Services in Schools, 27*, 385-387.

Mattes, L. J., & Omark, D. R. (1991). *Assessment of the bilingual bicultural child.* Baltimore: University Park Press.

Moran, M. J. (1993). Final consonant deletion in African American children speaking Black English: A closer look. *Language, Speech, and Hearing Services in Schools, 24*, 161–166.

Patterson, J. L. (1994). A tutorial on sociolinguistics for speech-language pathologists: An appreciation of variation. *National Student Speech-Language-Hearing Association Journal, 21*, 14–30.

Seymour, H., & Seymour, C. (1981). Black English and Standard American contrasts in communication development of 4- and 5-year-old children. *Journal of Speech and Hearing Disorders, 46*, 276–280.

Stockman, I. J. (1996). The promises and pitfalls of language sample analysis as an assessment tool for linguistic minority children. *Language, Speech, and Hearing Services in Schools, 27*, 355–366.

Taylor, O. L. (1972). An introduction to the historical development of Black English: Some implications for American education. *Language, Speech, and Hearing Services in Schools, 3*, 5–15.

Washington, J. A. (1996). Issues in assessing the language abilities of African American children. In A. G. Kamhi, K. E. Pollock, & J. L. Harris (Eds.), *Communication development and disorders in African American children* (pp. 35–54). Baltimore: Brooks.

Washington, J. A., & Craig, H. K. (1996). Dialectal forms during discourse of poor, urban, African American preschoolers. *Journal of Speech and Hearing Research, 37*, 816–823.

Williams, R., & Wolfram, W. (1976). *Social dialects: Differences versus disorders.* Rockville, MD: American Speech-Language-Hearing Association.

Wolfram, W. (1987). Are black and white vernaculars diverging? *American Speech, 62* (1), 40–48.

Wolfram, W. (1991). *Dialects and American English.* Englewood Cliffs, NJ: Prentice-Hall Regents.

Wolfram, W. (1993). A proactive role for speech-language pathologists in sociolinguistic education. *Language, Speech, and Hearing Services in Schools, 24*, 181–185.

Wolfram, W., & Fasold, R. W. (1974). *The study of social dialects in American English.* Englewood Cliffs, NJ: Prentice-Hall.

Wolfram, W. & Christian, D. (1989). *Dialects and education.* Englewood Cliffs, NJ: Prentice-Hall.

Wolfram, W., Detwyler, J., & Adger, C. (1992). *All about dialects: Instructor's manual.* Washington, DC: Center for Applied Linguistics.

# CULTURAL AND LINGUISTIC DIVERSITY: A DISCUSSION

# 1

# KEY TERMS and CONCEPTS

## THALIA J. COLEMAN and LINDA MCCABE-SMITH

Miscommunication and/or misunderstanding can occur when people attempt to communicate with each other using terminology that has not been clearly defined. Individuals sometimes debate issues until they realize they are not really disagreeing on the basic concept being discussed; they are simply using different words to talk about the same things. Sometimes terms, even though they refer to the same concept, are *loaded* with respect to underlying attitudes and implications. The purpose of this chapter is to offer definitions and/or explanations of some of the terms and concepts that are commonly used in discussions of cultural diversity. The terms are defined here as they are used by the contributors to this book.

**Cultural competence** as used in this text refers to the ability of service providers to recognize, honor, and respect the beliefs, interaction styles, and behaviors of the people we serve (Roberts, 1990, as cited in Battle, 1998). Other terms that are used interchangeably with cultural competence include *cultural sensitivity, cross-cultural competence, intercultural effectiveness,* and *ethnic competence.* They all refer to ways of thinking and behaving that enable members of one cultural, ethnic, or linguistic group to work effectively with members of another. Cultural competence is respect for difference, eagerness to learn, and a willingness to accept that there are many ways of viewing the world (Lynch & Hanson, 1992, p. 356). It actually involves movement along a continuum of achievements throughout a lifetime; it is an ongoing process. Cultural competence involves an awareness that people have different values, behaviors, and belief systems based on training and interactions encountered in their home communities. It also includes the willingness to respect those differences as just that—differences—without assigning judgments such as "right" or "wrong" to them. It also involves having specific knowledge of traditions/practices, preferences, social interaction patterns, and learning styles about groups from culturally different backgrounds. According to Green (1982, as cited by Lynch & Hanson, 1992), cross-cultural competence includes: (1) an awareness of one's own cultural limitations; (2) openness, appreciation, and respect for cultural differences; (3) a view of intercultural interactions as learning opportunities; (4) the ability to use cultural resources in interventions; and (5) an acknowledgment of the integrity and value of all cultures (p. 356).

Cultural competence is not adopting the values, attitudes, beliefs, customs, or behaviors of another culture. It does not suggest that one can categorize people into groups with no consideration for variability that exists within cultural groups. Finally, cultural competence does not mean knowing all there is to know about every culture (Lynch & Hanson, 1992). The National Maternal and Child Health Resource Center on Cultural Competency for Children with Special Health-Care Needs and Their Families presented a list of eight fundamentals of cultural competence. They are summarized in Table 1-1.

Anderson (1991) stated that it would be impossible for us to learn about all of the different cultures of our clients that we might encounter in our practice as speech-language pathologists. Anderson suggested that it would be more realistic to strive for increased cultural sensitivity toward people whose cultural background is different from our own. For example, it is important to know about major holidays, traditions, learning styles, general expectations for social interactions, and so forth, in order to establish and maintain appropriate clinical interactions. The sensitivity to and awareness of cultural differences combined with increasing knowledge of specific professional behaviors that are most appropriate when working with individuals from different cultures is what I mean when I use the term cultural competence. It does not mean knowing everything there is to know about everybody. Neither does it mean that culturally competent individuals will always do and say "the right thing" when interacting with people from backgrounds different from their own. It does mean that (1) the person is aware of and appreciative of differences across cultures, (2) he or she is willing to participate in activities designed to increase effectiveness when working with culturally diverse clientele, (3) he or she is willing to draw upon lessons learned about culturally based values, belief systems, and behaviors as he or she works with people, and (4) he or she always strives to work with families, and (when appropriate) respected members of the families' communities

**TABLE 1-1.   Fundamentals of Cultural Competence**

*We move forward along the continuum of cultural competence as we learn to honor the racial, cultural, ethnic, religious, and socioeconomic diversity of families by:*

1. Recognizing how important culture is in shaping people's values, beliefs, and experiences.
2. Understanding our own cultural values, beliefs, and behaviors and how we respond to individuals whose values and beliefs differ from our own.
3. Learning about the cultural norms of the communities of our clients and about the extent to which individual families share those norms.
4. Approaching each family with no judgments or preconceptions, enabling each family to define its own needs.
5. Helping families learn about the mainstream culture as it is reflected in the service system, so that they are able to use the system to meet their own needs.
6. Acknowledging that many families' previous experiences with racism and other forms of discrimination can affect future interactions with service providers.
7. Eliminating institutional policies and practices that may exclude families from services because of their race, ethnicity, beliefs, or practices.
8. Building on the strengths and resources of each child, family, community, and neighborhood.

Adapted from information provided by The National Maternal & Child Health Resource Center on Cultural Competency for Children with Special Health-Care Needs and Their Families, 1110 West 49th St., Austin, TX 78756, (800) 434-4453.

to develop intervention goals and strategies. Cultural competence incorporates the practice of providing services in the manner that is best understood and accepted by those who receive it (Roberts, 1990).

**Race** has traditionally been defined as that attribute that distinguishes one group of people from another based on physical characteristics (Kammey, Ritzer, & Yetman, 1990). Physical characteristics include such things as skin color, facial features (lips, nose, eyes, etc.), and texture of the hair. It is a socially defined concept that has now been discredited by some researchers because it is not a stable way of differentiating people. For example, African Americans have wide variations in skin color, hair texture, and facial features. Physical characteristics alone are not sufficient for categorization into a race (Gollnick & Chinn, 1998). The term *race* has no real meaning in a biological sense because there are no "pure" races. The crucial factor that designates any racial group is that the characteristics that distinguish it are socially defined. Criteria used to distinguish one racial group from another vary from one society to another (Kammey et al., 1990).

**Culture** is the shared beliefs, values, traditions, assumptions, and lifestyles of a group of people. It is an organization of objects, behaviors, and emotions that are learned through direct teaching, observation, or socialization. Its operation within individuals may be at varying levels of conscious or subconscious awareness. Culture consists of learned patterns of thoughts and behavior (Payne, 1986). Culture is the framework that guides and bounds life practices (Hanson, 1992, p. 3). It influences everything we do—from the way we dress for particular occasions to the way we think about issues and value people and things. It affects the way we dress, speak, act in various social settings and what we choose to eat. People of the same culture have shared beliefs (how we feel, think, and behave) and shared values (how we distinguish between right feelings, thoughts, and behavior and wrong feelings, thoughts, and behavior) (DeGaetano, Williams, & Volk, 1998). The culture of a group includes the entire way of life of a group. It includes the group's creativity and the way the group has given meaning to its existence through literature, language, music, art, philosophy, and technology (Grant & Sleeter, 1998).

Culture is associated with or influenced by factors such as age, gender, religion, education, child rearing practices, geographic region, and socioeconomic status. Many people use the terms *race* and *culture* synonymously, but culture is not the same as race. Two people may be of the same race and identify with two very different cultural groups.

**Ethnicity** is the social definition of groups of people based on certain cultural similarities. The term is sometimes confused with *race*. It is true that racial identity may be one aspect of ethnicity, but ethnicity also includes factors such as nationality, language, customs, and heritage. Members of ethnic groups are bound together by a common history. They may have distinct food habits, modes of dress, standards of beauty, political orientations, and patterns of recreation. Some ethnic groups in the United States are Chicanos, Italians, Jews, and white Anglo-Saxon Protestants (Kammey et al., 1990).

**Mainstream population,** as used in this book, refers to the group of Americans who are also known as the majority or dominant group. This group occupies a position of power and privilege. Traditional standards of "acceptable" behaviors, values, and belief systems have been established by this group of people.

**Minority group** is frequently used to refer to a group that is considered to be in a subordinate position of prestige, power, and privilege. People who belong to a minority group are often excluded from full participation in the life of a society (Kammey et al., 1990).

**Acculturation** is the process by which people assume attributes of a second culture (Battle, 1998). It is also called *enculturation* (Gollnick & Chinn, 1998) and involves varying levels of acceptance of selected rules for interactions and values of a culture other than one's own. People proceed through different stages of acculturation. These stages are just as recognizable as the stages of second language acquisition and the development of cognition. There are variations in the extent to which individuals adapt to a new culture and in the process of acculturation they experience (Hernandez, 1997). The process of acculturation may be emotionally challenging as individuals decide whether to adopt the language, values, and beliefs of a new culture and how many of the aspects of the new culture they will adopt. They may struggle between choosing loyalty to their own cultural heritage and taking on certain aspects of the new culture in order to be able to function successfully within mainstream society.

**Assimilation** is the process of abandoning one's own culture in favor of the values, behaviors, and belief systems of a new culture (Battle, 1998). It is characterized by acceptance of social codes, behaviors, and beliefs that were not part of the person's original culture. The American idea of assimilation carries with it the notion of a homogeneous society (Kammey et al., 1990). Battle (1998) discussed three models of assimilation and acculturation that have been used to explain cultural diversity in America.

- *Anglo-Conformity*. This model was the preferred model throughout much of this country's history. In this model, the "American way" was considered to be the only way. Immigrants were expected to abandon their unique cultural attributes, values, and practices and adopt traits of the dominant group (Kammey et al., 1990).
- *Melting Pot*. According to this model, citizens of this country form a new American culture in which no single culture is dominant. The new culture embodies a rich blend of all cultures. A new and different group that is distinct from any of the individual groups is formed (Kammey et al., 1990).
- *Cultural Pluralism*. This model promotes the idea of American citizens sharing a common citizenship and loyalty to this country while maintaining and fostering the unique languages, customs, and values of their own cultures.

**Bilingual** means having varying levels of functional proficiency in two languages. There is disagreement about how fluent speakers must be in each language (Gollnick & Chinn, 1998). True balanced bilingualism suggests equal proficiency in two languages (Owens, 1996). According to Owens, true bilingualism is rare. It is much more common for the individual to have more proficiency in one language than in the other.

**Value** is a standard used by people within a cultural group to assess the behavior of themselves and of others. Values are ideas about what is desirable, important, decent, and moral. They influence how we feel about prestige, family loyalty, status, our country, honor, and religion (Gollnick & Chinn, 1998).

**Learning style** (also called *cognitive style*) refers to the way individuals prefer to organize, classify, and assimilate information about their environment. It is a consistent pattern of behavior and performance that characterizes how individuals approach experimental events (Anderson & Adams, 1992; Swisher, 1992). Cognitive/learning style refers to the way people perceive, process, store, and retrieve information. Learning styles are culturally determined. Not all members of a cultural group learn in the same way, but patterns related to how members of different groups tend to approach tasks have been observed (Grant & Sleeter, 1998).

**Motivational style** is a preference for a set of goals and rewards that influence the behavior of individuals, and/or impact upon critical variables in their language and learning processes (Anderson & Adams, 1992).

**Ethnography** is the study of culture with the purpose of understanding why people live as they do and how they are alike or different from other cultures (Davis, Gentry, & Hubbard-Wiley, 1998). **Ethnographic approaches** to intervention help professionals learn what is most relevant to a family and facilitates improved professional–family relations. The ethnographic approach involves three methods for collecting data from families: literature reviews (e.g., medical records, therapy reports), interviews, and observations (Zarella, 1995).

**Ethnographic interview** is a process in which, from a sociocultural perspective, the interviewer comes to understand the social situations in which families exist and how the families perceive, feel about, and understand these situations (Westby, 1990, as cited in Moore & Beatty, 1992). Ethnographic interviewers tailor questions to the specific encounter, according to the needs of the situation (Moore & Beatty, 1992, p. 16).

**Ethnographic assessment** is dynamic. It requires examiners to

- Collect qualitative data through an initial interview and repeated observations
- Participate in the cultural context of the child being served
- Tap the multifaceted, complex patterns of verbal and nonverbal interpersonal communication across social contexts (Blackstone, 1993)

**Ethnocentrism** is the view held by people of a society that they are of central importance in the universe and therefore their ways of doing things are the right ways (Kammey et al., 1990, p. 680). Ethnocentricity is the tendency for one to believe that his or her way of doing things is better than that of those who do things differently.

**Service provision** is the sum total of agency and interagency actions and activities designed to meet an identified, perceived, or implied need. Service provision is the set of actions taken or followed by an agency in its effort to make services available to clients (Pullen-Smith, 1995).

**Cultural guides/mediators/brokers** are people from the cultural community who can guide service providers in culturally appropriate interactions with clients and their families. They could be community leaders, family members, friends of the family, or colleagues. Cultural mediators should be people who are trusted and respected by the families involved (Scott, 1998).

## STUDY QUESTIONS AND ACTIVITIES

1. Define the following terms:
   - cultural competence
   - race
   - culture
   - ethnicity
   - acculturation
   - assimilation
   - ethnographic assessment
   - ethnocentrism
2. React to the following statements. If the statement is true, explain why. If the statement is false, explain why.
   - Cultural competence is an ongoing process.
   - Cultural competence means adapting the values, attitudes, beliefs, customs, or behaviors of another culture.
   - A person's race can be determined by observing his or her skin tone, hair texture, and facial features.
3. Discuss Battle's (1998) models of assimilation and acculturation.
4. Read the following case example and complete the activity at the end.

   Lake View Academy is a prestigious private school (grades K–6) whose students had been white and middle-class until three years ago. The school administrators started experiencing problems in raising funds from local businesses due to their exclusivity. After several meetings to deal with the problem and in response to a mandate from their board of directors, the academy's admissions committee started admitting a few students from racially, ethnically, and socioeconomically diverse backgrounds. This year 25 of the 500 students enrolled at the academy were racially/ethnically different or from poor backgrounds. Some problems related to the diversity were noticed during the last academic year. For example, several of the teachers complained that it was much harder for them to teach their classes because the "minority" students were not as intelligent, did not show appropriate social behaviors, and had need of "cultural enrichment."

You have been asked to chair a committee to prepare a professional development activity for the faculty to help the teachers experience more success as they deal with culturally diverse students. Your committee has chosen the theme "Moving Toward Cultural Competence: Practical Applications for Classroom Teachers." Explain how you would develop your training session. Develop an outline showing the topics to be covered and describe activities you would include. What problems might you anticipate and how would you prepare to deal with them?

# REFERENCES

Anderson, N. B. (1991). Understanding cultural diversity. *American Journal of Speech-Language Pathology, 1,* 11–12.

Anderson, J. A., & Adams, M. (1992). Acknowledging the learning styles of diverse student populations: Implications for instructional design. In L. L. Border & N. V. Chism (Eds.), *New directions for teaching and learning: Teaching for diversity* (pp. 19–24). San Francisco: Jossey-Bass Publishers.

Battle, D. E. (1998). *Communication disorders in multicultural populations* (2nd ed.). Boston: Butterworth-Heinemann.

Blackstone, S. (1993). Clinical news: Cultural sensitivity and AAC services. *Augmentative Communication News, 6*(2), 3–5.

Davis, P. N., Gentry, B., & Hubbard-Wiley, P. (1998). Clinical practice issues. In D. E. Battle (Ed.), *Communication disorders in multicultural populations* (2nd ed., pp. 427–445). Boston: Butterworth-Heinemann.

DeGaetano, Y., Williams, L. R., & Volk, D. (1998). *Kaleidoscope: A multicultural approach for the primary school classroom.* Upper Saddle River, NJ: Prentice-Hall.

Gollnick, D. M., & Chinn, P.C. (1998). *Multicultural education in a pluralistic society.* Upper Saddle River, NJ: Prentice Hall.

Grant, C., & Sleeter, C. E. (1998). *Turning on learning: Five teaching plans for race, class, gender, and disability.* Upper Saddle River, NJ: Prentice Hall.

Hanson, M. J. (1992). Ethnic, cultural, and language diversity in intervention settings. In E. W. Lynch & M. J. Hanson (Eds.), *Developing cross-cultural competence: A guide for working with young children and their families* (pp. 3–18). Baltimore: Paul H. Brookes.

Hernandez, H. (1997). *Teaching in multilingual classrooms: A teacher's guide to context, process and content.* Upper Saddle River, NJ: Prentice Hall.

Kammey, K. C. W., Ritzer, G., & Yetman, N. R. (1990). *Sociology: Experiences changing society.* Boston: Allyn & Bacon.

Lynch, E. W., & Hanson, M. J. (1992). *Developing cross-cultural competence: A guide for working with young children and their families.* Baltimore: Paul H. Brooks.

Moore, S. M., & Beatty, J. (1995). *Developing cultural competence in early childhood assessment.* Boulder, CO: University of Colorado.

National Maternal and Child Health Resource Center on Cultural Competency for Children with Special Health-Care Needs and Their Families, 1100 West 49th St., Austin, TX.

Owens, R. E. (1996). Language differences: Bidialectism and bilingualism. In R. E. Owens, *Language development: An introduction* (pp. 398–426). Boston: Allyn & Bacon.

Payne, K. T. (1986). Cultural and linguistic groups in the United States. In O. L. Taylor (Ed.), *Nature of communication disorders in culturally diverse populations* (pp. 19–46). San Diego: College Hill Press.

Pullen-Smith, B. (1997). Provision of special services to culturally and linguistically diverse clientele. Workshop presented at Appalachian State University, Boone, NC. April, 1997.

Roberts, R. (1990). *Workbook for developing culturally competent programs for families of children with special needs* (2nd ed.). Washington, DC: Georgetown University Child Development Center.

Scott, D. M., (1994). Achieving excellence through diversity. It's a beginning. ASHA Convention Roundup: Asha supplement. Rockville, MD: American Speech-Language-Hearing Association.

Swisher, K. (1992). Learning styles: Implications for teachers. In C. Diaz (Ed.), *Multicultural education for the 21st century* (pp. 72–84). Washington, DC: National Education Association of the United States.

What is a real American? (1992, May 29). *USA Today.*

Zarella, S. (1995, January 23). Ethnographic approach to identifying client and family needs. *ADVANCE,* 6.

# 2

# CULTURALLY APPROPRIATE SERVICE DELIVERY: SOME CONSIDERATIONS

## THALIA J. COLEMAN and LINDA McCABE-SMITH

Several writers (e.g., ASHA, 1985; Battle, 1997; Cole, 1989; Crowe, 1997; Ellis, 1994; Gollnick & Chinn, 1998; Kammey, Ritzer, & Yetman, 1990; Lynch & Hanson, 1992; Owens, 1992; Taylor, 1986) have discussed the changing demographics of the United States. They contend that this country is no longer a "melting pot" where people from other countries come and leave behind the unique features of their individual cultures in order to blend with everyone who is called an "American." Some cultures work hard to maintain their individual identities. That enriches us all.

The 1990 Census reported that 61 million of the 248 million people in the United States were from culturally and linguistically diverse backgrounds. Thirty-two million Americans spoke one of many languages other than English (e.g., Spanish, Japanese, Laotian, Pakistani, Portuguese, Samoan, Russian). Over 6 million school-age children speak a language other than English at home (Hernandez, 1997). Of those coming from culturally and linguistically diverse backgrounds, the American Speech-Language-Hearing Association (ASHA) estimates that 10 percent have speech, language, or hearing disabilities (ASHA, 1996).

The speech-language pathologist or audiologist need not belong to a particular cultural group in order to provide the services needed by that group. Professionals whose cultural or linguistic backgrounds are different from their clients' can provide appropriate services if they have training and knowledge that enable them to distinguish between speech, language, or hearing disabilities and differences that are characteristic of a particular culture and language background (ASHA, 1996).

As mentioned in the introduction to this book, most ASHA-certified professionals believe that they do not have the knowledge base to provide appropriate intervention services to clients from culturally and/or linguistically diverse backgrounds. Each of the following chapters will address the "what" and "how" of culturally appropriate intervention practices. The focus of this chapter will be the "why" of the strategies we are suggesting for working with clients and families from nonmainstream backgrounds. We believe it is not enough to know "what to do." Our success as interventionists is grounded in our abilities to (1) show genuine interest in and concern for our clients, (2) establish effective professional relationships with them and their families, (3) adjust planned strategies to accommodate the motivation and abilities of our clients and/or their families, (4) adjust therapy and procedures to clients' culture and desires, (5) work effectively with professionals from a variety of other agencies, and (6) persuade others to joint us and/or support us as we try to implement innovations to traditional service delivery models. Before we can "sell" these innovations/modifications to others, *we* must first be firmly convinced that what we are doing is the right thing. The purpose of this chapter is to address issues that frequently surface during discussions about the clinical implications of the increasing cultural diversity among clients with communication disorders.

## THE NECESSITY OF ADDRESSING THE CLINICAL IMPLICATIONS OF CULTURAL DIVERSITY: HOW DOES CULTURAL DIVERSITY RELATE TO OUR PROFESSION?

For decades speech-language pathologists and audiologists have been engaged in discussions about the need for addressing issues of cultural diversity and the impact diversity may have on our traditional approaches and clinical intervention procedures. Current demographic trends have made it urgent that we increase our efforts to *do something* rather than just continue the discussions about the need (Adler, 1993).

Working with people on a personal level is a large part of what we do as speech-language pathologists and audiologists. To accomplish our goals, we must be able to establish effective relationships with clients, families, co-workers/team members, and professionals from other agencies.

What we think about the people with whom we interact on a regular basis, and how they perceive us, are important considerations as we strive to do our jobs better. Social and cultural factors are critical aspects of all clinical activities in speech-language pathology and audiology. They are present at the initial telephone clinical inquiry for information or scheduling and continue throughout the clinical process. Failure to recognize and take into account these factors can diminish the effectiveness of the services we provide to our clients. This is true even if we have state-of-the-art technology and use the most up-to-date clinical procedures (Taylor, 1992).

According to Cole (1989), numerous issues affect the service delivery process when differences across cultures are involved. She discussed eight multicultural imperatives that will affect the delivery of speech-language pathology and audiology services to multicultural populations when cultural or racial differences are involved. They are:

1. It is projected that one of every three children will be from a racial/ethnic minority by the turn of the century. It can be expected that at least one-third of the caseloads of SLPs and audiologists will be children from minority backgrounds.
2. Economically disadvantaged individuals are at greater risk for disabilities. The etiologies associated most frequently with many of these conditions overlap with conditions associated with poverty.
3. Individuals from culturally and linguistically different backgrounds have the same types of communication disorders as other groups, but the causes can be different.
4. Within each minority group there is considerable diversity. This makes it difficult to use standardized criteria to determine what is normal communicative behavior in any of these heterogeneous groups.
5. The degree to which traditional beliefs regarding disabilities and other health issues are retained by people in minority groups may vary considerably and could have significant impact on how certain treatment practices are perceived and received.
6. There is more potential for cultural conflict in clinical settings when the background of the service provider differs from that of the client.
7. Individuals from certain culturally diverse groups may have different preferences for service delivery than prevalent Western models.
8. There is much more linguistic heterogeneity in minority populations than there is in the mainstream group in America.

Cole (1989) concluded that the amount of success we experience in improving care and the quality of life to individuals with communications disorders from diverse backgrounds will depend on the "collective commitment and collective action at all levels: by ASHA, by state associations, within professional education programs, within local health service institutions, within local schools, and by each speech-language pathologist, audiologist, and communication scientist" (p. 70).

An additional imperative that has been addressed is the lack of ASHA-certified clinicians who are prepared to provide culturally appropriate service to an increasingly diverse population of clients and families. While the demographic characteristics of our nation are changing rapidly, the demographics of ASHA members who provide direct service have remained relatively constant. Individuals from diverse backgrounds comprise only 4 to 5 percent of the membership of ASHA. Consequently, middle-class white speech-language pathologists will be called upon to serve increasing numbers of individuals from diverse backgrounds who experience communication disorders (Campbell, Brennan, & Steckol, 1992; Keough, 1990). Although it is possible for white speech-language pathologists to be sensitive to the needs of clients from diverse backgrounds, cultural differences between speech-language pathologists and their clients may create barriers to appropriate and effective clinical practice (Cary, 1992). Diane Scott, a recent director of ASHA's Office of Multicultural Affairs, stated that it would be ideal if someone in need of our services received help from a knowledgeable and competent professional who speaks the same language and has similar cultural values. However, Scott explained that the cultural, language, and ethnic diversity that was once found only in the largest cities is now being found in smaller communities all over the country. She stated that these population changes may be creating a "cultural mismatch" between service providers and those they serve (Scott, 1994).

Some middle-class white Americans who speak English assume that the manner in which they think or speak is the only way or the right way (Owens, 1992). More than ever before, however, individuals from culturally different backgrounds are electing to retain their own values and belief systems. Those who are called upon to serve individuals from cultures different from their own are now challenged to reexamine the validity (or lack of it) of traditional assessment and intervention strategies. The increasing diversity of our society carries with it a need to prepare professionals who are able to provide quality services to racial/ethnic minorities with speech, language, and hearing impairments (Anderson, 1992; Scott, 1994). We must be aware of the possible impact of different values and beliefs on the success or failure of our clinical, professional, and educational interactions. Awareness of those differences will help us make necessary adjustments to facilitate cooperation, enhance positive interactions, and promote implementation of recommendations.

# THE INTERPERSONAL DIMENSION
# OF SERVICE DELIVERY

## *Ethnocentricity and Service Delivery*

The interpersonal dimension is a vital component of effective clinical management of any type of communication disorders (Taylor, 1990). Taylor believes that differences in the verbal and nonverbal rules used by speech-language pathologists and their clients can cause unintended episodes of insult, discomfort, or hypersensitivity. These episodes could adversely affect the interpersonal dynamics needed in order for us to effectively engage in professional activities with culturally or linguistically diverse clients. It is imperative, therefore, for us to make every effort to learn as much as we can about appropriate social and professional behaviors to use when we are serving individuals from cultures other than our own. One way to enhance our interpersonal skills is by being good observers. For example, we can observe clients' reactions to statements and make appropriate adjustments to our words and behavior. We can also seek the advice of cultural mediators when we are not sure about expectations regarding social interactions.

Ethnocentrism is the tendency for people of a society to believe they are of central importance in the universe and that their way of thinking and behaving is the "right way" (Kammey et al., 1990). There is a natural tendency for us to be ethnocentric; it helps us to organize our world, providing a consistent pattern to follow. Our own culture is treated as if it were *the* natural way to function in the world. We view the rest of the world through our cultural perspective, compare other cultures to ours, and evaluate others according to our standards (Gollnick & Chinn, 1988). We may assume that our values, belief systems, and behaviors are the "right way" of doing things. Consequently, those who exhibit different behaviors are assumed to be operating in a manner that is less admirable, not right, nonsensical, or substandard. Assumptions we make about people lead to attitudes that may have a negative impact upon our interactions with them and on the way we interpret behaviors we observe. For example, as professionals observe caregiver–child interactions, their own values or preferences could influence how they interpret interactions they see. If the interactions are not interpreted within the context of the family's culture, the conclusions could be inaccurate. Therefore, intervention strategies based on those conclusions would be inappropriate. For example, in some cultures, lack of direct eye contact is considered polite; direct eye contact is considered to be a challenge, especially to authority figures. A professional who believes direct eye contact is desirable might incorrectly assume that the family he or she is observing feels the same way. The interventionist might determine that "good" eye contact should be a therapy goal. This would not be an appropriate goal for that family because it conflicts with natural behavior within the family's culture.

## Bias, Stereotypes, and Prejudice

To comprehend the significance of ethnocentrism on the formation of assumptions, it is important to understand the nature of bias and prejudice. *Prejudice* is an adverse judgment or opinion formed beforehand or without knowledge or examination of the facts. It is the act of holding unreasonable preconceived judgments or convictions and may involve irrational suspicion or hatred of a particular group on the basis of factors such as race, gender, or religion (*American Heritage Dictionary,* 1996). Prejudice manifests itself in feelings of anger, fear, hatred, and distrust about certain groups of people (Gollnick & Chinn, 1998). Persons who are prejudiced may show bias in their actions regarding certain people and in interactions with those people. *Bias* is a preference or an inclination, especially one that inhibits impartial judgment. It may also be an unfair act or policy stemming from prejudice and may involve favoring some people or things over others (*American Heritage Dictionary,* 1996).

All of us have biases. We have preferences and dislikes (DeGaetano, Williams, & Volk, 1998). For example, we have favorite foods, music, relatives, sports, or friends. We show preferences for style of clothing, types of entertainment, or occupations. However, our own biases about how one should behave in certain situations could influence how we interpret the behavior of other people if we use our bias as "the norm" or for making judgments. On that basis, any behavior that is not compatible with what we deem to be the "right way" of behaving or performing may be misinterpreted by us as abnormal or substandard.

A *stereotype* is a belief that all people who belong to a particular group have similar characteristics (Kammey et al., 1990). Stereotypes are oversimplified opinions or images of entire groups of people. They are categorizations individuals make about other people to justify negative or positive feelings that they have about those people. There are stereotypes about people based on their race, gender, sexual orientation, profession, age, disability, and other factors (DeGaetano et al., 1998). Some examples of stereotypical beliefs are (1) Westerners are trend-setters, (2) Midwesterners are dull, (3) Northeasterners are brainy, and (4) Southerners are lazy (*American Heritage Dictionary,* 1996). There are common stereotypes regarding gender. For example, females are often thought of as emotional and not "in control" during stressful situations. Many people consider males to be better leaders, more objective, logical, and strong (Kammey et al., 1990). Such stereotypical beliefs lead to preferential treatment of males in some situations. People who believe men are better leaders and more "in control" might be inclined to give certain jobs to men, even when women with equal or better qualifications are available (DeGaetano et al., 1998). Pinkney (1984) stated that stereotypes result from our need for coherence, simplicity, and predictability in our lives. Pinkney believes that without stereotypes we would be faced with the necessity of having to interpret each new social situation as if it were the first time we had encountered such a situation. According to Pinkney (1984), stereotypes are a way of organizing information and observations. Stereotypes are not necessarily negative. As a person who is "Southern-born-and-bred," I rather enjoy the stereotypical notion of Southern hospitality. Pinkney (1984) believes prejudice is the consequence of negative feelings being attached to a stereotype.

People have stereotypical notions about people, places, and things. We may form these ideas based on what has been presented in the mass media (television, magazines, etc.) and based on our own limited experiences. It is always a mistake to generalize influence of culture (expressions, images, behaviors) about any particular member of a group, whether the group affiliation is based on race/ethnicity, gender, geographical region, or any other factor. Many variables significantly bear on individual variations within groups. One of those variables is the degree of acculturation or how much the individual has taken on the cultural characteristics of the dominant group. Some variations are the length of time spent in a given country, the nature and amount of interactions with people outside one's own group, socioeconomic status, extent of education, age, gender, and geographical region.

## Assumptions, Attitudes, and Adjustments

### Assumptions

Assumptions are ideas that are taken for granted or believed to be true without any proof (*American Heritage Dictionary*, 1996). Assumptions may develop based on hearsay, direct or indirect learning, or by a combination of those factors. Assumptions serve useful purposes. For example, many accurate clinical judgments are made based on observations after numerous experiences in similar situations. However, assumptions about individuals with whom we have had no previous contact should be avoided. Those assumptions could result in inappropriate professional interactions and/or inaccurate interpretation of data/behaviors. One real-life example involved a student clinician who conducted a diagnostic session with an African American male preschool child. The child had severe articulation errors. The student told the boy's parents that they should not worry about the errors because they were "probably just Black dialect." The clinician had become aware of some features of Black English and had made the assumption that all African Americans speak it. She made no attempt to discover whether the child was in fact a speaker of Black English. Neither did she seek to determine if all of the child's "different" speech sound productions were features of that particular dialect. In that particular instance, the student clinician's assumptions were wrong. The child's parents did not use Black English. The child's speech and sound errors were not features of a dialect. They were symptoms of a disorder.

Although assumptions about a group of people can be formed without interacting with anyone from that particular group, a negative encounter with an individual who is a member of a culture, race, or ethnic group different from our own can lead to the making of generalizations about that entire group. That is especially true when we have not had the opportunity to interact with many others with that particular background. Assumptions formed as a result of undesirable experiences, but in the wake of little or no opportunity to have positive interactions with people of the same group, may lead to experientially based assumptions. These assumptions may seem logical, especially if they are consistent with common stereotypes about the group in question.

Assumptions may also result from direct or indirect learning. *Direct learning* refers to those beliefs we are intentionally taught by parents, teachers, and significant others. They include what we read in textbooks, research articles, and other professional literature, and products of the popular press. They encompass what we glean from seminars, classes, talk shows or news broadcasts on radio and television, and other sources such as political speeches. For direct learning to occur, there must be someone who purposefully functions as an instructor and imparts specific knowledge to another person. The knowledge imparted does not have to be factual, but it must be presented in a manner that convinces the learner(s) that the information is important enough to understand and retain. That is, there must be a successful effort on the part of one or more individuals to have the learner(s) accept an idea as being truthful. *Indirect learning* may occur without any intentional use of words or actions on the part of one individual to teach another. A person may learn indirectly by observing a pattern of behaviors or hearing remarks repeated in similar contexts over a period of time. For example, if a child notices that a parent always locks the car doors when riding on certain streets or in certain neighborhoods, the child may interpret that behavior to mean those streets or neighborhoods are more dangerous than others. The child may further associate the streets or neighborhoods with the same group(s) of people who live there and conclude that those people are more dangerous than others.

### Attitudes

Cross-cultural interactions present a special challenge because they require us to work with clients who have different values and belief systems from our own and to avoid making judgments as to the superiority of one set of values/beliefs over another. We must be willing to engage in self-reflection in order to become more culturally aware. We must honestly assess where we are along the continuum of understanding, because we cannot afford to *assume* a degree of competency that we have not achieved. It is not enough for us to believe we are sufficiently aware of and sensitive to cultural differences. We need some means by which we can objectively evaluate our status as culturally competent service providers. Some tools are available to help us in this effort, such as the *Cultural Competence Tool For Self-Reflection* (Moore & Beatty, 1995); *The Self-Assessment Checklist for Personnel Providing Services and Supports in Early Childhood Settings* (Taylor, 1995); *Assessing Your Tolerance for Controversial Issues: An Exercise for Awareness and Growth* (Fromkin & Sherwood, 1976); and *Self-Appraisal: Cross-Cultural Counseling and Communication* (McFadden, 1995).

An attitude is a state of mind, feeling, orientation, or disposition (*American Heritage Dictionary,* 1996). According to Harris (1986), attitudes evolve from individuals' value systems and culture. She believes that these value systems are often

> so ingrained in a person's mind that his or her values become truth, usually not only for that particular person but for all humans. Practitioners must acknowledge the potential for differences in perception of the causes and meaning of disabilities, the elements necessary for and differences in the value of rehabilitation, and the differences between their own belief systems and those of their clients. (p. 229)

The United States is one of the most culturally diverse nations in the world. The United States is also a country in which conformity is valued and rewarded; diversity is sometimes discouraged or even feared. Prejudiced attitudes can emerge as discriminatory behavior that adversely affects some minority groups (Pinkney, 1984).

It is my belief that we may have acquired certain attitudes about certain groups of people based on common stereotypes and/or previous experiences with a few members of those groups. We may have acquired those attitudes without being conscious of their presence. However, those attitudes may have subtle, and not so subtle, influences on our behavior and on expectations we have regarding academic performance, social behavior, communication skills, and so forth. These attitudes may also be based on false assumptions. Some of the more common false assumptions that may lead to inappropriate attitudes and, consequently, to ineffective clinical interactions are:

- *We are all alike; people are people.* Current research on issues of cultural diversity focus on identifying cultural behaviors and important dimensions that are not related to categorizations of inferiority versus superiority. Perhaps, in an attempt to correct or compensate for some of the negative beliefs that emerged from research trends of an earlier era, some people have sought to minimize the differences between diverse populations. One current way of expressing this notion is the concept of a culture-blind or color-blind society. Although it is true that humans probably share many more similarities than differences across cultures, it would be a mistake to assume that all people share the same values and belief systems. If we assume that all individuals are alike, we may also assume that everyone's values and belief systems are the same. Thiederman (1991) believes that this attitude amounts to a negation of the uniqueness of individuals from culturally different groups and to denying the existence of other cultures. There are differences that would be important for us to be aware of as we strive to build professional relationships with individuals who do not share our own background. For example, not all people appreciate being addressed by their first names by people who are meeting them for the first time. In some cultures people of opposite genders do not shake hands with each other. Roles of family members differ considerably based on culture. If we are unaware of differences such as these, we will make mistakes that will hinder our professional interactions.
- *People of cultural backgrounds different from my own must have values and beliefs that are different from mine.* This is the opposite viewpoint from the one just discussed. The truth is along a continuum between the two extremes. There are many variables (education, SES, religion, geographic region, gender, etc.) within groups that have an impact on individuals' belief systems. People from different cultural backgrounds may share common experiences that have helped shape similar values and beliefs. For example, two people from the same racial or ethnic group may have very different standards for acceptable child rearing practices and may have opposing political viewpoints. On the other hand, two people of different genders, from different races, and from different geographical regions may share similar political perspectives and agree about how children should be raised within the family unit.

- *Racial or ethnic diversity is the same as cultural diversity.* It would also be a mistake to assume that we can determine whether people believe as we do about certain issues by looking at them. As was discussed in chapter 1, race, culture, and ethnicity are different factors. We must be careful not to assume sameness or difference based on group identity.
- *Difference equals deficiency.* Individuals who do not "conform to the norm" are not always appreciated for their differences. When nearly all of the norms have been established based on one group, all other groups who show different performance may be considered to be subjects for intervention. The purpose of the intervention would likely be to help members of the "deviant" group perform in a way that is closer to that of the dominant group and to adopt values and belief systems that are more consistent with its "acceptable behavior." The major problem with that approach is that it makes no allowance for culturally different behavior patterns, learning styles, and so forth. Furthermore, it does not take into account the fact that normalcy in one culture does not necessarily equate with normalcy in a different culture. Finally, we are still trying to determine what is normal in selected groups. For many diverse groups, no reported attempts have been made to determine "normalcy." There is an emerging database on some aspects of normal development for a few groups (Goldstein, 1995; Quinn, 1995; Seymour & Bland, 1991; Stockman, 1986). Until we can say with certainty what is or is not normal behavior for various cultural groups, we are continuing to compare apples to oranges and then proceeding to try to make apples more like oranges or vice versa.
- *The "common sense" syndrome.* Terms such as uncooperative, noncompliant, withdrawn, and "strange" have frequently been used to describe individuals. Often, when I have asked if the complainer had explained in detail his or her expectations to the "uncooperative" individuals, the response was, "Well, I just thought that was common sense!" As we work with individuals whose backgrounds are different from ours, we would do well to remember that what is "common sense" to us may not be "common sense" to others. That is especially true when we are working with individuals whose culture is not the same as ours.
- *What's right for me is right for you.* This is another example of ethnocentrism at work in our thinking and attitudes. Professionals base their perceptions of the client and the client's problems on assumptions that are relevant to the majority culture. They measure reality against

their own assumptions and values and by only superficially accepting cultural variations in clients (Battle, 1997). A conscious effort is required to overcome the effects of this attitude.

- *This is the way I have always done it.* This argument may be one of the most powerful reasons for us to reexamine traditional models of service delivery we provided to all populations, including those who belong to the dominant culture. Continuous expansion in knowledge of how speech and language is acquired is having significant impact on our understanding of normal communication skills and models of service delivery to people who have disabling conditions. Within the last decade alone, there has been an explosion of information available to us. This is an exciting time to take advantage of new information to become increasingly successful in our clinical and educational endeavors. However, it requires a willingness to change, to consider the possibility that some of the newer, different approaches to service delivery may be better for our clients and their families, and even for us! If we adopt this attitude for all our clinical activities, it will be much easier to make suggested modifications to traditional intervention strategies as we work with people from backgrounds that are different from our own.

### Adjustments to Old Attitudes

There are activities we can incorporate into classroom instruction and personal-growth activities to address change of old attitudes as we move along the continuum toward cultural competence. Some suggestions are to

1. Focus on both similarities among groups of people and areas of difference to facilitate a balanced approach and culturally appropriate strategies for clients and their families. One strategy to aid in facilitating a balanced approach is to discuss the topics: What is a typical family? How many families represented in the classroom consist of two-parent households, grandmother and grandchildren, and so on? Make a list of the different family structures. This, of course, can be modified to fit a particular environment or situation.

2. Continue to evaluate our own personal prejudices and biases and seek ways to minimize their impact on service provision to clients who do not share our cultural background. This can be done by utilizing tools such as those developed by Moore and Beatty (1995), Fromkin and Sherwood (1976), and McFadden (1995). One tool is the establishment of Diversity Learning Circles. These circles consist of small groups of individuals who know and trust each other

well enough to have frank discussions about diversity issues. They could read books or articles on the subject; view movies, films, and television shows; attend lectures on multicultural themes; and interview and/or interact with people from culturally different backgrounds. The group would then meet to discuss members' feelings about the selected experiences. A key element to the success of any such group would be a commitment on the part of each member to becoming more culturally competent. Without that commitment, the group could become just a means to complain about what upsets individuals about people who are not like them. Group members must feel free to openly discuss how they feel about issues being discussed. However, the focus of the group should be to help each member increase levels of cultural competency. Another version of this would be the buddy system approach. That approach would work in a similar manner to the learning circles but would involve only two or three people. Those "buddies" would become partners in an effort to increase their cultural awareness and sensitivity. They would be a support system for each other—monitoring each other's progress, encouraging participation in activities that would enhance cultural competency, listening to concerns, and offering advice.

3. Seek ongoing interactions with individuals from a variety of backgrounds and experiences. The more frequently we interact with people and situations that are unfamiliar to us, the more familiar (comfortable) we may feel in those encounters: for example, attend a local church, organize an international food day, conduct an informal interview with someone from a culturally different group. These interactions also help us learn the rules of social engagement (using first names versus formal forms of address, touching, proximity, etc.) used by people from culturally diverse groups. As we increase our familiarity with more and more people from certain cultures, we will recognize individual and group variations.

4. Engage in formal discussions about issues related to cultural diversity. Some people suggest that these discussions would be more open and productive if they are engaged in by people from "like" groups discussing an outside culture. Others believe it is important to include people in the discussions who are representative of the group being discussed. It is my belief that there is no one answer that would be applicable to every situation. The situation in which the discussion takes place should be comfortable enough for open and honest dialogue as we strive to grow in personal ways as culturally competent professionals.

5. Avoid generalizations. Generalization is a natural behavior in the growing process. Most generalizations that are made about people tend to be stereotypes, because they bind the massive diversity of humanity into a homogeneous society. The results are dehumanizing. Stereotyping is impossible to eliminate (Lynch & Hanson, 1992), but we can increase awareness of usage of generalized statements. To at least minimize this behavior professionals must first understand and define the term *stereotype* for themselves. Educators or in-service trainers could have participants write a stereotypical statement as they understand the term. Instruct individuals that the written statement may be a stereotypical statement they have heard or used. They should not use their names. The responses can be put in a basket. Following the writing activity have a discussion about stereotypes and the written responses. This activity may be used in training students and other professionals in diversity awareness and stereotyping.

6. Realize that developing cultural competence is an ongoing process. Educators are expected to guide students' awareness of their own thinking and that of others. Our purpose is not to impose our values on students; instead, we guide them in making choices based on expressed reasoning, problem solving, and decision making (Tiedt & Tiedt, 1990). Transformation in attitudes and the development of empathy take time; therefore, acquiring cultural competence is not possible within a short span of time. All of this is an ongoing process.

## Other Suggestions

Speech-language pathologists, audiologists, and other special-service providers can engage in a wide variety of activities to enhance their awareness and sensitivity to cultural differences. Some suggestions are:

1. Take a course in cultural diversity.
2. Take a foreign language. It would be especially helpful to take a course in conversational Spanish if, for example, there is a large Hispanic population in your community.
3. Attend cultural festivals and other events sponsored by minority groups.
4. Participate in organizations such as Habit for Humanity. People from many different backgrounds have opportunity to interact with each other while engaging in projects for this and similar organizations.
5. Visit a church, synagogue, or other place of worship where many of the members' backgrounds differ from your own.

## SUMMARY AND CONCLUSIONS

The focus of this chapter has been a discussion of several issues related to providing culturally appropriate service to people whose backgrounds are different from our own. We must consistently take these issues into consideration as we strive to establish effective professional relationships with clients and their families, speech-language pathologists and audiologists, and our professional colleagues from other disciplines. Regardless of our different backgrounds, people have many things in common. Because of our different backgrounds, we may differ in the way we think, cope with stress, celebrate events, rear our children, feel about our government, define family roles and responsibilities, access health care, interact with authority figures, and engage in social interactions.

The population of the United States is becoming more and more diverse. Most of us will interact more frequently with individuals from backgrounds that are different from our own. Special service providers will have to take into account culturally based behaviors, values, and belief systems if they are to be effective in meeting their professional goals. The issues addressed in this chapter comprise a basis upon which we can continue to build as we move further along the continuum of being culturally competent service providers.

## STUDY QUESTIONS AND ACTIVITIES

1. Discuss why acculturation and assimilation may be important factors to consider as we work with some clients and families from culturally and linguistically diverse backgrounds.
2. What are some stereotypes that are commonly held by Americans?
3. React to the following statements.
   - All people are alike. We should treat everyone the same.
   - Social and cultural factors are critical components of all clinical activities in speech-language pathology and audiology.
   - If people just use common sense, we would not have to study about other cultures in order to conduct effective and appropriate clinical interactions.
   - Techniques that have been used for years in our profession should not be altered just because we are working with people who are from different backgrounds.
4. Read the following case example and answer the questions at the end.
   Ambrea Clark is an African American educator whose skin tone is very fair (light). She has hazel eyes and long, brunette hair. Ambrea recently accepted a position at Altec High School. She was well received by her colleagues and attended many social functions with them. The issue of race was never dis-

cussed. One day in the teachers' lounge a co-worker made the following comments to Ambrea.

"I had the most awful experience yesterday during an afterschool conference with the parents of one of my black students. I knew we were going to have a problem as soon as they came into the room. They were not at all friendly like my other parents are. But you know how those people are. They always seem to have chips on their shoulders. Anyway, I told them my name was Mrs. Smith and then, in an effort to be friendly, I addressed them by their first names. That usually lets people feel more comfortable and accepted. I suddenly realized that the CD I had playing in the background was "easy listening" music and decided they would probably not want to listen to that. I happened to have one of Miles Davis' CDs in my collection. I discreetly changed the music so it would more accurately reflect the music of their culture. Then I proceeded to talk to them about their child's problems. Can you believe they actually got upset with me and suggested that I am a racist? Honestly! After all I did to show them how accepting I am. It just goes to show that you just can't please those people. Every time something does not go their way they start talking about race. I know there have been some problems in the past, but things are much better now. I am not responsible for what my ancestors did. It just makes me so furious!"

- What are some of the assumptions that may have been made by Ambrea's co-worker?
- How do you think Ambrea should have responded to her co-worker?
- How do you think Ambrea felt as she was listening to the comments?
- If you were charged with the responsibility of designing a training activity to increase the co-worker's level of cultural awareness and sensitivity, what are some of the things you would include?
- If you have overheard the comments from the co-worker, what, if anything, would you say to Ambrea?

## REFERENCES

Adler, S. (1993). *Multicultural communication skills in the classroom*. Boston: Allyn & Bacon.

*American Heritage Dictionary of the English Language* (3rd ed.) (1996). Boston: Houghton Mifflin Company.

American Speech-Language-Hearing Association (ASHA). (1985). Clinical management of communicatively handicapped minority language populations. *Asha, 27*(6), 29–32.

American Speech-Language-Hearing Association (ASHA). (1996). LET'S TALK: I know the answer, I just didn't recognize the question! *Asha, 61*, 51–52.

Anderson, N. B. (1992). Understanding cultural diversity. *American Journal of Speech-Language Pathology, 1*, 11–12.

Battle, D. E. (1997). Multicultural considerations in counseling communicatively disordered persons and their families. In T. A. Crowe (Ed.), *Applications of counseling in speech language pathology and audiology*. Baltimore: Williams and Wilkins.

Cole, L. (1989). E Pluribus Pluribus: Multicultural imperatives for the 1990s and beyond. *Asha, 31,* 65–70.

Campbell, L. R., Brennan, D. G., & Steckol, K. F. (1992). Preservice training to meet the needs of people from diverse cultural backgrounds. *Asha, 34,* 29–32.

Cary, A. L. (1992). Get involved: Multiculturally. *Asha, 34,* 3–4.

Crowe, T. A. (1997). *Applications of counseling in speech language pathology and audiology*. Baltimore: Williams and Wilkins.

DeGaetano, Y., Williams, L. R., & Volk, D. (1998). *Kaleidoscope: A multicultural approach for the primary school classroom*. Upper Saddle River, NJ: Prentice Hall.

Ellis, D. M. (1994). *Trends, projections and practices for developing cultural sensitivity*. Multicultural Institute, American Speech-Language-Hearing Association. Sea Island, GA.

Fromkin, H., & Sherwood, J. (1976). *Intergroup and minority relations*. La Jolla, CA: University Press.

Goldstein, B. A. (1995). Spanish phonological development. In H. Kayser (Ed.), *Bilingual speech-language pathology: A Hispanic focus* (pp. 17–40). San Diego: Singular.

Gollnick, D. M., & Chinn, P. C. (1998). *Multicultural education in a pluralistic society*. Upper Saddle River, NJ: Prentice Hall.

Harris, L. (1986). Barriers to the delivery of speech, language, and hearing services to Native Americans. In O. L. Taylor (Ed.), *Nature of communication disorders in culturally and linguistically diverse populations* (pp. 219–236). San Diego, CA: College Hill.

Hernandez, H. (1997). *Teaching in multilingual classrooms: A teacher's guide to context, process, and content*. Upper Saddle River, NJ: Prentice Hall.

Kammey, K. C. W., Ritzer, G., & Yetman, N. R. (1990). *Sociology: Experiencing changing societies*. Boston: Allyn & Bacon.

Keough, K. (1990). Emerging issues for the professions in the 1990s. *Asha, 32,* 55–58.

Lynch, E. W., & Hanson, M. J. (1992). Steps in the right direction: Implications for interventionists. In E. W. Lynch & M. J. Hanson (Eds.), *Developing cross-cultural competence: A guide for working with young children and their families* (pp. 355–377). Baltimore: Paul H. Brookes.

McFadden, J. (1995). *Self-appraisal: Cross-cultural counseling and communication*. Columbia: University of South Carolina–Columbia.

Moore, S. M., & Beatty, J. (1995). *Developing cultural competence in early childhood assessment*. Boulder: University of Colorado–Boulder.

Owens, R. (1992). Language differences: Bidialectalism and bilingualism. In *Language development: An introduction* (3rd ed., pp. xx). Boston: Allyn & Bacon.

Pinkney, A. (1984). *The myth of black progress*. New York: Cambridge University Press.

Quinn, R. (1995). Early intervention? . . . What does it mean? In H. Kayser (Ed.), *Bilingual speech-language pathology: A Hispanic focus*. San Diego: Singular.

Scott, D. M. (1994). Are we ready for the 21st century? *Asha, 47,* 50.

Seymour, H. N., & Bland, L. (1991). A minority perspective in the diagnosis of child language disorders. *Clinical Communication Disorders, 1,* 39–50.

Stockman, I. J. (1986). Language acquisition in culturally diverse populations: The black child as a case study. In O. Taylor (Ed.), *Nature of communication disorders in culturally and linguistically diverse populations* (pp. 117–156). San Diego: College Hill.

Taylor, O. L. (1986). Historical perspectives and conceptual framework. In *Nature of communication disorders in culturally diverse populations*. San Diego: College Hill.

Taylor, O. L. (1990). Language and communication differences. In G. H. Shames & E. H. Wiig (Eds.), *Human communication disorders* (3rd ed., pp. xx). Columbus, OH: Merrill Publishing Company.

Taylor, O. L. (1992). Clinical practice as a social occasion. In L. Cole & V. Deal (Eds.), *Communication disorders in multicultural populations*. Rockville, MD: American Speech-Language-Hearing Association.

Taylor, T. D. (1995). *Promoting cultural diversity and cultural competence: Self-assessment checklist for personnel providing services and support in early childhood settings.* Georgetown University Child Development Center, University Affiliated Program.

Thiederman, S. (1991). *Bridging cultural barriers for corporate success.* New York: Lexington Books.

Tiedt, P. L., & Tiedt, I. M. (1990). *Multicultural teachings: A handbook of activities, information and resources* (3rd ed.). Boston: Allyn & Bacon.

# CULTURAL CONSIDERATIONS FOR DEVELOPING COLLABORATIVE RELATIONSHIPS

# 3

# LANGUAGE LEARNING AND BEHAVIORAL DIFFERENCES IN CULTURALLY DIVERSE POPULATIONS

W. FREDA WILSON and JOHNNY R. WILSON

Speech-language pathologists, audiologists, special educators and other allied health professionals who manage communication disorders do not always realize that individuals vary in the way they process and understand information (Anderson & Adams, 1992). There is considerable research that suggests that individuals learn various behavioral styles that are embedded in culture, ethnicity, and language diversity. The complex mosaic of meanings, perceptions, actions, adaptations, and symbols that make people who they are also serve as influence to their learning preferences (Lynch, 1997). In order to deliver speech, language, and hearing services to children from culturally diverse backgrounds, it is critical to recognize the intricate relationship between language, learning, and communication backgrounds. Acknowledging the dynamic correspondence between language, learning, and cultural diversity will nurture and improve the quality of speech, language, and hearing services to all aspects of a multicultural society (Battle, 1997; Diaz, 1992).

We are aware that the multitudes of cultures coexisting in our society create a quilt of language, learning, and behavioral styles that are often misunderstood and inaccurately interpreted. It is essential that professional behaviors of individuals involved in the management of the communication of children and their families from diverse populations confirm language, learning, and behavioral style differences as legitimate entities.

## LANGUAGE, LEARNING, AND BEHAVIORAL STYLES

Not all humans learn language and social behavior in the same way. Where you come from, who you are, and the cultural, social and environmental circumstances of your life play significant roles in the way you communicate, learn, and behave. Dunn and Griggs (1988) described learning, communicative, and behavioral styles in terms of how the individual's ability to learn, communicate, and behave is influenced by the following factors:

1. Psychological orientations such as analytical and global strengths
2. Physical characteristics, which include auditory, visual, tactile, and kinesthetic skills
3. Sociological needs, such as need for group or individual social situations
4. Emotionality, which includes degrees of motivation, persistence, responsibility, and need for structure
5. Environment, which refers to the role that noise level, temperature, light, and space play in one's style of communication, learning, and behavior

Although most Americans' learning, language, and behavioral styles have been influenced by a majority culture Eurocentric perspective, there is no one communicative, learning, and behavioral style that is best for all people. It is important to determine what communicative, learning, and/or behavioral style is best for a particular individual.

### Definitions and Explanations

The terms *cognitive style* and *learning style* are often used interchangeably. Although some scholars use the terms differently, Anderson (1988) defines **learning style** as a preferred mode of organizing, classifying, and assimilating information about the environment. **Cognitive style** is a general preference for certain modes of operation that incorporate culturally specified dimensions that generalize to other aspects of social, communicative, and general behavior. Anderson and Adams (1992) also discussed *motivational styles,* which they define as preference for a set of goals and rewards that influence the behavior of individuals and/or impact upon critical variables in people's language and learning process. Anderson and Adams (1992) and Swisher (1992) defined learning style as a consistent pattern of behavior and performance that characterizes how individuals approach experimental events. According to Keefe and Languis (1983), language, learning, and behavioral style differences impact on cognitive, affective, and physiological factors that play a significant role in how a leaner perceives, interacts with, and responds to any learning and/or experimental environment.

Chamberlain and Medeiros-Landurand (1991) point out that cognitive style is the way in which individuals process information in particular tasks. Cognitive style refers to global, relational, and intuitive language learning and behavioral processing versus reflective, methodical, and analytical language. Statistically, cultural and language features frequently found to impact behavioral style are dependent versus independent learning, analytical versus spontaneous learning, global perception analysis of details, stimulation and variety, activity level, pace, and response style.

Learning, language, and behavioral preferences are culturally determined. Anderson and Adams (1992) found that people of the same cultural background share similar patterns of intellectual abilities, thinking styles, and interests. Anderson (1988) suggested that sociocultural and environmental factors are critical variables in the development of any cultural behavioral, learning, or language style. He postulated the notion that child rearing, systems of rewards and punishment in the family, value and belief systems, and sex role development are important sociocultural factors in language, learning, and behavioral style development. Cultural values have an impact on socialization practices, which, in turn, affect the ways children prefer to learn, communicate, and behave. If we assume that all students are the same when they are not, those children from multicultural and nontraditional backgrounds are most affected (Collett & Serrance, 1992). There are multiple ways of perceiving, evaluating, believing, and behaving. How people have learned to learn about their world is a result of language, learning, and behavioral practices typical of the cultures from which they come (Swisher, 1992). For example, if children are expected to behave in a particular way and are placed in situations where this behavior is reinforced, their preference for that particular style is reinforced (Anderson & Adams, 1992).

Effective therapeutic or educational intervention is more than just the delivery of information. It involves finding the best culturally sensitive means of successfully engaging our children in the process of acquiring new information (Anderson & Adams, 1992).

Professional involved in the delivery of communication and special education management to diverse populations must impart information to clients and their families. These professionals, through a variety of clinical procedures and paradigms, must facilitate techniques that will allow children to learn and acquire skills in natural culturally and stylistically comfortable ways. We must share linguistic, behavioral, and learning style information with parents and other team members to facilitate successful implementation of intervention strategies. As we engage in those practices, we must learn how to make culturally appropriate decisions about what is the best method to impart information with respect to cultural diversity (Gay, 1992). Since, according to current demographic data, our country is rapidly becoming more culturally and linguistically diverse, clinical and educational case loads will reflect a broader spectrum of diversity. A more diverse population of children means there is and will be variability in language behavior and learning styles that will generate conflicts when individuals are asked to perform in a manner, or setting that is foreign to their composite style(s) (Anderson, 1988).

## VARIATIONS IN LANGUAGE, LEARNING, AND BEHAVIORAL STYLES

### *Field-Dependent or Field-Sensitive*

Anderson and Adams (1992) described the field-dependent or field-sensitive orientation to language, learning, and behavior. Field-dependent persons process information from their entire surroundings. They are as concerned about the human relational interaction and communication style of an information or stimulus sources as they are about the message or behavior presented. They also expect the provider or source of a stimulus event to relate to them in a holistic way as individuals. People with this orientation are not comfortable in situations where the source of stimulation or provider of information—that is, the teacher or clinician— does not use styles consistent with their expectations. According to Swisher (1992), field-dependent children have a global perspective and tend to be highly sensitive to the social environment. Field-dependent people do best on verbal tasks. They learn material better that has human social content and is characterized by innovative, creativity, and humor. Their performance is influenced by an authority figure's expression of confidence or doubt in their ability to do well in given situations. They can be described as relational/holistic/affective–oriented children (Anderson & Adams, 1992). Wilkerson (1994) presented additional features of persons characterized by field-dependent styles. She reported that they

- Like to work with others to achieve a common goal.
- Like to assist others.
- Selectively attend to humans or socially oriented materials.
- Learn best when materials are structured and organized and when objectives are clearly stated.
- Learn best when instructions are explicit.
- Rely on perceptual field stimuli to facilitate information processing.

## Field-Independent

Field-independent children are analytic and nonaffective in their orientation. They do best on analytic tasks and tend to learn material more easily that is inanimate. These individuals' performance is not greatly affected by the opinions of others (Anderson, 1988). According to Wilkerson (1994), field independent children

- Like to compete to gain individual recognition.
- Are task oriented.
- Like interactions with teachers that are formal and controlled.
- Seek nonsocial rewards.
- Learn best when material is unstructured.
- Respond better to material with an impersonal content and that is theoretical in nature and noncreative.
- Perceive objects as separate from the field.

Swisher (1992) described field-independent children as individualistic and less sensitive to the emotions of others. These children favor inquiry and independent study and can provide their own structure to facilitate learning. They are intrinsically motivated.

## Cautions About Stereotyping

According to Grossman (1995), no group or individual is completely field-independent or field-dependent. Although selected individuals or racial/ethnic groups may appear to utilize primarily certain language, learning, and behavioral styles, practitioners, educators, and clinicians should note that aspects of opposite styles will also exist in their composite personalities. Cognitive language, learning, and behavioral styles operate along a continuum. Although certain groups seem to cluster at one end or the other, individuals can be anywhere along the continuum. Similarities in world views and cognitive styles of certain racial/ethnic groups affect their perceptions of the world, how they choose to think about it, and how they interact with it. Consequently, in order to maximize the efficacy and success of clinical service delivery to persons from multicultural backgrounds, service providers must acknowledge a child's age, race, *cultural* background, language, disability, family income, or place of origin, and other variables. Information about culturally based learning and behavior styles must utilized carefully (Lynch, 1997).

Hilliard (1989, as cited in Lynch, 1997) stated that we do not have to avoid addressing preferred styles of interaction because of fear that we may stereotype individuals. Empirical observations, when interpreted properly, help us become more sensitive to the needs/preferences of the children and families we serve, thereby increasing the effectiveness of our work with them. According to Grossman (1995), some generalizations have the potential to be helpful. They are helpful if they facilitate our sensitivity to the possibility that individuals may have certain typical attitudes, preferences, values, learning styles, and behavior patterns. He also emphasized the importance of not overgeneralizing characteristics that are typical in a particular group of people to *all* members of that group.

## HOW COGNITIVE/LEARNING STYLES INFLUENCE ASSESSMENT RESULTS

Grossman (1995) described the following aspects of learning style that may influence how a child performs while being assessed. The author presents examples of cautions and behaviors to avoid for each aspect of learning style presented by Grossman.

### Dependent versus Independent Learners

Independent learners are relatively self-reliant during the assessment process. Dependent learners require considerable guidance and feedback to perform at their optimum level.

### Reflective/Analytical versus Spontaneous/Intuitive/Impulsive

Some children's cultures stress the importance of analyzing and reflecting on questions and problems. They are encouraged to be sure that they know the answer before responding. Other cultures emphasize responses that are intuitive and responsive in nature. For learners who are reflective or analytical, examiners should allow sufficient time for them to prepare their answers. Examiners should not call on someone else or move on to the next item as a result of assuming that the student does not know the answer because he or she is slow in responding.

## Risk Taking

Differences exist between how sure individuals have to be that they know the answer, can complete a task, or have the appropriate opinion before they will risk a response during assessment. Examiners should determine prior to testing if the child is a risk-taker. If the child is not, he or she may need to be reassured that it is appropriate to take guesses in that particular situation.

## Global Perception versus Analysis of Details

Individuals who use a global approach to learning perceive things in a holistic manner. They see everything as a part of the whole and notice few differences among the parts. Analytic learners divide the whole into subcategories based on differences.

## Stimulation and Variety

Individuals show differences in their tolerance for assessment tasks that are boring, monotonous, tedious, and repetitious. Some students will be more willing to continue those tasks than others will.

## Activity Level

Almanza and Mosely (1980, as cited by Grossman, 1995) reported that a student's ethnic and socioeconomic backgrounds greatly influence his or her willingness to sit still for long periods of time. Hale-Benson (1995) discussed similar findings with specific reference to African American children.

## Pace

People show cultural differences in the pace they use for work and play. Some individuals try to accomplish as much as possible within a specified time period. Other people would rather work at a relaxed, steady pace. Children who are used to working at a slower pace may make more errors when they are required or encouraged to work as fast as they can.

## Response Style

All people do not react in the same way to life situations. Cultural and individual differences exist regarding whether there are intense or subdued responses to various types of encounters.

## MISPERCEPTIONS AND BEHAVIORAL STYLES

Hilliard (1989, as cited in Lynch, 1997) suggests four ways in which a child's behavioral style may result in misperceptions. They are

1. Underestimating student's intellectual ability. Some students prefer to focus on the global aspects of a problem rather than the specifics. A child's efforts to deal with problems in a holistic way may not be valued as much as another child who uses a more analytical approach to problem solving. According to Hilliard, educators should strive to have all students learn to apply both methods without making negative judgments about students who have a holistic orientation to learning.

2. Behavioral style in storytelling. Hilliard describes the mainstream approach to storytelling as very linear with a clearly defined beginning, middle, and end. There are few departures from the central points. Culturally different children show variation from this approach. For example, African American children often appear to depart from the main point, each time returning or "spiraling" back to create the enriched whole. According to Hilliard, these differences may be assumed to be lack of skill or competence rather than a different approach that has been learned over the years. Professionals should not underestimate a child's overall level of competence because he or she has had more practice with one style than with another.

3. Expectations in relation to behavioral styles. According to Hilliard, professionals may have more difficulty communicating with and establishing effective working relationships with individuals who differ significantly from themselves in variables such as race, culture, ethnicity, language, race, gender, and socioeconomic status. People may sense this lack of communication and rapport and perform less well and feel less adequate than they would in situations where they and professionals working with them share a similar background.

4. Language differences. Cheng (1993, as cited in Lynch, 1997, p. 62), suggested that "the cultural, language, and ideological differences that occur in communication can lead to a 'difficult discourse,' and difficult discourse can lead to misperceptions and misunderstandings between students and [professionals]."

## CULTURALLY DIFFERENT BEHAVIOR STYLES

### Verbal Communication Styles

When professionals, children, and family members from different cultural backgrounds interact with each other, there are multiple opportunities for miscommunication. Professionals who are unaware of children's culturally influenced communication styles may mistakenly believe the children are shy, insecure, disrespectful, and so forth. Children may misinterpret communication from teachers and other professionals. For example, they may not be able to distinguish between times when their teachers are serious and when they are joking. Therefore, to communicate effectively with culturally diverse individuals, professionals should be aware of communication style differences that exist between them and their students or clients (Grossman, 1995). If service providers and their clients and families do not share the same background and understanding of interactional patterns, they may misinterpret attempts at communication. Lessons and other activities that are embedded within the professional's culture may be confusing or understood differently to individuals from backgrounds that are different (Chamberlain & Medeiros-Landurand, 1991).

Grossman (1995) discussed several examples of typical communication style differences. They are

1. *Formal versus Informal Communication.* Expectations of some cultures relative to communication are much more flexible than others. Some groups expect strict adherence to specific conventions in certain situations. Other cultures are much more relaxed and informal about rules for communication.
2. *Emotional versus Subdued Communication.* Some cultures protect the rights of individuals to express their feelings and expect their members to learn to tolerate, accept, and deal with the expression of intense feelings. There are other cultures that are more concerned with protecting people's sensibilities. They expect feelings to be communicated in a subdued way.
3. *Direct versus Indirect Communication.* People in some cultures are expected to speak directly, openly, and frankly. The emphasis in other cultures is for communication that is perceived as indirect and polite in order to maintain smooth interpersonal relationships. Instructors/clinicians must know which would be the preferred method to use when providing feedback concerning a child's work.
4. *Poetic and Analogous Communication.* Some people use a communication style that is poetic and analogous rather than clear and concise.

Professionals who are not aware of these style differences may assume the speaker is "beating around the bush," being evasive, or unsure of his or her response.

5. *Honesty.* Cultures have very different ideas about exactly what is and is not honest communication. They also differ in whether honest communication is desirable. There are issues that influence a group's opinion about how honest communication should be. Some of those issues are the relative importance placed by the culture on maintaining one's honor or one's "face," avoiding disagreement and conflict, avoiding personal responsibility, and so on.

6. *Responses to Guilt and Accusations.* In some cultures lowered eyes are interpreted as an admission of guilt; in others, as a sign of respect. Avoiding direct eye contact with authority figures or elders is viewed as a sign of respect and submission in some cultures. Direct eye contact can also be viewed as challenging.

7. *Themes Discussed.* There are certain topics that are avoided in certain situations and when talking with certain people. All cultures have unwritten rules that apply to when it is appropriate to talk about what and to whom. These rules vary between groups.

8. *Needs.* Professionals should determine whether individuals from a child's cultural background express their needs openly or expect others to be sensitive to nonverbal cues about their feelings and problems.

9. *Admission of Errors and Mistakes.* Professionals should be aware that individuals from some cultures may be unwilling to accept the consequences of their behavior. Culturally based attitudes would make some people resistant to admitting their responsibility to others.

10. *Disagreement, Unwillingness, and Inability.* Individuals in some cultures are brought up to believe there are some situations in which it is appropriate to break promises or to say something that is not true. Two such situations might be when doing so contributes to interpersonal harmony or to help someone "save face."

11. *Conflict Resolution.* Professionals should seek to determine how conflicts are handled in their client's culture—whether they are dealt with in a straightforward manner or "swept under the rug." They should also know whether it is better to intervene when students have conflicts or permit them to settle the conflicts themselves.

12. *Turn Taking.* The rules of turn taking vary across cultures. When working with individuals from culturally different backgrounds, it is important to know the length of time a person must wait before he or she begins to respond or introduce a new topic after another person has completed a statement. Table 3-1 presents a summary of information about culturally based verbal communication skills.

## TABLE 3-1   Culturally Based Communication Styles: Verbal

1. *Formal versus Informal Communication.* Expectations of some cultures are much more flexible than others.
2. *Emotional versus Subdued Communication.* Some cultures express their feeling and require their members to learn to tolerate, accept, and deal with the expression of intense feelings. Others expect feelings to be communicated in a subdued way.
3. *Direct versus Indirect Communication.* Some people speak directly, openly, and frankly while others prefer to speak indirectly and politely in order to maintain smooth interpersonal relationships.
4. *Poetic and Analogous Communication.* Some people use a more poetic communication style or explain things by means of analogies rather than clear and concise terms and relationships.
5. *Honesty.* Issues such as the relative importance placed by the culture on maintaining one's honor or one's face, avoiding disagreement and conflict, and avoiding personal responsibility influence a group's opinion about how honest communication should be.
6. *Responses to Guilt and Accusations.* The same behaviors may have different meanings across cultures. For example, lowered eyes would indicate an admission of guilt in some cultures, but it would be a sign of respect in others.
7. *Themes Discussed.* All cultures have unwritten rules about what should or should not be talked about in specific situations.
8. *Needs.* It is important to ask whether individuals from a student's culture express their needs openly or expect others to be sensitive to their feeling and problems.
9. *Admission of Errors and Mistakes.* Some students may be willing to accept the consequences of their behavior, whereas others resist admitting their responsibility to others.
10. *Disagreement, Unwillingness, and Inability.* Some students are brought up to believe that not following through on promises and saying something that is not true are acceptable behaviors when doing so contributes to interpersonal harmony or helps someone save face.
11. *Conflict Resolution.* Conflicts may be faced and dealt with in a straightforward manner by some, but swept under the rug by others.
12. *Turn Taking.* The length of time a person must wait to begin to respond or to introduce a new topic after another person has completed a statement varies with different cultures.

Adapted from Grossman (1995).

## Nonverbal Communication

Grossman (1995) also discusses several aspects of nonverbal communication that can result in miscommunication across cultures. In some cultures

- Individuals laugh or giggle when they are embarrassed.
- There are gender differences in emotional expression.
- Defiance can be expressed by silent stares, forced smiles, rolling the eyes, or putting hands on hips.
- Looking adults in the eyes is a sign of submission.
- Avoiding eye contact with adults is a sign of submission.
- Touching is very common; it is avoided with strangers in other cultures.
- Head nods, raising of the eyebrows, and so on have different meanings in different groups.
- Head and finger use that is commonly accepted in one culture would be offensive in others.

A summary of some culturally based nonverbal communication style differences is presented in Table 3-2.

### TABLE 3-2.   Culturally Based Communication Styles: Nonverbal

Some examples:
1. *Emotion.* Some cultures laugh or giggle when they are embarrassed.
2. *Defiance.* Defiance can be expressed by silent stares, eye rolling, forced smiles, placing hands on hips, etc.
3. *Submissiveness.* In some cultures, looking at an adult in the eye shows respect; in others avoiding eye contact communicates the same message.
4. *Physical Contact.* Some groups are more likely to touch people than others.
5. *Agreement and Disagreement.* The ways people express agreement and disagreement may vary among cultures (head nods, eyebrow raising).
6. *Beckoning.* A hand or finger gesture commonly accepted in one culture may be offensive to another.

Adapted from Grossman (1995).

## Relationship Style

The way in which we relate to others is based on cultural rules. Culturally based differences in relationship style have implications for those of us who teach or provide instructions to others on a regular basis. Grossman (1995) discussed several relationship styles: participatory versus passive, aloof, distant versus involved personal relations, dependent versus independent learning, peer versus adult-oriented, and individualistic versus group-oriented. A summary of Grossman's discussion follows.

### Participatory versus Passive Learning
Children who are brought up to be active learners are expected to ask questions, discuss ideas, and so on. They regard educators as guides who lead and stimulate them to learn. Other children are less active and more passive in the learning process. To them, teachers are fountains of information from which students can drink and be filled.

### Aloof, Distant versus Involved Personal Relations
Some children expect their teachers to restrict their involvement with them to their functioning in school. In other cultures children expect teachers to be interested and involved with them as people who are also students. There are also gender differences involved in this issue. Females usually show a preference for closer personal relationships with their teachers than males.

### Dependent versus Independent Learning
More nonmainstream students tend to want more direction and feedback from their teachers than do their mainstream counterparts.

### Peer- versus Adult-Oriented
Whether children look primarily to adults for guidance, support, and direction, or tend to learn from and be guided by other children and youth is a culturally determined behavior.

### Individualistic versus Group-Oriented
Children who are brought up to be relatively individualistic show a preference to work alone even when they are assigned to work in groups. They would need to be taught how to work on projects with others. Other children prefer to work cooperatively and would not function as well independently. Children would not fit neatly in one category or the other. It is a matter of degree of preference. A summary of culturally based relationships presented in Table 3-3.

## Motivational Style

A child's motivation to succeed in school is determined by a number of cultural variables including gender and socioeconomic factors. Many children from culturally different backgrounds may be alienated, distrustful, angry, and disillusioned about schools. These feelings are precipitated and/or facilitated by prejudice and discrimination they experience in their schools and in society. They do not believe their accomplishments in school will actually make a real difference in their lives. Some of the children may also have to deal with pressure from their peers not to conform or to do well. Professionals working with children must assess each child's

## TABLE 3-3   Culturally Based Relationship Styles

1. *Participatory versus Passive Learning.* Some children are brought up to be active participants in the learning process. They are expected to ask questions of adults, discuss ideas, and so on. Other children are expected to be less active and more passive recipients of instruction and information.

2. *Aloof, Distant versus Involved Personal Relations.* In some cultures educators are expected to be restricted to their functioning in school. In other cultures, they are expected to be interested and involved in them as persons, who are also students. There are also gender differences, with females often preferring more personal involvement with their teachers than males do.

3. *Dependent versus Independent Learning.* Many students from nonmainstream backgrounds tend to be more interested in obtaining their teacher's direction and feedback than do mainstream students.

4. *Peer- versus Adult-Oriented.* In some cultures children look primarily to adults for support and direction. Children in others cultures tend to learn better from other children.

5. *Individualistic versus Group-Oriented.* Children who are brought up to be relatively individualistic prefer to work alone. They are likely to continue working alone even when assigned to work in groups.

6. *Aural, Visual, and Verbal Learners.* Students show preferences for aural, visual, or verbal cognitive styles. Educators should use a multisensory approach when they instruct diverse learners.

7. *Kinesthetic/Active/Energetic Learning versus Calm, Inactive Verbal Learning.* Some students learn best by doing, manipulating, touching, and experiencing, and others prefer more sedentary approaches such as lectures, reading, written, and oral explanations, and discussions of ideas. Students also differ in terms of whether they function better in highly stimulating or more calm learning environments.

8. *Nonverbal Cues.* Some students' learning would be enhanced (or adversely affected) by perceptions—not by what is said.

9. *Trial and Error versus "Watch and Do."* Students from some cultures can usually take in stride the mistakes they make in public when they volunteer answers or are called on. Others have greater difficulty exposing themselves in public while they are learning from their mistakes.

10. *Argumentative/Forensic Instruction versus Direct Instruction.* In some cultures adults teach children by asking questions about their beliefs in order to guide them to a more correct or accurate understanding of things. In other cultures, children are unaccustomed to having their beliefs questioned critically.

11. *Learning from Examples, Stories, and Morals versus Direct Instruction.* In some cultures, in addition to being told things directly, children are led to an understanding of life through the legends they learn, the morals of the stories they are told, and the examples they are shown. Direct instruction can be supplemented by using these strategies.

Adapted from Grossman (1995).

motivation to learn what they are trying to teach. Adjustments may have to be made in instructional strategies and activities in order to increase the child's level of motivation (Grossman, 1995).

Some students have been brought up in cultures that allow them to learn what is useful and interesting to them instead of what someone has decided they should learn. Other students arrive at school with the mental set to learn whatever teachers present to them (Grossman, 1995).

Children from some cultures choose tasks that are challenging and novel. The risk of failure or rejection does not discourage them from attempting new things. Other children choose to "play it safe" and stick with familiar tasks, toys, and materials, for example (Grossman, 1995).

A summary of culturally based motivational styles/issues is summarized in Table 3-4.

## CONCLUDING STATEMENT

There is no one communication, learning, or behavioral style that is used by all people. Many cultural variables have a significant impact on how and when we choose to communicate, how we behave in various settings, and how we prefer to learn. Even individuals from the same background may differ in those areas. We do not fit neatly in any one category but tend to lean more heavily in one direction than in others. It is important for service providers to determine preferred styles of our students/clients if our professional interactions are to be successful. Research is ongoing in this very important area and we still have much to learn. In this chapter we have presented an overview of information that is available to help us as we strive to become more competent in our provision of services to individuals from culturally and linguistically diverse backgrounds.

## STUDY QUESTIONS AND ACTIVITIES

1. Define cognitive or learning style.
2. Explain the following learning styles
   - dependent or field-sensitive
   - field-independent
3. Discuss how cognitive/learning styles may influence assessment results.
4. What are some ways in which behavior styles may be influenced by culture? What are some culturally determined behavior styles?
5. Discuss some aspects of nonverbal communication that may result in miscommunication across cultures.

## TABLE 3-4   Culturally Based Motivational Styles/Issues

1. *Motivation.* Some students in various groups are pressured by their peers not to conform or to do well in school because to do so is to "act white" (Grossman, 1995, p. 272). Some females may also have mixed feeling about academic success because it may make them less popular with males. Also, in some cultures, educational success is more of a male "thing" than females. Therefore, educators should not assume that all students are equally motivated to succeed academically. They must assess each individual's motivation and make appropriate adjustments in their strategies.

2. *Learning on Demand versus Learning What Is Relevant or Interesting.* All cultures require all children to learn many things whether they want to or not. However, some students have been brought up in cultures in which they have considerable leeway to learn what is useful and interesting to them rather than what some others have decided they should learn. Others students are better prepared to study whatever teachers present to them.

3. *Risk Taking.* Will students choose tasks that are challenging and novel if these also involve risk of failure or rejection, or will they stick to those that are familiar?

4. *Time Orientation, Punctuality, and Pace.* Although all ethnic groups are concerned about and prepare for the future, there are significant differences in the extent to which people sacrifice present satisfactions for future goals. Because individuals differ in these respect, it is important to know whether students can work toward the accomplishment of long-term goals and rewards or are more responsive to short-term goals, immediate satisfaction, and immediate reinforcement. In some cultures, when a person is late it reflects primarily on the late person, who is seen as irresponsible. In others, lateness is perceived as a statement about the late person's disrespectful attitude toward those who have been kept waiting. Students who are accustomed to working at a slower pace make more errors when instructed to work as fast as they can.

5. *Self-Confidence.* Ethnic and socioeconomic differences appear to be important in the students' beliefs about their abilities to control their lives.

6. *Acceptable and Unacceptable Learning Activities.* Some students may be unable to participate in various school activities because of religious or moral upbringing or because of other responsibilities at home.

Adapted from Grossman (1995).

6. Read the following case example and answer the questions at the end.

Carnella Ellison has been a successful teacher in rural South Carolina for many years. She has earned several awards for teaching including "1996 Teacher of the Year." Her students like her and often bring little gifts to show their appreciation for her. Carnella puts a lot of effort into developing materials and activities to make learning interesting for her students. She believes that students learn best by being active participants in their learning and seeks to involve students in a variety of learning tasks. She gives awards to individual students who make the highest grades on exams and/or earn the highest number of points on projects.

The community in which Carnella works had been a rather homogeneous one until two years ago when two large factories opened in the county, offering hundreds of jobs. That led to an influx of new residents seeking jobs at the factory and in other areas related to the new industry (construction needs, health care, fast food, etc.). The demographics of the population in the community surrounding Carnella's school have drastically changed. The community would now be described as a multiracial/multicultural community of working-class families. The families have a strong sense of pride in their racial and ethnic backgrounds and have many celebrations reflecting their heritage. They are hard workers and support the efforts of others in the community to be successful. Many of the families believe in the concept of "working for the whole." Selfish acts for personal gain are not appreciated. Extended families are very active in helping with family decision making about child rearing and other issues.

This past school year Carnella began to notice changes in the behavior of some of the students in her classes. Some of them seemed to be uncomfortable when participating in the activities her other students had always loved. They preferred to work on collaborative tasks in groups rather than to participate in contests to win prizes. Many of the students seemed to enjoy hands-on activities and readily engaged in projects that included physical activity. Some of the students did not pay attention when she read stories to them, did not ask questions during discussions, nor did they seek clarification about instructions they did not understand. They seemed to be hesitant to take guesses and only responded when they were confident they knew the right answers to questions. Carnella began to feel that the students did not like her because some of them did not exhibit direct eye contact when she talked to them. A few of them pulled away when she tried to hug them. She became very despondent and began to consider herself to be a failure as a teacher. She decided to seek help from the staff counselor. You are the counselor who has been assigned to help her.

- What do you think are some of the major problems/challenges Carnella is facing as a teacher?
- What are some of the recommendations you would make to her regarding the strategies she might consider using in her classroom?
- How would you attempt to explain some of the students' behaviors that have puzzled Carnella?

## REFERENCES

Anderson, J. (1988). Cognitive styles and multicultural populations. *Journal of Teacher Education, 39,* 2–9.

Anderson, J. A., & Adams, M. (1992). Acknowledging the learning styles of diverse student populations: Implications for instructional design. In L. L. Border &

N. V. Chism (Eds.), *New directions for teaching and learning: Teaching for diversity* (pp. 19–24). San Francisco: Jossey-Bass Publishers.

Battle, D. E. (1997). Multicultural considerations in counseling communicatively disordered persons and their families. In T. A. Crowe (Ed.), *Applications of counseling in speech-language pathology and audiology* (pp. 118–141). Baltimore: Williams & Wilkins.

Chamberlain, P., & Medeiros-Landurand, P. (1991). Practical considerations for the assessment of LEP students with special needs. In E. V. Hamayan & J. S. Damico (Eds.), *Limiting bias in the assessment of bilingual students* (pp. 111–156). Austin, TX: Pro-Ed.

Collett, J., & Serrance, B. (1992). Stirring it up: The inclusive classroom. In L. L. Borders & N. V. Chism (Eds.), *New directions for teaching and learning: Teaching for diversity* (pp. 38–39). San Francisco: Jossey-Bass Publishers.

Diaz, C. (1992). The next millennium: A multicultural imperative. In C. Diaz (Ed.), *Multicultural education for the 21st century* (p. 15). Washington, DC: National Education Association of the United States.

Dunn, R., & Griggs, S. A. (1988). The learning styles of multicultural groups and counseling implications. *Journal of Multi-Cultural Counseling and Development, 17,* 146–153.

Gay, G. (1992). Effective teaching practice for multicultural classrooms. In C. Diaz (Ed.), *Multicultural education for the 21st century* (pp. 39–55). Washington, DC: National Education Association of the United States.

Grossman, H. (1995). *Teaching in a diverse society.* Boston: Allyn & Bacon.

Hale-Benson, J. (1995). *Educating African-American children in the context of their culture.* Annual Convention of the National Black Association for Speech, Language and Hearing. Washington, DC.

Keefe, J. W., & Languis, M. (1983). *Learning Stages Network Newsletter, 4*(2), 1.

Lynch, E. W. (1997). Instructional strategies. In A. I. Morey & M. K. Kitano, *Multicultural course transformations in higher education: A broader truth* (pp. 56–70). Boston: Allyn & Bacon.

Swisher, K. (1992). Learning styles: Implications for teachers. In C. Diaz (Ed.), *Multicultural education for the 21st century* (pp. 73–80). Washington, DC: National Education Association of the United States.

Wilkerson, D. (1994). Differences in learning styles. In Multicultural Institute, *Challenges in the expansion of cultural diversity in communication sciences and disorders.* American Speech Language-Hearing Association. Sea Island, GA.

# 4

# INTERAGENCY SERVICE PROVISION: IMPLICATIONS FOR CULTURALLY DIVERSE CLIENTS

## BARBARA PULLEN-SMITH and WANDA WOODS

Health-care reform, education reform, welfare reform, downsizing, and total quality management (TQM) are but a few phrases that evoke images of change. In the past decade, our nation's efforts to improve the systems represented by these constructs have and will tremendously alter access to and provision of health and human services, particularly in public health. Individuals, families, and communities who "fall through the cracks" have always been a concern, but the total impact on all families and communities when major systems *simultaneously* change has yet to be measured. The very systems and institutions that are causing change will be challenged to redefine and reshape their own service provision arenas. Many health and human service agencies and organizations will find it beneficial to develop and/or strengthen the kind(s) of associations, partnerships, and alliances with each other that will produce generous profit margins and revenues as designated bottom lines indicative of success. Already, interagency service provision efforts focusing on asthma, early intervention, child abuse prevention, attention deficit disorder, managed care, and primary care service delivery offer strong proof of the feasibility of collaborative relationships for successful health and human service provision outcomes (Marsland, 1994; Peterken & Bonynge, 1995; Shea, Rahmanic, & Morris, 1996; Solberg, Isham, Kottke,

Magman, Nelson, Reed, & Richards, 1995). However, the development of partnerships for some health and human service agencies and organizations will present a challenge.

It is the premise of this chapter that health and human service agencies and organizations (systems) can better serve children, other clients, and their families through interagency service provision efforts. Challenges are certainly a part of such efforts, but benefits are available for both the client and the agency. Speech-language pathologists and other special service providers regularly work with professionals from many different agencies and organizations. Coordination of our efforts with other professionals is essential if our service delivery efforts are to be successful. It is important for all who work with families of children with special needs to identify ways in which we can more effectively provide the help they need. The more we understand how systems work, how efforts may overlap, and common barriers to accomplishing goals, the more likely we are to increase our efficiency and effectiveness while providing clients the services they require. Subsequently, the purpose of this chapter is to identify and discuss a few key issues and factors related to interagency service provision from a public health perspective and provide practical insights into overcoming some of these issues/factors using a model that addresses culture as a specific issue of consideration in interagency service provision.

## SOME CHALLENGES OF INTERAGENCY SERVICE PROVISION

"A child is a member of a family system" (MacPhee, 1995, p. 417). Regardless of whether the family is a capable unit having resources, order, and mutually reciprocating relationships, or is struggling to cope, needing many resources, having strained, nonreciprocating allegiances and interactions, a family orients the child to its environment and prepares him or her for the world. Like any other system, the family system has inputs, outputs, controls, and feedback mechanisms that operate via a prescribed pattern (Lilley & Guanci, 1995). MacPhee (1995) describes the family as "a system of interdependent, interacting individuals related to one another by blood or consent. Families are open living systems constantly exchanging information and energy with the environment" (p. 417). However, while the family system can often successfully compensate for life changes such as birth, marriage, moving, job changes, and even death, acute, unknown, and chronic illnesses or debilitating conditions can present overwhelming challenges, particularly when the disease or condition affects a child. It is generally at the juncture of sickness and disease that families venture outside of their systems to look for and to receive care from the formal health-care system. Pursuing this need brings the family in contact with any of several health and human service agencies or organizations.

Like the family, health and human service agencies function as a system. But, because of the type of inputs, controls, feedback mechanisms, and outputs that drive the system, and the way these items are introduced into the system, health and human service agencies can be more restrictive than a family. It is this difference—a generally restrictive system trying to accommodate a flexible system at a point of crisis imposed by a chronic illness or a debilitating condition—that requires a closer examination of interagency service provision. As an illness or condition is addressed, it is possible that several health and human service agencies will be brought together to meet the needs of the client and family. It is the coordination of services between and among agencies that frequently presents a challenge for the client and family as well as the agencies involved.

## A Working Definition of Service Provision

The term *service provision* is the sum total of agency and interagency actions and activities designed to meet an identified, perceived, or implied need. Service provision is the set of actions taken or followed by an agency (including all processes of implementation) in its effort to make services available to clients who are in and outside of the service provision system. Effective interagency service provision connects clients and their social support networks to the appropriate resources. This linking process can be achieved through the provision of different levels of service provision, including:

- *Direct Service.* Providing hands-on or immediate outcome service that may be clinical, medical, or psychosocial in nature.
- *Referral.* Sending the client to other resources that meet the client's needs more effectively than the initial agency of contact.
- *Coordination.* Pulling together different resources to address specific needs identified through both an initial and ongoing assessment with the client.
- *Skill-building.* Identifying and implementing educational opportunities for the client that enhance the client's and family's ability to maneuver within the system and negotiate for resources and services needed.

- *Collaboration.* The working together of several systems, and with several agencies, toward the common aim of meeting the client's needs.

The parameters for service provision (and interagency service provision) are determined by each agency's mission statement. In theory, the mission statement—a written philosophy and accompanying policies—sets the course, attitude, and tone of the agency's direction. Also, it outlines standards of practice, authorizes and defines boundaries for relationships within the agency and with other agencies/organizations, and provides clients with an idea of what to expect in the service provision process. The real mission of an agency is often revealed not just by the actual services it provides, but by other factors including: (1) perceptions and experiences of the clients served, (2) the relationship(s) and interaction(s) with other agencies/organizations on behalf of the client, and (3) the products or outcomes of both the agency's internal and external activities. Providers and systems must be cognizant of these and other factors that can impact the level and quality of services received by clients.

## ACCESS TO SERVICES: COMMON BARRIERS FOR CLIENTS/FAMILIES

Health and human service agencies should be mechanisms for exchanging information, services, and resources both within agencies and between agencies in ways that are most effective to meet the needs of clients and their families. This exchange is not as effective if families run into real or perceived barriers. Barriers, such as actions or activities that impede the provision of services that adequately, appropriately, and specifically meet the needs of the client, create real problems for families trying to access services.

Gaining entry into a system is one of the simplest ways to define "access," but for some clients, it is among the hardest things to accomplish. Access issues that influence one's ability to get needed health and human services can involve a variety of independent and interrelated factors, including, but not limited to: (1) socioeconomic status, (2) insurance, (3) ability to pay, (4) awareness, (5) availability, (6) support systems, (7) ability to negotiate the system, (8) history/experience, (9) transportation, and (10) cultural influences. Seldom does one factor operate alone. Usually multiple factors impact a client's or family's ability to get needed services at any given time. For the purposes of this chapter, these factors will be discussed in the context of five categories: lack of awareness of the service, value/priority of the service, cultural influences, history/experience, and lack of resources/support.

## Lack of Awareness of the Service

Agencies must assume responsibility to ensure that the population for which the service is intended is aware of the available services and know how to access them. Frequently, doors to a clinic or hospital are open and the clients do not show. Health and human service professionals may perceive the absence of the client and family as an indicator of the absence of need or a lack of interest. However, clients and their families simply may not be aware of the service in the way that providers are. For many clients and their families, little is known about prerequisites for accessing services.

The perceived lack of awareness on the client's part may be a reflection of the agency's lack of skill in identifying and locating pathways of communication for that client and his or her family. Many agencies and organizations spend large sums of money in public awareness campaigns only to discover that most of their clients were referred by a friend. This fact is certainly consistent with communication patterns for culturally diverse individuals. In most racial and ethnic populations, oral and face-to-face communication is both significant and important. It permits the conveyance of intent, which is a key factor in the establishment of trust. And as with any consumer, the development of trust increases the likelihood that the client and their family will return, follow through on the prescribed regimen, and refer others to the agency (American Heart Association, 1993; Davis & Voegtle, 1994).

Understanding a client's cultural communication networks is key to developing messages that will reach racial and ethnic minorities in a meaningful way. As health and human service agencies consider lack of awareness as a barrier for clients and their families, asking the following six questions will provide insight into how to increase awareness of the agency's services among the population(s) it serve(s):

1. What is the *real* message of the agency?
2. What is the *intent* of the message?
3. What *communication mechanism* does the agency use to get the message to the intended audience?
4. Is there a mechanism in place to get *feedback* from the clients regarding their understanding of the message or need for services? Is the client feedback valued and used?
5. What *action* does the message encourage clients to take? Is the message *promoted* in such a way that the intended client will use the service?
6. Are the *services provided* in a way that is *consistent* with the agency's message?

If these questions and their subsequent answers are addressed in a clear, ongoing, and inclusive fashion, agencies stand to reap three key benefits:

- An atmosphere of trust is created.
- Clients will feel that they are valued by the agency and will be more comfortable approaching the agency.
- Diverse clients will use the service.

As well, such a questioning process may also help agencies finetune the parameters of their service provision efforts while increasing the knowledge and confidence of clients when using the agency's services.

## Value/Priority of the Service

Frequently, providers in health and human service settings become frustrated when clients are late for appointments or miss them altogether, do not follow recommended actions for care, or are not responsive as defined by the providers. It is important to recognize and understand the client's perspective. Clients may have a totally different understanding and perception of the value of the service for themselves or family members. Whether the client values a service is influenced by factors such as socioeconomic status, barriers present in accessing the service, knowledge about the service, acceptability of the service, information received from informal/formal networks about the service, and other pressing family needs. However, the perceived *need* for the service will have substantial influence on both the value and priority of the service for the client, as supported in the following statement by MacPhee (1995).

> A need is defined as the family's perceptions of what is important for them to acquire. Family members will allot time, energy, and resources to meeting a need. Unmet needs are hierarchically ordered from most to least important, and family need hierarchies are highly unique. Often professionals describe families that fail to adhere to their child's treatment regimen as resistant and noncompliant. Actually, these families may be attending to other important needs and a professionally prescribed treatment regimen is a low priority. (pp. 418–419)

Therefore, the family's perception of what occurred and the provider's perception may be totally different. For example, a family may value speech therapy, but may choose not to keep an appointment because it is a low priority in the context of addressing other basic needs. Some providers may label them as noncompliant. The family, however, may perceive this action as doing what they had to do at the moment and that there was little harm done to the child in the process. In some instances the client and family may value the service, see it as a priority, but are unable to accomplish the action or activity. This inability to act may be influenced by a lack of knowledge, skill, support, or resources. Furthermore, the family's functioning style (i.e., how a family copes with life challenges) influences where, when, and how a family will seek services.

It is essential for providers to understand the clients' and/or their family's motivation for initially seeking the services: Was the problem or concern for which the client is being treated diagnosed by the parent, client, teacher, health provider, or a child care worker? What was the client's/family's point of entry into the system? Were they self-referred or referred by another agency/individual? What are the cultural influences and perceptions related to receiving help outside of the family? What are the family's perceptions and history regarding systems? How long has the family been a part of the system? How long has the family been attempting to resolve specific issues to get its needs met?

The answers to these questions will increase the provider's understanding of the family's strengths, needs, insights, support systems, decision-making processes, coping skills, experiences, and expectations. These answers will also assist the providers in developing interventions and recommending resources that respond more appropriately to the need presented.

## Cultural Influences

Culture is not something tangible; it cannot be touched. It is an invisible component of our lives that has a powerful influence on every aspect of ours lives. It is shaped by numerous social factors that are constantly changing. Many clients, their families, and the agency or system that serves them are all touched and significantly influenced by some type of cultural orientation. Culture is the conceptual framework from which an individual views and orients him- or herself to the world. Cross, Bazron, Dennis, and Isaacs (1989) see culture as the composite of human behavior that includes the way we think, communicate, and act. It encompasses the customs, beliefs, values, and institutions of a racial, ethnic, religious, or social group. According to Abbey, Brindis, and Casas (1990), "culture serves as a road map for both perceiving and interacting with the world. Because culture is dynamic and ever changing, the road map can lead in different directions" (p. 8).

Culture profoundly affects a family's understanding of, interactions with, and decisions made related to health, wellness, illness, and death

(Kinsman, Mitchell, & Fox, 1996). More specifically, "health assumptions and practices are directly influenced by life experiences and culture" (Galvis, 1995, p. 1104). As health and human service professionals encounter more clients from diverse cultures, it will be critical for the individual, the health/human service professional, and the system in which he or she works to develop ways to accommodate these differences as the agency/organization moves toward effective service provision as a bottom line product. A culturally sensitive approach to service delivery ensures that clients will come away from the agency with the services they want and not just the ones that the agency deems important or useful for the clients.

## History/Experience

Clients and their families bring more to an intake interview than themselves. A history is present for every client and family member that a health and human service agency or organization serves. This history includes perceptions/information about (1) being a member of the family, (2) the illness or disease, (3) the agency providing the service, (4) the act of going outside of the family for help, and (5) how the illness, health condition, and other needs are to be addressed. All mental, physical, spiritual, and social experiences are a part of this history and have some impact on both client and family well-being. A provider's ability to identify and understand a client's history is important as the professional seeks to locate services to address the need presented. It is essential that providers view families as an extension of the agency and as facilitators in the provision of services. Clients and families have valuable information locked away within individual members as well as spread throughout the relationship in the family (Cox, 1994). Appropriate identification and utilization of this historical information can indeed help diminish the possibility of having it function as a barrier to access.

## Lack of Resources/Support Needed to Access the Service

Opportunity is America's calling card and has been since the great immigration of Europeans to Ellis Island in the early 1900s (Adler, 1996). Success stories from many first-generation families, as well as those of some of the most recent immigrants, promote the particular ethos or mindset that individuals, families, and communities are successful or unsuccessful, resourceful or unresourceful. Many clients and families put forth commendable efforts, but still find themselves without adequate resources and unable to access services.

Chronic illnesses and debilitating conditions take their toll on families. The absence of material resources such as money, insurance, transportation, and child care are real access issues and can determine whether parents will stay overnight at the hospital after a child's surgery and/or return the next week for a clinic appointment. The management of stress, brought on by illness or any particular change in the family's routine, can stimulate a need for coping skills that may or may not be present. The family in the following scenario is facing some of the access issues previously noted. As well, the health/medical condition of the child has brought new stresses, challenges, and the need for coping mechanisms.

---

**Case Example 4.1**

A family of six (mother, father, son, grandparents, child having surgery) arrived at a hospital for their child's first ear surgery to correct a hearing problem. The child needed surgery approximately six months ago, but the family did not have the $15,000 needed to cover the cost of the surgery (insurance provided partial coverage). Benevolent sources of income were available to the family earlier, but a series of paperwork had to be signed and notarized. Also, the family could not get clarity from the hospital as to what accepting money from the benevolent source would mean for them. The family was very hesitant to use this as an option and proceeded to mobilize its community to contribute financially to their need. It took six months with community and family support to raise the $15,000.

Admission testing reveals that the child's hearing loss had continued to worsen. The patient chart revealed only two out of six follow-up appointments were completed. Given the length of time it had taken for the family to get this child into surgery and the pattern of follow-up, the multidisciplinary team is concerned about the family's understanding of how critical timing is in follow-up care for this child. They considered the family's ability to follow up a risk factor in their consideration of whether surgery should be done.

---

Case Example 4.1 resulted in additional stresses and challenges for both the family and the hospital. Initial resolution of these stresses and challenges could have begun by considering the following questions:

1. What are some of the stressors for the family?
2. What are some of the stressors for the hospital?
3. What can be identified as the family's strengths/needs?
4. What can be identified as the hospital's strengths/needs?
5. What could be done to turn the needs of both the family and the hospital into strengths?

It is likely that a health or human service professional may perceive a family in the preceding situation as one lacking resources and support (e.g., hospital's concern that family missed four of six appointments). Given the nature of health and human service provision systems, many families who lack specific material or tangible resources are viewed as deficient. However, the family may have other social and nontangible resources that can help them access services (e.g., family's ability to raise the $15,000). Professionals working with clients and families who appear to lack resources would do well to examine the possibility of converting the family's needs into strengths—every deficit should be mapped with a strength (Kretzmann & McKnight, 1993; Parks & Straker, 1996). The ability of the professional to see the family as a "glass half-full rather than half-empty" could be the motivation needed to promote confidence within the family. Dunst, Trivette, and Deal (cited in MacPhee, 1995) support this thought, noting that "positive effects from informal supports are generally greater than those derived from formal support resources" (p. 419). Operating out of such a viewpoint, health and human service professionals may more effectively serve a client and his or her family by identifying formal agency resources to address needs that are not covered by the family's informal support system.

## COMMON BARRIERS FOR SYSTEMS

There are multiple barriers in systems that keep clients from getting services. While clients and families must make an effort to negotiate the system in order to get their needs met, health and human service agencies must bear some responsibility as well. Systems must take steps to ensure that services are readily accessible to all clients. Some of the most common access barriers are created when systems (1) lack adequate knowledge about their clients' culture, (2) lack knowledge of existing intra- and interagency resources, and (3) lack interagency collaboration. These systematic inadequacies become more prolific when one takes into account the current and significant shift of the racial/ethnic make-up of the nation.

### Lack of Adequate Knowledge About Their Clients' Cultures

Most of the states in the United States do not reflect as much diversity in population as do California, New York, and Texas. However, many localities across the nation are experiencing an increased level of diversity in their respective populations. Toms and Hobbs (1997) noted that between

1980 and 1990 the Asian/Pacific Islander population grew by 107.8%; the Hispanic/Latino population grew by 53%; the American Indian population grew by 37.9%; blacks [African Americans] grew by 13.2%; and whites grew by 6% Their analysis of the United States' future population(s) indicates that by the year 2050 all racial/ethnic groups will constitute 47% of the population. The breakdown of that percentage is as follows: African Americans, 14.1%; Asian/Pacific Islanders, 8.2%; American Indian-Eskimos, Aleuts, 1.0%; others, 22.6%; and white Americans, 52% (p. 9).

Let's discuss the significance of increasing cultural diversity on service provision in just one state in this country. North Carolina's increasing racial and ethnic diversity mirrors the image reflected in the national data. The 1990 census reports that 1.6 million people or one in every four persons in North Carolina is a member of a minority group. African Americans constitute the largest minority group at 22% of the total population. This is nearly twice the national average of 12%. American Indians and Hispanics/Latinos each make up about 1.2% of the population, while Asians represent about .8%. Between 1980 and 1990 the Native American population in North Carolina increased by 11.2%. During that same ten-year period the African American population increased by 10.4%, and the white population increased by 12.4%. Population projections over the twenty-year period between 1990 to 2010 estimate that North Carolina's total population will grow by 21%. The Hispanic/Latino population is growing at three times the rate of other groups (Surles, 1993).

Such a colorful picture of diversity for both America and North Carolina means that many health and human service professionals will be faced with providing services to clients and families who come from a variety of cultural backgrounds (Adler, 1996; Toms & Hobbs, 1997). With these significant demographic changes, the probability increases that cultural and language challenges will function as barriers in a system unprepared to handle these diverse groups. Agencies that have not acknowledged and incorporated strategies to respond appropriately to their increasingly diverse client base may find themselves to be culturally incompetent.

Cultural incompetence (the lack of cultural competence) in an agency is operationalized in many ways: (1) dehumanizing minority clients, (2) discriminatory practices, (3) believing that one approach to service delivery will meet the needs of and be appropriate for all clients, or (4) hiring "token" minority staff (Cross et al., 1989). Cultural incompetence in agencies can keep people from diverse backgrounds away from the system and the services. Administrators and managers must understand this important connection between their approach to service provision and their clients' success in receiving all or part of the services offered. An agency's or system's ability to recognize, understand, plan for, and accommodate cultural differences has a significant impact on the family's ability to access the services.

"Attaining some level of cultural competence may be viewed as a goal towards which professionals, agencies, and systems can strive; thus becoming culturally competent is a developmental process" (Cross et al., 1989, p. 13). According to Cross and colleagues (1989), the cultural competence continuum defines six phases, with the most competent level being cultural proficiency. The first four phases describe the levels of cultural incompetence that can exist in agencies. These phases are defined below.

- *Cultural destructiveness:* Attitudes, policies, and practices that are harmful to cultures and hence to individuals within the culture. Historically, some agencies have been actively involved in services that have denied people of color access to their natural helpers or healers, removed children of color from their families on the basis of race, or purposely risked the well-being of minority individuals in social or medical experiments without their knowledge or consent (p. 14).
- *Cultural incapacity:* The system or agencies lack the capacity to help minority clients or communities. The system remains extremely biased, believes in the racial superiority of the dominant group, and assumes a paternal posture towards "lesser" races. The characteristics of cultural incapacity include discriminatory hiring practices, subtle messages to people of color that they are not valued or welcome, and generally lower expectations for minority clients (p. 15).
- *Cultural blindness:* The system and agencies provide services with the belief they are unbiased. They function with the belief that color or culture makes no difference and that all people are the same. The premise is that services are universally applicable. Such services ignore cultural strengths, encourage assimilation, and blame the victims for their problems (p. 15).
- *Cultural pre-competence:* The agency recognizes its limitations in serving minorities and tries to improve services for a specific population (p. 16).

The final two phases describe culturally competent and culturally proficient agencies.

- *Cultural competence:* A set of congruent behaviors, attitudes, and policies that come together in a system, agency, or among professionals and enable that system, agency, and professionals to work effectively in cross-cultural situations. Agencies are characterized by acceptance and respect for difference, continuing self-assessment regarding culture, careful attention to the dynamics of difference, continual expansion of cultural knowledge and resources, and various adaptations to service models to better meet the needs of minority populations. Such agencies view minority groups as distinctly different from one another and as having numerous subgroups, each with important cultural characteristics. Further, culturally competent agencies understand the interplay between policy and practice and are committed to policies that enhance services to diverse clientele. Cultural competence is developed over time through training, experience, guidance, and self-evaluation (p. 17).

- *Cultural proficiency:* This point on the continuum is characterized by holding culture in high esteem. Culturally proficient agencies seek to add to the knowledge base of culturally competent practice by conducting research, developing new therapeutic approaches based on culture, and publishing and disseminating the results of demonstration projects. Culturally proficient agencies hire staff who are specialists in culturally competent practice. Such agencies advocate for cultural competence throughout the system and for improved relationships between cultures throughout society (p. 17).

While the cultural competence continuum defines the process and various stages for agencies, it is a challenge for agencies to progress along the continuum because efforts must be strategic, comprehensive, systemic, and long-term. Agencies must address a key question, "How far are we willing to go to accommodate and serve our clients?" Top level agency administrators and providers have to assume responsibility for developing culturally appropriate services. They must recognize, acknowledge, and plan for the reality that each staff person will be at a different level in his or her understanding of and appreciation for cultural differences. There will also be differences in each staff person's understanding and interpretation of how cultural differences directly impact job performance and the agency's ability to provide effective services. Training is one key to ensuring that administrators recognize that there is a connection between understanding cultural differences and the provision of quality services. Cultural competence training, communication workshops, and staff development opportunities are vehicles available to agency administrators and their staff to increase their level of understanding.

Top-level administrators must be willing to put the agency's commitment to cultural competence in writing. The agency's mission statement, policies, programs, and services must reflect an understanding of and value for diversity. The agency's position must be communicated clearly, consistently, and on an ongoing basis. The agency administrators set the tone in this systems change process. Administrators must be willing to do more than make staff responsible for developing and implementing strategies for moving the agency along the cultural competence continuum. They must set an example for staff by (1) increasing their own knowledge of other cultures, (2) participating in skill-building training, and (3) taking the lead in implementing specific strategies to promote change.

Likewise, providers must understand how culture and history impact social issues and health-seeking behaviors. It is unrealistic to think that providers will become experts on all of the nuances of the different cultures. However, it is important that providers have a general understanding of cultural beliefs, practices, perceptions, and coping strategies for dealing with issues relating to their clients. In order to meet the health and human service needs of all clients, systems must make some adjustments. Some of the other common system barriers have little to do with the culture of clients but are directly related to the culture of organizations themselves.

Health service agencies are described as both social and cultural systems; a system of meanings and behavioral norms attached to particular social relationships and institutional settings (Jezewski, 1993). "Health care systems are like other cultural systems; they are symbolic systems built out of meanings, values, and behavioral norms. The culture of the health care system can be recognized as different from the lay culture of the person entering that system as a patient or client" (Jezewski, 1993, p. 80). Because an agency has its own culture, it frequently cannot, and sometimes does not, pay attention to clients who do not fit the agency's culture. An ongoing review/assessment of services is essential to ensure that the agency's needs are not totally driving the service provision system. It would be wise for an agency to achieve an equitable balance between the needs of the agency and needs of the clients.

## Lack of Knowledge of Existing Intra- and Interagency Resources and Other System Challenges

Lack of knowledge of existing intra- and interagency resources is a common problem in health and human service agencies that creates major barriers for providers. Sometimes providers lack a general knowledge of the resources and services around them because there is limited time and limited opportunity to learn about or to become comfortably familiar with resources outside of the realm of their area of responsibility or expertise. In the course of carrying out day-to-day activities there are few opportunities to communicate program and service information within and between agencies. Regular staff meetings are often devoted to program updates or relaying any changes in policies, administrative procedures, or program directions. The communication that does occur outside of meetings usually is (1) focused on a specific client or program, (2) in response to a specific case or request, or (3) initiated simply to retrieve needed information or resources. Because of such a limited sphere of communication, it is not uncommon for colleagues in the same system to be unaware of each other skills, expertise, needs, and/or difficulties in serving clients/ families who are culturally different. The result is that human and material resources within and among agencies are underutilized.

Few orientation programs adequately prepare new staff for the implementation and operational challenges inherent in health and human service agencies. Staff orientations do not include in-depth information about the intricacies of agency operations, organizational relationships, existing resources, and what staff members need to know in order to successfully negotiate the system to get the job done. Unless agencies offer training and create opportunities for dialogue, staff do not have a sense of where the organization has been, where it wants to go, who within the agency can help it get to its destination, or a vision of the agency's mission beyond staff members' individual divisions or programs.

It is easy for systems, and the people in them, to get comfortable doing business the same way year in and year out. Generally speaking, systems do not support innovation. The inability of most service provision systems to accommodate innovation is one of the most challenging traps for health and human service providers. Literally, the traps are the organizational boxes that define reporting relationships and group people, programs, and services together. Providers need to be innovative to meet the needs of their clients. Often times being innovative means stepping "outside of the box." Those providers who do step outside of the box may find themselves in a position of having to convince administrators that the new approach to service provision will benefit both the clients and the agency. All of these factors are far too often the reality for agencies and health and human services providers. An environment is created and perpetuated that is not conducive to interagency collaboration or service provision. This environment is plagued with duplication of services, an inefficient use of limited resources, and the absence of a central entry point for clients. To avoid these situations, an organized approach such as strategic planning to intra- and interagency collaboration is necessary. Strategic planning occurs infrequently in health and human service agencies. When it does occur, other agencies are seldom invited to participate in the process. Consequently, long-range plans are developed for agencies without thinking through service provision issues with other agencies that serve the same clients. Conducting joint strategic planning is a good first step to effective interagency service provision. This is a way for agencies to figure out a central point for client access to services and pivotal points for interagency collaboration.

### Lack of Interagency Collaboration and Its Influence on Clients/Families

Frequently, bringing all of the agencies serving a family together to address a health or social need can in and of itself function as a barrier to clients and their families. The following are a few barriers that can make interagency service provision a challenge:

1. Nonexistent to poor communication between and among agency and staff
2. Absence of a shared vision regarding the quality of service provision
3. The absence of a shared vision regarding expected outcomes for the client or family
4. Exclusion of key participants who have a stake in the service provision process
5. Past working relationship with the family
6. Level and intensity of coordination and collaboration
7. Lack of clarification and understanding of role delineation, responsibilities, and outcomes among and across agencies

The degree to which an agency can address and/or eliminate any one or all of these barriers will determine that agency's ability to provide effective services to its clients. Clients can have multiple needs and require multiple services. But who is responsible for ensuring that the client can successfully access needed services within and across agencies? Administrators must train staff using modeling and coaching techniques on how to be advocates for both the agency and clients. This balance is important to ensure that client-driven, quality services are provided. A provider who works collaboratively with his or her counterparts in other agencies, and one who functions as an advocate, is in a better position to successfully meet the needs of the client and his or her family. Brower (as cited in Jezewski, 1993) states that "an advocate is one who defends, pleads the cause of, promotes the rights of, or attempts to change the systems on behalf of an individual or group" (p. 78). Providers must be willing to function as advocates for their clients' needs and rights.

Jezewski (1993) affirms the importance of an advocate in her article "Culture Brokering as a Model for Advocacy." She states,

> In a perfect world with equal access to health care and patients who are powerful players in the health care system, advocacy would be unnecessary or, at most, an entity that more fully empowers patients to be autonomous, self-determining, informed consumers of health care services. Many times institutional, so-

cial, political, economic, and cultural constraints prevent patients from accessing health care they determine to be appropriate. When these constraints are present, an advocate is necessary to facilitate the acquisition of health care. (p. 79)

This notion is extended to health and human service agencies as well because the same constraints exist to keep clients from needed services. As an advocate for clients, providers must assume a lead role in addressing system barriers created by ineffective interagency collaboration. The responsibility for or burden of successfully negotiating the system should not rest solely with the client and his or her family.

## BUILDING BRIDGES: CLIENT-FOCUSED STRATEGIES AND SOLUTIONS WITHIN SYSTEMS

Bureaucracy can be as burdensome on systems as it frequently is on clients/families seeking services. The reality is that services are often provided in spite of the system. Some very practical steps can be taken to improve access and help systems advocate more efficiently on behalf of clients.

### *Involving Clients in Developing Solutions*

Interagency service provision can be an effective, efficient, appropriate, and mutually beneficial venture if:

1. Players have a joint goal or aim as a single focus rather than a secondary focus.
2. The needs of those being served are accurately assessed.
3. Individuals involved in the service provision process are clear about their roles, the latitude that these roles permit, and the responsibilities that their roles require.
4. Differences of clients and families are recognized and addressed in service provision.
5. The interagency collaborative efforts are natural and not forced.
6. Conflict resolution mechanisms are put into place up front. (Peterken & Bonynge, 1995)

Client-focused services somehow must include clients and their families in the process. Providers must engage clients and families as partners in the service provision process and be careful not to (1) make premature assumptions about the family's strengths or weaknesses, (2) make decisions for the family, or (3) rush a family through the decision-making process in an effort to meet the agency's service provision goal(s). Only through mutual respect and understanding can a successful provider/client partnership for change be developed and maintained. This partnership for change must be mutually defined. This mutual agreement is the foundation for establishing effective communication, respect, cooperation, and trust. Feeling empowered is important for a family that is dealing with a child's health condition.

According to MacPhee (1995), empowerment of families occurs when the following four basic principles are implemented:

Principle 1. Focus intervention/prevention on the family, not the child.

Principle 2. Work with the family to create opportunities for ALL family members to acquire and employ competencies that strengthen the family.

Principle 3. Respect the family's rightful role to decide what is important to family members. The provider role is to strengthen and support the family decisions and actions.

Principle 4. Acknowledge the positive aspects of the child and family. "Too often professionals search for things that must be wrong, especially in families who have children with severe handicaps or significant chronic illness" (p. 418).

Once a client enters the system of care, several outcomes are possible. The client and family may buy into the service, relate to the provider, and agree with the defined outcomes. The other possibility is that they never return and are unresponsive to follow-up attempts. The provider must strive to get the client and family to value the service as much as it is valued by the provider/agency. Good communication, mutual respect, and common understanding are critical in this interaction. Sometimes providers will need to function as translators. They must be able to translate technical, clinical, and medical terms into a language that clients can understand and appreciate. Providers must not only be able to translate words, but concepts as well.

On the other hand, some clients and families arrive in the provider's office fully expecting the health/human service professional to make all the necessary decisions regarding the medical/or health-related condition or social need (MacPhee, 1995; Rappaport, 1981). A provider who functions as an advocate is able to spot such internal relinquishing of power and turn some aspects of the decision-making process over to the client and/or the family.

Clients and their families frequently have ideas and information that, if incorporated into the system, can improve the level and quality of an agency's service provision process. Therefore, agencies that are really serious about meeting the needs of the client must see client feedback as essential. Agencies should outline a process for how this feedback is incorporated into agency policies, practices, and plans of operation.

Case Example 4.2 will give the reader some clues about the traps agencies fall into when they prejudge the needs of clients, families, and communities. The agency highlighted in this scenario is a local hospital that decided to expand its service area and attempted to build a relationship with the African American community at the same time.

---

**Case Example 4.2**

A local African American community was the site for a new satellite clinic. This community had a documented history of chronic and acute health problems, a substantial elderly population, and very few health care providers. The hospital conglomerate planning the clinic did some analysis of demographic and income information, but minimal contact was made with the people who lived in the community. Interestingly enough, the hospital had no past history of working with or providing services in this African American community. Subsequently, services were determined before knowing much about the community to be served. When an official presentation was made to the community leadership that the clinic was going to be built, the idea was not received well. Some community leaders sought the advice from African American health professionals in their churches, but the input provided came a little late.

---

The hospital's approach is an example for how service delivery is planned FOR rather than WITH the community. Before deciding on the services, it is important to involve the clients and their families up front to develop solutions. It is important to have a clear understanding of the target population in the service area and its service needs. The right questions must be asked of the right people. In this scenario, statistics on the demographics of the community were documented; however, the agency did not have a good understanding of people in the community or their perception of service needs.

A comprehensive community assessment would have included not only health status data and information on employment and socioeconomic status, but it would have well included input from formal and informal leadership from the targeted community. This assessment would have identified other relevant information about the community such as:

- Existing resources (human, material, social)
- Current health care practices
- Current patterns for accessing needed health care services
- Health care service needs from the community's perspective

Some key questions should have been asked of the community during the planning process, such as: Where do members currently go for services? How do they get there? Do you think your community needs a clinic? If yes, what services should be provided? When should they be offered? Who should be able to use them? These and other questions should have been presented to the formal and informal leadership of the community. Formal and informal leaders play different roles, but both are keys to understanding and working with the community. It is important to understand how these leaders influence and represent a community.

The hospital in this scenario talked to "formal" leaders in the community. Formal leaders were identified as "professionals" or "experts" in their fields or individuals who maintained high social status. Formal leaders were recommended to the hospital staff by others from the broader community rather than from members of the targeted community. The majority of the formal leaders identified did not live in the targeted community, nor did they necessarily personally know anyone who lived in the target community. Therefore, their input and perceptions were usually second-hand and may have been based on speculation rather than fact. These individuals may have defined themselves as leaders or representatives of particular groups. Their designation of such status may not have been supported by the entire community. This created a communication gap between the agency and the community before the services were put in place.

It is necessary for agencies to reach the informal leaders in the community. Informal leaders do not necessarily maintain a high profile, but they have influence in the community. These are those indigenous members who have a history in the community, the power to make or break the formal leadership, the ability to move the community, and the power to limit "outsider" access to the community if they choose.

Understanding the importance of reaching and engaging both formal and informal leaders is a significant first step. The challenge lies in identifying effective and efficient strategies to access key leaders in the community. Each community is unique. Multiple approaches may be implemented before an agency has access to the community and to its formal and informal leaders.

According to Bell, Hill, and Wright (1961), some approaches for reaching formal and informal leaders of the target community are as follows:

- *Positional approach:* Persons who occupy formal positions of leadership in the target group, such as ministers, rabbis, mayors, public agency directors, business owners, officers of voluntary organizations, and elected leaders of labor organizations (p. 6).
- *Social participation approach:* People who join or participate in voluntary and community organizations. They may be excellent sources of information about the culture and organization of the target community or public (p. 21).
- *Reputational approach:* Members of a group can also be identified as leaders by the extent to which others within the group regard them as leaders. Members of a group are asked to tell who they think their most influential leaders are. Those leaders that are mentioned most often are considered the reputational leaders.
- *Decision-making approach:* Actual involvement in making decisions is the basis for identifying leaders. Investigating one or more specific policy decisions can identify the individuals who influenced the decision (p. 22).
- *Opinion leadership approach:* Members of a group are asked to name those persons from whom they would ask advice on a topic of concern. The persons identified most often may be regarded as the opinion leaders on that topic (Bell et al., 1961, p. 23).

Once leaders have been contacted it is essential that they are directly involved in the planning and decision-making process.

While the hospital scenario focused on an agency and the strategies for building a trusting and cooperative relationship with an entire community, the same principles apply for agencies and providers when dealing with individual clients and their families. Agencies and providers must understand the role(s) of each family member by seeking answers to the following questions: Who is defined as the "leader" of the family? Who makes the major health care decisions? Who should be involved in the care of the client?

## SUMMARY

Public health. Minority health. Organizational health. Interagency service provision is the basis for success in each of these arenas. Designing programs and services that reach minority children, families, and communities is not hard to do, but it takes interest, commitment, skill, and perseverance. Those agencies that build trust by looking into and then moving out into the places of our society where cultures come alive strengthen both their integrity and skill. Agencies that provide culturally based services create an environment for effective service provision to racial and ethnic minorities. It lays a foundation for building trust, promoting effective communication, and creating supportive relationships. In order for interagency service provision to be culturally appropriate for clients, each health and human service agency must make a commitment to cultural competence. The approach must be both comprehensive and long-term. All levels of the organization must be included and all staff adequately trained. Training and practice are needed to develop the necessary skills to promote effective systems change. Only when all health and human service agencies become culturally competent can the true power of effective interagency service provision be realized (Pullen-Smith, in preparation).

## STUDY QUESTIONS AND ACTIVITIES

1. Discuss some challenges to interagency service provision.
2. Explain the following levels of service provision:
   • direct service
   • referral
   • coordination
   • skill building
   • collaboration
3. What are some common barriers for clients/families in accessing services provided by health and human service agencies?
4. What are some of the aspects of family history/experience that may have an impact on how agency services are perceived and received?
5. Discuss seven barriers that can make interagency service provision a challenge.
6. What are some ways in which interagency service provision can be effective, efficient, appropriate, and mutually beneficial?

## REFERENCES

Abbey, N., Brindis, C., & Casas, M. (1990). *Practical guidelines: Family life education in multicultural classrooms*. Santa Cruz: Network Publication.

Adler, M. M. (1996). The Beth Israel health care system addresses the challenge of cultural diversity. *Journal of Nursing Administration, 26*(9), 3–4.

American Heart Association (North Carolina Affiliate, Inc.). (1993). *Developing AHA initiatives in culturally diverse communities*. Chapel Hill, NC: Author.

Bell, W., Hill, R., & Wright, C. (1961). *Public leadership: A critical review with special reference to adult education*. San Francisco: Chandler.

Cox, R. P. (1994). Systematic circularity: Working with individuals for family level change. *Journal of Psychosocial Nursing, 32*(7), 33–39.

Cross, T. L., Bazron, B. J., Dennis, K. W., & Isaacs, M. R. (1989). *Towards a culturally competent system of care* (Vol. 1). Washington, DC: Child and Adolescent Service Systems Program CASSP Technical Assistance Center.

Davis, B. J., & Voegtle, K. H. (1994). *Culturally competent health care for adolescents: A guide for primary care providers*. Chicago: American Medical Association.

Deane, B. R. (1995). Effecting change: Diversity affects personal and organizational development. *Journal of Dental Education, 59*(12), 1099–1102.

Galvis, D. L. M. (1995). Clinical contexts for diversity and intercultural competence. *Journal of Dental Education, 59,* 1103–1105.

Jezewski, M. (1993). Culture brokering as a model for advocacy. *Nursing and Health Care, 14*(2), 78–84.

Kinsman, S. B., Mitchell, S., & Fox, K. (1996). Multicultural issues in pediatric practice. *Pediatrics in Review, 17*(10), 349–355.

Kretzmann, J. P., & McKnight, J. L. (1993). *Building communities from the inside out: A path toward finding and mobilizing a community's assets*. Evanston, IL: Center for Urban Affairs and Policy Research, Neighborhood Innovations Network, Northwestern University.

Lilley, L., & Guanci, R. (1995, November). Applying systems theory. *American Journal of Nursing,* 14–15.

MacPhee, M. (1995). The family systems approach and pediatric nursing care. *Pediatric Nursing, 21*(5), 417–437.

Marsland, K. (1994). Child protection: The interagency approach. *Nursing Standard, 8*(33), 25–28.

Parks, C., & Straker, H. (1996). Community assets mapping: Community health assessment with a different twist. *Journal of Health Education, 27*(5), 321–22.

Peterken, C., & Bonynge, S. (1995). Improving care for children in a multi-agency alliance. *Nursing Times, 91*(30), 31–32.

Pullen-Smith, B. (in preparation). *Cultural diversity training: Laying a foundation for change in public health*. Manuscript in preparation.

Rappaport, J. (1981). In praise of paradox: A social policy of empowerment over prevention. *American Journal of Community Psychology, 9*(1), 1–25.

Shea, K., Rahmanic, C., & Morris, P. (1996). Diagnosing children with attention deficit disorders through a health department public school partnership. *American Journal of Public Health, 86*(8), 1168–1189.

Solberg, L., Isham, G., Kottke, T., Magman, S., Nelson, A., Reed, M., & Richards, S. (1995). Competing HMOs collaborate to improve preventive services. *The Joint Commission Journal on Quality Improvement, 21*(11), 600–610.

Surles, K. B. (1993). *North Carolina's minorities: Who and where,* SCHS Studies No. 72. Raleigh, NC: State Center for Health Statistics.

Toms, F. D., & Hobbs, A. (1997). *Who are we?* Forrestville, MD: Diverse Books.

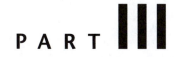

PART **III**

# CULTURALLY APPROPRIATE ASSESSMENT AND INTERVENTION PRACTICES

# 5

# EARLY INTERVENTION: WORKING WITH CHILDREN WITHIN THE CONTEXT OF THEIR FAMILIES AND COMMUNITIES

## LEMMIETTA G. MCNEILLY and THALIA J. COLEMAN

### MOVING TOWARD FAMILY-CENTERED INTERVENTION

The family is a system in which all of the components are interdependent; that is, what happens to one member of a family affects other members of the family. Speech-language pathologists and other special service providers work with families that are under a great deal of stress because they include at least one person with special needs (Luterman, 1991). Families from culturally and linguistically diverse populations present with some unique features that service providers are not always competent to handle effectively. This chapter will present some factors to consider and methodology for providing family-centered intervention for families of culturally diverse groups.

In many cases, family members are the significant communication partners for language development with young children. If early intervention is going to be successful, it is critical to build partnerships with family members (Robinson, 1997). Family members teach young children by demonstration. Often family members are unaware of the impact they have upon young children. Because young children are so impressionable, it is important that we empower family members to facilitate language development in the home and community to reinforce the foundations we build in the clinical/school settings.

Donahue-Kilburg (1992) characterized the traditional model of intervention as one in which service providers focus on what they perceive as the client's strengths and needs with little or no attention given to the family's perspective. It is one in which clients are often separated from the rest of the family in order to be given assessment tools and therapy. In addition, traditional therapy is planned and carried out by the interventionist alone or aided by parents who are given specific instructions. Clinicians need to be more facilitative and encourage family members to play a participatory role in both the assessment and the treatment rendered to young children. Clinicians can learn a lot from the family as well as offer specific language facilitation strategies that are consistent with the family's cultural values and beliefs and that can be utilized in the family and community.

The focus of service provision for clinicians providing early intervention services has shifted from child-centered to family-centered or family-directed. In family-centered intervention, families participate as decision makers and partners in all aspects of service delivery. The goals of intervention focus on strengthening and supporting the family (Noonan & McCormick, 1993). The ultimate responsibility for managing a child's health, developmental, social, and emotional needs lies with the family. Therefore, it is our responsibility, as special service providers, to enable families to function as primary decision makers, teachers, caregivers, and advocates for their children (Shelton, Jeppson, & Johnson, 1992). Some of the families will need to access special services for children beyond the early years. Therefore, early intervention service providers have the unique opportunity to give families the tools that they can utilize for as long as they need to access various systems as their children's needs change and the children get older.

## Building Collaborative Relationships with Families

McLean and Crais (1996) discussed several reasons for building collaborative relationships with families. The family holds a central position in the child's life and development. Families have unique knowledge about the child that is unavailable to professionals if not disclosed by the family. Families are usually reliable in performing activities such as completing screening tools or developmental checklists of their children's behavior. This leads to increased participation in other aspects of intervention. Working in collaboration with families can improve the ecological validity of assessment. It also helps family members understand their importance in the overall intervention process and increases the level of family satisfaction about the entire process. McLean and Crais concluded that building collaborative relationships not only recognizes family rights, but may also improve the efficiency and validity of assessment activities. The focus of this chapter will be a discussion of the nature and importance of family-centered intervention. Suggestions for working with families from nonmainstream backgrounds will be presented.

## *Family-Centered Intervention: A Description*

The family-centered approach to intervention is unique in at least three ways. It (1) focuses on the client in the context of his or her family, (2) considers the strengths and needs of the entire family, and (3) involves family members in assessment and treatment planning. Family-centered intervention requires the professional to relinquish a certain amount of control over the intervention process (Donahue-Kilburg, 1992).

Shelton, Jeppson, and Johnson (1992) summarized the key elements of family-centered care. The first element is the recognition that the family is the constant in the child's life. Personnel from various agencies who work with the child and family at any given time may change, but the family will always be the family. A second element of family-centered care is family/professional collaboration at all levels of care. Exchanging complete and unbiased information between families and professionals is another element of this type of care. Sharing of information is a critical factor in enabling parents to participate fully in the decision-making process. Even parents who have had professional training in related areas prior to the birth of a child with special needs require information (Shelton et al., 1992). When information is exchanged, it should always be done in a supportive, professional, and respectful manner.

Family-centered care also involves the recognition and honoring of cultural diversity. There must be recognition of strengths and individuality within and across families, including ethnic, racial, spiritual, social, economic, educational, and geographic diversity. Interventionists must also be able to recognize and respect different modes of coping exhibited by parents. In order to facilitate achievement of targeted outcomes, service providers must be capable of implementing comprehensive policies and programs that provide various types of support to meet the diverse needs of families. Interventionists should encourage and facilitate support networks for families. Another responsibility of persons providing special services to children and their families is to ensure that service and support systems are flexible, accessible, and comprehensive in responding to needs identified by diverse families. A final element of family-centered care identified by Shelton, Jeppson, and Johnson (1992) is appreciation of families as family units and children as children. Interventionists should recognize that families and children possess a wide range of strengths, concerns, emotions, and aspirations apart from their need for special services and support.

Trout and Foley (1989) also discussed characteristics of a family-centered approach. They describe the family-centered approach as one that

1. *Acknowledges the complex and transactional nature of development.* Language and communication skills do not develop in a vacuum. Children acquire skills in many areas at the same time. Development in any one of those areas will have an impact on development in other areas. Each developmental gain or loss affects the family. There may be developmental concerns about areas other than or in addition to speech and language. *Arena assessment* is one way of ensuring that a professional does not limit focus of intervention to his or her discipline alone.
2. *Respects diversity and the developmental nature of parenthood.* Parenting is not a simple process. It is further complicated when there are children with disabilities. Parents of children with disabilities experience grief for the loss of the perfect child that they expected. Also, parenting is not static. It is not a matter of either having "good" parenting skills or not having them. There is continuing development over time. Parenting skills or attainments are also culturally based and may be expressed in different ways. For example, the way parents show attachment to their children varies across cultures. Early interventionists must resist the urge to teach parents how to act "normal," since this label does not neatly transfer from one culture to another.
3. *Respects the decision making and autonomy of each family.* Relationships between families and service providers should be a supportive partnership of learning, growth, and adaptation. Professionals should not be offended if families choose to seek second opinions and to investigate alternative treatments. Service providers should promote the rights of families to state their rights and to say "no" when they choose to. Furthermore, interventionists must understand that as families are making decisions about services for children with special needs, they have the right to focus on needs of the entire family unit. Interventionists must help to ensure that programs and policies address the long-term needs of the total family, not just the immediate needs of the child with special needs (Shelton et al., 1992).
4. *Is enabling for the family.* Service provider relationships with families should promote the self-sufficiency and self-esteem of the families.

Service providers should build upon behaviors that are already a part of the observed parent-child interactions. Interventionists must reinforce and enhance pleasurable reciprocal behavior observed between parent and child. Special service providers must support families without undermining their confidence in their ability to care for their own children (Shelton et al., 1992). Often parents of children with special needs require reinforcement that they are making the right choices for their children. Service providers should also help families access various aspects of health care systems and support networks. According to Donahue-Kilburg (1992), one of the major components of the empowerment process is the provision of information. Donahue-Kilburg suggested that professionals can help families to feel empowered by giving them, or helping them to gather, needed information. Also, interventionists can help family members feel competent by creating opportunities for competence to be displayed or acquired. Noonan and McCormick (1993) discussed expectations parents have of program staff. Parents expect staff to be supportive, accepting, and nonjudgmental. They also desire trust, commitment, and honest communication. Additionally, they want to feel that they are being heard. Finally, they want assessment and intervention to focus on the child as a member of the family unit.

5. *Recognizes the central role of relationships and the inner life in promoting optimal development.* Team members must know the fundamentals of relationship building that is characterized by consistency, predictability, warmth, positive regard, and empathy.

According to Anderson and McNeilly (1992), professionals must keep in mind that there is considerable diversity in cultural groups. They also emphasized the fact that the extent to which any family can be characterized by any set of cultural values and practices varies with each individual family. There are issues that are common to families who have children with special needs. However, interventionists must remember at all times that each family is different. Consequently, they will show differences in coping skills, the ability to adapt to the needs of the child, and in the amount of involvement they desire in the intervention process. At all times interventionists must remember that they are working with individuals. Individuals are a composite of their real-life experiences. Even people who are from backgrounds that are similar may have very different ways of dealing with various aspects of life because many of their experiences might have been different.

Robinson (1997) stated that the most critical elements of family-centered care are understanding that children are parts of families and realizing that effective intervention must be built on positive relationships with members of the individual families. Robinson believes family-centered approaches provide opportunities to establish positive relationship with families of the children served. They also facilitate the creation of interventions that fit into natural settings where families and children live. In addition, family-centered care encourages interventionists to use more flexible categories when describing children. In family-centered care, interventionists are likely to look for *profiles of strengths and needs* rather than just numerical scores. Furthermore, as services are provided in a family-centered environment, interventionists tend to realize that many children with special needs and their families have far more strengths than needs.

## BECOMING MORE FAMILY-CENTERED IN PROFESSIONAL PRACTICE

Bailey (1996) recommended the following steps interventionists should take as they strive to develop goals that include family concerns and preferences:

- Develop a relationship with the parents or primary caregivers and other key members of the immediate and extended family
- Identify strengths and needs of the child
- Identify concerns of the family
- Identify family members' view of the problem

According to Robinson (1997), as professionals attempt to comply with Part H of IDEA, developing goals with family members is a natural part of the process. Working with families means to involve them as partners in all aspects of intervention, including assessment, developing goals and establishing priorities for implementation of those goals, and choosing the most appropriate strategies for accomplishing those goals.

### Family-Centered Intervention Practices

Development of family-centered goals is facilitated by the framework of the Individual Family Service Plan (IFSP). Under the provisions of PL 99-457, a multidisciplinary team including the child's parents or guardians must develop a written IFSP. Federal law mandates that the IFSP must (1) be developed jointly by the family and professional interventionists, (2) be based on multidisciplinary assessment of child and family (family assessment is voluntary), and (3) include services to enhance the development of the child and empower the family to meet the special needs of the child (Donahue-Kilburg, 1992).

Donahue-Kilburg (1992) developed the following eight-step process for IFSP development based on the work of Campbell (1990) and McGonigel, Kaufmann, and Hurth (1990):

1. Statement of philosophy and values
2. First contacts with families
3. Assessment planning
4. Child assessment/evaluation
5. Determining desired outcomes
6. Ongoing child and family assessment
7. Implementation
8. Reviews and update of the IFSP document

These eight steps are discussed throughout this text. Steps two through seven are discussed in chapters 3 through 9 and will not be dealt with here. Step one addresses program philosophy. Members of early intervention teams should have written statements concerning families and the various aspects of the early intervention process. Step eight is concerned with periodic reviews of program outcomes. The IFSP should be reviewed and updated at least once every six months. There should also be an annual meeting to revise the IFSP. Family members and the service coordinator should be participants in these program reviews. When the child is about to become eligible for preschool services (3 years old), a plan for transition to those services must be a part of the IFSP (Donahue-Kilburg, 1992). The school-based services are mandated by Part B of IDEA and the individual elements are documented in an Individualized Educational Plan (IEP).

## Levels of Family Involvement

Not all families choose to get involved in the assessment and treatment process at the same levels. Alexander, Kroth, Simpson, and Poppelreiter (1982) identified four levels at which parents or guardians can be involved in the intervention process:

1. *Awareness level:* Parents are made aware of the goals that have been established for the child, how the goals will be accomplished, and the progress the child is making toward those goals.
2. *Knowledge and information level:* Parents are provided specific and extensive information about all aspects of the child's program.

3. *Meaningful exchanges and interaction level:* Family members participate at some level in program-related activities.
4. *Skill acquisition and training level:* Family members are directly involved in carrying out specific therapeutic activities for the child.

According to Donahue-Kilburg (1992), the nature and amount of family involvement may change over time. Job changes, illnesses, and other factors may force family members to readjust time commitments. Families are likely to be more eager about involvement in the intervention process if they know the clinician understands and supports their need for flexibility.

## THE SEQUENCE OF INSTRUCTION IN EARLY INTERVENTION

Families and interventionists need to communicate about the systematic plans for instruction to young children. Donahue-Kilburg (1992) suggested an instructional sequence, adapted from clinical practice and based on the work of Guitar, Kopff, Kilburg, and Conway (1981); Girolametto, Greenberg, and Manolson (1986); McDade and Simpson (1984); and McDade and Varnedoe (1987). It is a comprehensive approach to helping families facilitate communication development in at-risk or language-deficient infants and toddlers. The steps of the process are:

1. Evaluate videotaped parent-child interactions in a culturally sensitive manner.
2. Verbally present information on language-facilitation techniques tailored to the culture and education level of the family.
3. Give the same information in a written form so that it can be read and shared with other family members.
4. Arrange to view professionally prepared instructional videos that illustrate language-facilitation techniques with family members or lend them copies to be viewed at home.
5. View portions of the original assessment video with the parents looking for examples of behaviors that work with their children. The clinician may select portions of these tapes prior to the session with the family. The clinician takes the lead in pointing out positive parent behaviors. Parents should be allowed to take the lead concerning behaviors that are not so facilitative. If the clinician agrees with the parents that the behavior was not helpful, a brief acknowledgment is appropriate.

6. The parents and clinician can mutually decide on facilitative behaviors to increase or begin using.
7. Parents can first try these behaviors by role playing them with each other or with the clinician.
8. Once parents understand the use of the behaviors, they can practice them one at a time in videotaped play interaction with their children.
9. In the next session with the clinician, the parents and clinician can view all or clinician-selected portions of the video from the last session, again emphasizing behaviors that work with their children. Parents can critique their own use of techniques and discuss their progress with the clinician.
10. The parents again practice behaviors in videotaped interaction.
11. Between sessions, parents can practice the facilitative behaviors with the children.
12. The clinician assesses parent and child progress toward desired outcomes from the videotaped interaction.

According to Donahue-Kilburg (1992), steps nine, ten, eleven, and twelve are repeated until they are mastered. This approach helps parents quickly see how the techniques work and, therefore, increases their eagerness to use them. The clinician can then function in the role of consultant to the family members and family members can enjoy the experience of promoting language growth as they maintain their normal roles in the family.

## CHALLENGES IN FAMILY-CENTERED INTERVENTION

One of the primary challenges to move from client or child-centered approaches to family-centered approaches requires interventionists to relinquish "professional" decision making about services for the child. Bailey and Simmeonson (1988) stated that the major goals for early interventionists are to support families as they care for their children, to enhance child development outcomes, and to facilitate effective interactions between caregivers and children in the family context.

Another challenge to engaging in family-centered intervention is the reluctance of some families to participate in early intervention services. For some, there is a high degree of shame associated with receiving certain types of services, especially if those services are offered through government agencies such as the health department or social services. Some people may have religious convictions that make them hesitant to participate in services offered by various agencies. Furthermore, families who are from wealthy backgrounds may be embarrassed about receiving help from public agencies. Therefore, we should have clear open discussions about service delivery options with families. Families can then deal with their concerns and prioritize them.

At times service providers have inappropriately labeled parents noncompliant or uncooperative. For example, the perceived lack of cooperation could have been a result of inappropriate interactions, poorly explained recommendations, or other mistakes made by professionals during the course of meetings with parents. When family needs and values are not considered, less than favorable consequences are likely (Caldman, Shurvell, Davies, & Bradfield, 1984). Thus, we need to facilitate intervention that is compatible with the family's cultural values. Open communication will be helpful in this instance.

## FAMILY ASSESSMENT

Bailey (1991, p. 27) defined family assessment as "the ongoing and interactive process by which professionals gather information in order to determine family priorities for goals and services." He described the process as one that is continuous, involving professionals and family members. Bailey discussed four types of family assessment strategies: informal communication, semi-structured interviews, surveys and rating scales, and direct observation procedures. The most commonly used of the four procedures is *informal assessment.* Some examples of opportunities for informal assessment include telephone calls, notes, and chance interactions that occur in the community. According to Bailey, the key strategy is for professionals to take advantage of these situations to gain insight into how the family operates in given situations and what they may expect of us in our interactions with them. *Semi-structured interviews or discussions* are usually planned and conducted in order to achieve certain goals. The goals may be very specific or very global. The discussion, although structured, must be flexible enough to adjust itself according to the interactions that occur. *Caregiver-completed surveys and rating scales* are typically completed by the caregiver. These scales fall into two general categories, nonstandardized instruments with the primary purpose being that of determining parents' perceived needs for services and standardized measures for the purpose of assessing various domains. There are also *standardized measures completed by professionals.* Although these measures are similar to those discussed in the previous category, the major difference is that these instruments are completed by professionals rather than by families. Service providers should exercise caution in the using these measures because some people may be resentful about a person outside of the family making judgments about aspects of the family.

Service providers may determine that a cultural mediator is needed for the assessment process. Suggestions for including a cultural mediator in the assessment process are presented in Table 5-1.

## FAMILY-CENTERED CARE AND DIVERSE BACKGROUNDS

When addressing the child's needs, one of the professional's responsibilities is to conduct an assessment of family interactions, strengths, and resources. As we engage in those activities we should look to determine what the families *could* do rather than what they cannot do as our partners in intervention. We must also remember that we bring our values to our interactions with families. We do not have to change our value and belief systems in order to relate appropriately to people from backgrounds other than ours. However, we as interventionists must be diligent in our efforts not to impose those values into interpretations of assessment findings. We have to acknowledge and appreciate the right of families to believe as they do.

### TABLE  5-1    Roles of a Cultural Mediator

- Referral source for the culturally different community.
- Liaison between parents and other members of the intervention team.
- Community link between staff and parents to ensure parents are part of the team.
- Advocate for parents.
- Resource person to help team members determine goals/strategies that are relevant for the cultural community.
- Source of information from parents.
- Interpreter during assessments and meetings with parents.
- Translator of written summaries, reports, informal tests, and checklists.

   The mediator may also:

- Be the primary person who interacts with the child (with guidance from team members), providing informal interpretation during play assessment.

Adapted from Moore & Beatty (1995).

## Working with Families from Culturally Different Backgrounds

A family-centered approach involves respecting cultural and socioeconomic differences. That involves considering family values in planning assessment, determining appropriateness of a child's skill development, developing goals/objectives for intervention, and implementing the intervention strategies. It really complicates matters when programs designed to assist families present conflicting values that are important within the family and its community. Therefore, service providers need to offer services that are rendered culturally appropriate. Suggestions for establishing effective working relationships with families from culturally diverse backgrounds are presented in Table 5-2.

## Culturally Competent Service Provision

Lynch and Hanson (1996) stated that the ability to work with children and families from culturally diverse backgrounds requires a commitment to gaining new information and becoming aware of the ways in which one thinks and behaves. Green (1982) presented five personal attributes needed by culturally competent service providers that include awareness of one's own cultural limitations; openness to cultural differences; adoption of a learning style that is client-oriented, interactive, and flexible; ability to help someone recognize and use resources; and recognition of the integrity of all cultures (p. 74).

Professionals who work with nonmainstream children with special needs are challenged to understand and respect different cultural styles, values, and preferences regarding child rearing. All people do not share the same values or belief systems, even people who are of the same race or ethnic group. Professionals should demonstrate understanding of culturally acceptable learning styles with children, as well as culturally based attitudes that families have toward children with special needs such as communication disorders (Robinson, 1997). Hanson, Lynch, and Wayman (1990) provided several guidelines that will help interventionists increase cultural competence in supporting families of children with special needs. The professional should be able to

- Describe the ethnic background with which the family identifies.
- Identify how the ethnic community is organized socially.
- Describe the values, ceremonies, and symbols of the family's current belief system.
- Learn about the group's history and current events that directly affect family life.

**Table  5-2     Suggestions for Establishing Effective Working Relationships with Families from Culturally Diverse Backgrounds**

1. Describe the ethnic group with which the family identifies.
2. Identify the social organizations of the community, such as family and peer networks, religious organizations, and resources available.
3. Determine how members of the community gain access to and use social services.
4. Determine whether questions about any of the following issues might be sensitive to members of that culture: health, illness, pregnancy, birth, family relationships, child-rearing practices, time orientation, schools, health care providers, employment, level of education.
5. Identify how people in the family's community treats issues related to privacy and courtesy.
6. Describe prevailing cultural traditions that relate to the expression of emotions, feelings, religious expressions; and response to handicapping conditions, illness, and death.
7. Identify the healing systems used by this culture.
8. Determine whether medical or nonmedical intervention would compromise beliefs in these healing systems, raising the potential for conflict between the family and the rest of the team.
9. Determine how families in this community typically participate in caring for and making decisions about family members.
10. Identify prevailing attitudes toward health and illness and how these attitudes might affect people's responses to team member inquiries, intervention, or seeking help.
11. Describe attitudes of the community toward the dominant culture and how these might affect the acculturation process.
12. Describe how members of the community demonstrate respect or express status, age, and gender.
13. Identify ways in which adults and children typically interact with one another.
14. Determine how members of the community typically interact with members of the teaching and medical professions.
15. Determine typical first words in this language.
16. Identify typical interactive games and rituals.
17. Identify significant features of this community's language that are different from English.
18. Identify the best communication style for team members in regards to tempo of conversation, eye or body contact, and distance between speakers.
19. Determine how the team member's gender may affect interactions.
20. Describe the history of the group and current events that affect the family.

Adapted from Eliades & Suitor (1994).

- Make a determination of how members of the community access and use social services.
- Determine the attitudes of the ethnic community toward seeking help.

Open and honest communication will facilitate usage of these guidelines with families of young children from culturally diverse populations.

Robinson (1997) discussed some advantages of working closely with families prior to testing the child. The clinician's knowledge and understanding will be enhanced as a result of this practice and that will facilitate the assessment process. The advantages discussed by Robinson include:

1. Minimizing test bias
2. Obtaining valid information about the child's language/dialect and communication development status
3. Gaining knowledge of possible cultural expectations parents may have of the child
4. Gathering information about perceptions of the child's abilities in the first language/dialect
5. Determining the need for an interpreter prior to the assessment
6. Understanding of family concerns and values regarding the child's use of English or vernacular variations of English and the degree to which the native language/dialect and/or English are spoken in the home setting
7. Assisting professionals in understanding parent-child interaction patterns in the home
8. Helping professionals design appropriate intervention with family input

### Learning from the Parents

Families can provide interventionists with information that may enhance the service delivery process for children and families from culturally diverse populations. Trout and Foley (1989) stated that families have a lot to teach interventionists about the best way to do their jobs. Parents and professionals may have different perspectives, but weaving intervention strategies together representing those different perspectives results in more positive outcomes. Professionals can offer the expertise of their discipline and knowledge gained from working with many children. Parents can contribute information on their particular child in various settings. Parents can also offer a valuable perspective on the range of services they need and how these services could be more accessible and supportive to them. In addition, family members may bring fresh, innovative, and creative solutions to long-standing service delivery problems (Shelton et al., 1992). It is especially important to take advantage of the opportunity to learn from families when we are working with cultures other than our own. Be honest and ask parents questions about cultural practices for their family. Observe how parents and children interact with each other and ask if these behaviors are typical of their normal interactions. Parents can also describe various social expectations for children within their own culture.

Specific areas of information parents can address include the following: (1) the issue of deficit or difference, as the child may not be considered to have a deficit in the native language; (2) information regarding resources in the home to follow through on language development in English (Are there any other English speakers in the home?); (3) family resources and expectations of the child (Who are primary caregivers in daily routines?); and (4) paralinguistic information on communication (How does the child communicate nonverbally?) (Robinson, 1997, pp. 127–128).

## Initial Contacts with Families

During initial meetings, such as the preassessment conference, family members can provide important information that will guide future interactions with them and their children, such as family expectations for communication. The first contact should be brief and not overwhelming with too much information for the family members. During those initial contacts family members can convey important information in many areas.

## Communicating with Culturally Diverse Clients and Families

Many people have their own conception of what constitutes a family. For them, a family is a group of people brought together by marriage or birth, usually including a mother, father, and one or more children. However, the reality of life in the United States forces us to have to revisit that conception. A less restrictive definition is more appropriate in order to fit the wide range of traditional and nontraditional family units we see today. In addition to awareness of the fact that the nuclear family unit may not be the same as it once was, special service providers need to explore the possible involvement of members of the extended family as decision makers (Donahue-Kilburg, 1992). Kenkel (1977) reported that what each family member is and will become is affected by the family group to which he or she belongs. One of the functions of a family is to pass on to children the skills, norms, and values of their culture. Those cultural skills include its language, attitudes, beliefs, and patterns of behavior (Donahue-Kilburg, 1992). Clearly, when working with families from nontraditional backgrounds, special service providers must consider their value and belief systems as they interact with them as partners in the intervention process. Not everyone in this country, including people of the same racial or ethnic background, shares the same values. To provide culturally sensitive, family-centered services, service providers must be aware of the family's values. That is especially true when these values differ from those of the professional and when they may be at odds with the traditional approach to intervention (Donahue-Kilburg, 1992).

Improving communication with family members could eliminate many of the problems previously discussed regarding provision of family-centered care. As early interventionists, we must learn to listen to parents and let them know we are interested in what they have to say.

## *Working with Interpreters/Translators*

Service providers who work with families who do not speak English or whose proficiency in English is limited should work with interpreters if they do not speak the language of the family. The first crucial decision is selection of appropriate translators or interpreters. Prior to the interpreter meeting the family, the service provider should interview the person. The service provider should feel comfortable communicating with the interpreter and vice versa. The interpreter should be clear about the communication process and role expectations. Some disciplines and some states have specific qualifications for individuals serving as translators. Consult your professional organization for this type of information. Service providers who lack experience working with interpreters need to prepare for the first meeting by gaining information about rules for communicating with the interpreter. Anderson (1991) addresses cultural considerations. Service providers need to be aware that all persons who speak a particular language are not necessarily qualified to interpret for members of various cultural groups that also speak the same language.

Some public health agencies have developed guidelines for interpreter services. The Office of Minority Health in the North Carolina Department of Environment, Health, and Natural Resources developed specific guidelines for interpreter services, which are presented in Table 5-3.

Discussions with family members regarding assimilation and acculturation of the family can provide the service provider with useful information. The amount of time a family has lived in a country and/or the level of English proficiency are not direct indicators of acculturation

## TABLE 5-3    Guidelines for Interpreter Services in Public Health Agencies

The role of the interpreter is to serve as the conduit of all communication between the provider and the client, and additionally, to convey communication between the provider and the client, while converting the exchange from one language into another. Unless other duties are specified in a job description (e.g., nurse/interpreter), the interpreter does not provide health services. Therefore, the interpreter should not explain health care procedures, outcomes, or recommendations to the client without the provider present.

***Interpretation Functions.*** This refers primarily to spoken language services. The interpreter

- Responds to requests for interpreter services in a variety of settings, such as maternity clinics, immunizations, and HIV testing and counseling.
- Interprets information regarding the patient's needs. This may include consent for care, screening, treatment, recommendations, instructions for follow-up, and future appointments.
- Interprets as accurately and directly as possible, given the idiomatic differences between languages, and keeps the spirit and letter of the original communication.
- Communicates possible misunderstandings by the client to the provider. The interpreter should not explain health care issues or procedures to the client, other than what is communicated by the provider. This is important to assure consistent quality for all clients.
- Assists providers in understanding the client's culture, especially as it relates to health service interactions. This includes nonverbal communications, health practices, and social relationships.

***Translation Functions.*** This refers to written work only. If translation of materials is considered part of the job, certain guidelines should be followed.

- If any changes are needed in the material regarding the content or the literacy level, the authorized health provider should make these in English first, then give them to the interpreter/translator.
- The supervisor of the clinic or department should determine the accuracy and currency of materials used before the translation is done.
- Written translations should be done as literally or directly as possible, given the idiomatic differences between languages. Every attempt should be made to maintain the meaning and length of the English language version.

***Ethics and Confidentiality.*** The interpreter

- Maintains strict confidentiality regarding any patient-provider communication.
- Acknowledges own limitations in language or subject matter.
- Does not accept an assignment for which he or she is not qualified. The limiting factor may be language skill or subject matter knowledge. In an emergency, the interpreter will inform the parties involved of his or her own limitation.
- Refrains from counseling clients and from inserting own opinion or judgment when communicating.

*Continued*

**TABLE 5-3** *Continued*

***Community Volunteers.*** These people are assumed to be untrained in health care terminology or the interpretation process. They may also have limited skills in one of the two needed languages. However, they can help in making appointments and in giving directions and instructions. If these people have the knowledge and skills of paraprofessional interpreters, then they could interpret for some services.

***Language Fluency.*** All interpreters should be fluent in both languages. In the case of English-Spanish interpreters, native Spanish speakers should have completed high school or the equivalent with Spanish as the primary language. Non-native speakers of Spanish could be those who majored in Spanish in college or had equivalent experience such as being in the Peace Corps. Ideally, second language competency should be determined through oral and written examinations.

***Paraprofessionals.*** This group includes student workers who earn money or course credit, clinical providers with some skill in a second language, and other employees who use their skills in more than one language. Minimum requirements include:

• Good skills in both languages.
• Basic knowledge of medical interpretation.
• Training in ethical issue.

***Professional Interpreters.*** These people can interpret for all services, including clinical services. They should have:

• A college degree or the equivalent in experience.
• Advanced language skills in both the spoken and written forms.
• Advanced knowledge of medical interpretation.
• Training in ethical issues.
• Experience in interpretation. They need to be able to use their language skills on a variety of levels to communicate between providers and clients or patients.

Source: Office of Minority Health, North Carolina Department of Environment, Health, and Natural Resources. Raleigh, NC. Used with permission.

level. Avoid making assumptions about families based on these variables. Open and honest discussions about specific areas will help the service provider make reasonable conclusions regarding the family's level of acculturation.

## SUMMARY AND CONCLUSIONS

Working with families from culturally and linguistically diverse families presents some unique challenges and opportunities for speech-language pathologists. It was our intent to present both new and experienced clinicians with some viable options and rationales for selection of strategies. Communication and education in family-centered care is a two-way street. Families will gain significant information from service providers who will in turn learn a great deal from families. Some keys to successful work with families include:

- Observe behaviors as families interact with each other.
- Listen to concerns/interests/desired outcomes expressed by family members.
- Ask questions. Avoid making assumptions regarding parental expectations for their children.
- Avoid making generalizations about cultural values, beliefs, and practices, especially based on perceived ethnicity.
- Ask families about their cultural values, beliefs, and practices that are relative to the communication development of their children.
- Maintain open and frequent lines of communication with parents/guardians.
- When necessary, access an interpreter who is a member of the same culture. For example, don't assume that all persons who speak Spanish are members of the same Hispanic culture.
- Discuss with bidialectal/bilingual parents of young children their decisions regarding using standard American English in the home as well as their attitudes toward English-only instruction in the school/clinical setting.
- Discuss oral and written language differences and similarities for culturally and linguistically diverse individuals.

The information presented in this chapter is not meant to be totally exclusive for working with culturally and linguistically diverse families. However, it is our belief that a number of special considerations need to be made when working with all families, and we have presented the options known to the authors at the time this chapter was written. As interventionists develop successful interactions with families, the list of options available will increase. We also recommend continuous collaboration and communication with co-workers regarding the success of various strategies.

## STUDY QUESTIONS AND ACTIVITIES

1. Describe the process of selecting and working with an interpreter.
2. Compare and contrast the variables of working with an African American family who has lived in the same rural community for forty years versus an

African American migrant family that moves to a different community every four to five months. Both families have two-year-old children. The children speak primarily in single word utterances. What recommendations would you make for intervention for each family?

3. Describe some of the benefits and disadvantages of including a cultural mediator in the assessment process.

4. Describe ways in which intervention planning may be enhanced by information provided to the early interventionist by family members. If family members failed to provide any information regarding the nature of communication within their community, how would you vary your approach to treatment for a young bilingual child with language delays?

5. The following case studies may be used to stimulate discussions in interactive learning activities in the classroom. Some questions that might be suggested for discussion include:

   • How would you seek to include families as partners in the intervention process?

   • What challenges might there be to the intervention process?

   • What intervention goals and strategies would you develop?

**Case Study 5.1**

Jason is a two-year-old African American boy living with a foster mother. His history is positive for prenatal exposure to crack cocaine. His mother is a teenager and his father is thirty years old. He receives early intervention services and his biological parents are permitted visitation at the Early Intervention center two days per week only. He cried when his father left the room.

Jason's communication skills are characterized by 4- to 5-word spontaneous productions. Most of his responses to yes/no questions are "no." He enjoys playing with cars, trucks, and airplanes alone or with an adult. After six months of classroom-based speech language services he is beginning to play with peers and to say "yes" appropriately. He responded very well to the facilitating strategies of modeling (suggest to say "Yes, I want . . .") and positive reinforcement of verbal praise and clapping in response to appropriate communication with peers and adults. He also smiles in response to something he likes. He now separates very well from Dad when he leaves. He gives him a hug and says "Daddy it's time for you to go that way."

**Case Study 5.2**

Marcus is a two-year-old boy whose family is from Haiti. He presents with feeding problems and some sensory integration difficulties. His utterances are primarily 1 to 2 words. His speech is characterized by a number of phonological processes. At home he eats mashed foods and drinks liquids from a bottle. At this time the family is not interested in home-based speech services and is comfortable with the feeding practices presently utilized in the home.

Marcus receives classroom-based services in the center. The physical therapist is addressing sensory integration concerns, and the speech-language pathologist is addressing feeding and communication skills. He accepts oral motor stimulation before snack from the SLP. He is given a cup to drink with physical assistance with lip seal around the cup. He is offered a variety of tastes, smells, and textures for exploration during snack. The discussions during snack center around verbal praise for putting food in his mouth. He is positively reinforced for all eating and is not required to remain at the snack table until all other children have completed their snacks. He enjoys licking or sucking salt from crackers and goldfish. He likes taking a bite of a cracker and smashing it within his mouth before he swallows it. His expressive skills have increased with intervention. He initiates some comments about the environment and says some simple routine phrases, for example, Thank you, Time to go, No, Mine.

**Case Study 5.3**

Mario is a two-year-old boy. Spanish is the primary language spoken in the home. Mario lives with his parents and one older brother enrolled in special education at school. Mario's physical size is that of a seven-year-old boy for height and weight, his head circumference is in the 90th percentile for a sixteen-year-old boy. Results of genetic testing have not identified a syndrome to date. His language skills are characterized by single word utterances in both English and Spanish. He makes little contact with others. He enjoys looking at pictures in books and playing with blocks and cars/trucks. His attention to tasks is limited and his play with toys is often bizarre or atypical. No toys are available in the home, because his mother reported that the children keep breaking the toys. Recommendations for intervention included home- and center-based intervention with a bilingual case manager. Family assistance with the selection of developmentally appropriate play activities and materials was deemed a priority. Services from occupational therapy and speech and language are also delineated.

# REFERENCES

Alexander, R., Kroth, R., Simpson, R., & Poppelreiter, T. (1982). The parent role in special education. In R. McDowell, G. Adamson, & F. Woods (Eds.), *Teaching emotionally disturbed children.* Boston: Little-Brown.

Anderson, N. (1991). Understanding cultural diversity. *American Journal of Speech-Language Pathology, 1,* 9–10.

Anderson, N. B., & McNeilly, L. G. (1992). Meeting the needs of special populations. In M. Bender & C. Baglin (Eds.), *Infants and toddlers: A resource guide for practitioners.* San Diego: Singular Publishing Group

Bailey, D. (1991). Issues and perspectives on family assessment. *Infants and young children, 4,* 26–34.

Bailey, D. B. (1996). Assessing family resources, priorities, and concerns. In M. McLean, D. B. Bailey, Jr., & M. Wolery (Eds.). *Assessing infants and preschoolers with special needs.* Englewood Cliffs, NJ: Prentice Hall.

Bailey, D., & Simeonsson, R. (1988). *Family assessment in early intervention.* Columbus, OH: Merrill.

Caldman, D., Shurvell, B., Davies, P., & Bradfield, S. (1984). Compliance in the community with consultants' recommendations for developmentally handicapped children. *Developmental Medicine and Child Neurology, 26,* 40–46.

Campbell, P. (1990). *The individualized family service plan: A guide for families and early intervention professionals.* Unpublished manuscript. Tallmadge, OH: Family Child Learning Center.

Donahue-Kilburg, G. (1992). *Family-centered early intervention for communication disorders: Prevention and treatment.* Gaithersburg, MD: Aspen Publishers.

Eliades, D. C., & Suiter, C. W. (1994). *Celebrating diversity: Approaching families through their food.* Arlington, VA: National Center for Education in Maternal and Child Health.

Girolametto, L., Greenberg, J., & Manolson, H. A. (1986). Developing dialogue skills: The Hanen early language parent program. *Seminars in Speech and Language, 7,* 367–381.

Green, J. W. (1982). *Cultural awareness in the human services.* Englewood Cliffs, NJ: Prentice-Hall.

Guitar, B., Kopff, H., Kilburg, G., & Conway, P. (1981). *Parent verbal interactions and speech rate: A case study in stuttering.* Paper presented at the annual convention of the American Speech-Language-Hearing Association, Los Angeles, CA.

Hanson, M., Lynch, E., & Wayman, K. (1990). Honoring the cultural diversity of families when gathering data. *Topics in Early Childhood Special Education, 10,* 112–131.

Kenkel, W. (1977). *The family in perspective* (4th ed.). Santa Monica, CA: Goodyear Publishing Co.

Luterman, D. M. (1991). *Counseling the communicatively disordered and their families.* Austin, TX: Pro-Ed.

Lynch, E. W., & Hanson, M. J. (1996). Ensuring cultural competence. In M. McLean, D. B. Bailey, Jr., & M. Wolery (Eds.), *Assessing infants and preschoolers with special needs.* Englewood Cliffs, NJ: Prentice Hall.

McDade, H., & Simpson, M. (1984). Use of instruction, modeling, and videotape feedback to modify parent behavior: A strategy for facilitating language development in the home. *Seminars in Speech and Language, 5,* 229–240.

McDade, H., & Varnedoe, D. (1987). Training parents to be language facilitators. *Topics in Language Disorders, 7,* 19–30.

McGonigel, M., Kaufmann, R., & Hurth, J. (1991). The IFSP sequence. In M. McGonigel, R. Kaufmann, & B. Johnson (Eds.), *Guidelines and recommended practices for the individualized family service plan* (2nd ed., pp. 15–28). Bethesda, MD: Association for the Care of Children's Health.

McLean, M., & Crais, E. R. (1996). Procedural considerations in assessing infants and preschoolers with disabilities. In M. McLean, D. B. Bailey, Jr., & M. Wolery (Eds.), *Assessing infants and preschoolers with special needs* (pp. 46–68). Englewood Cliffs, NJ: Prentice Hall.

Moore, S. M., & Beatty, J. (1995). *Developing cultural competence in early childhood assessment.* Boulder: University of Colorado.

Noonan, M. J., & McCormick, L. (1993). *Early intervention in natural environments: Methods and procedures.* Pacific Grove, CA: Brooks/Cole Publishing Company.

Robinson, N. (1997). Working with families. In L. McCormick, D. F. Loeb, & R. L. Schiefelbusch (Eds.), *Supporting children with communication difficulties in inclusive settings: School-based intervention.* Boston: Allyn & Bacon.

Shelton, T. L., Jeppson, E. S., & Johnson, B. H. (1992). *Family-centered care for children with special health care needs.* Bethesda, MD: Association for the Care of Children's Health.

Trout, M., & Foley, G. (1989). Working with families of handicapped infants and toddlers. *Topics in Language Disorders, 10*(1), 57–67.

## SUGGESTED READINGS

Anderson, N., & McNeilly, L. (1992). Meeting the needs of special populations. In M. Bender & C. Baglin (Eds.), *Infants and toddlers: A resource guide for practitioners* (pp. 49–68). San Diego, CA: Singular.

Crais, E. R. (1992). Moving from "parent involvement" to family centered services. *American Journal of Speech-Language Pathology, 1*(1), 5–8.

Donahue-Kilburg, G. (1992). *Family-centered early intervention for communication disorders: Prevention and treatment.* Gaithersburg, MD: Aspen.

Langdon, H. W., & Cheng, L. L. (1992). *Hispanic children and adults with communication disorders: Assessment and intervention.* Gaithersburg, MD: Aspen Publishers.

Webster, E., & Ward, L. (1993). *Working with parents of young children with disabilities.* San Diego, CA: Singular.

# 6

# CULTURALLY APPROPRIATE ASSESSMENT: ISSUES AND STRATEGIES

## W. FREDA WILSON, JOHNNY R. WILSON,

## and THALIA J. COLEMAN

Special service providers, such as speech-language pathologists, must become culturally sensitive diagnosticians in order to be able to offer appropriate services to their clients. Culturally, linguistically, and behaviorally different children cannot receive appropriate management unless they receive comprehensive culturally, linguistically, and behaviorally appropriate assessment. Haynes, Pindzola, and Emerick (1992) outline several requirements of a good assessment, which includes detailed synthesis of information from all aspects of the phenomenon being evaluated. A good diagnostician must have a knowledge of norms, an understanding of testing techniques, good observation skills, and the ability to establish effective working relationships with clients and their families (Haynes et al., 1992).

There is growing disenchantment with the use of standardized tests *alone* as the way to determine the strengths and needs of individuals. Damico, Smith, and Augustine (1996), Secord and Wiig (1992), and Taylor (1986, 1990) state that our responsibility to children is to create and/or utilize appropriate assessment tools that accurately index the communication behavior and language of individuals. Culturally, linguistically, and behaviorally specific descriptions of what children say, how children behave, and what types of materials children use are the means to reliable assessment.

Lewis (1997) defined assessment as the process of gathering information about children's performance in order to determine their communicative, educational, behavioral, and psychosocial status. According to Lewis, traditional assessment tools may not always be the best choice for children who are not from "traditional" backgrounds. Large numbers of children from diverse culturally/linguistically different backgrounds are referred to special educators, psychologists, pediatric healthcare providers, and speech-language pathologists. Many of these children do not have speech or language disorders, only *differences*. Consequently, one of the major responsibilities of the speech-language clinician is to accurately diagnose communication disorders and distinguish them from communication differences (Paul, 1995).

Wolfram (1983), Taylor (1986, 1990), and Wyatt (1995) questioned the validity of tests when they are used across different cultural groups. Leonard and Weiss (1983) and Wyatt (1995) support the idea that many available standardized language tests may penalize children who are culturally, linguistically, and/or behaviorally different. According to Vaughn-Cooke (1986), one of the most critical and urgent problems facing speech-language pathologists and other healthcare providers is the absence of adequate culturally, linguistically, and behaviorally sensitive assessment tools that provide valid and reliable evaluations of people from culturally diverse backgrounds. Teachers, researchers, healthcare providers, and others from different segments of the world community have addressed the growing dissatisfaction with traditional tests and testing procedures, especially when they are used with individuals from nonmainstream backgrounds (e.g., Adler, 1993; Adler & Birdsong, 1983; Andersen & Battle, 1993; Battle, 1998; Holland, 1983; Juarez, 1983; Stockman, 1986).

## CRITICAL CONCEPTS

The term *diagnosis* refers to the act of describing and determining precisely the type, nature, and scope of a person's problem. When an individual enters the assessment process, he or she may present characteristics that could be similar to someone else who has a very different diagnosis. It is the responsibility of the diagnostician to determine how a client's particular characteristics and resultant problem is different from many other possibilities. According to Haynes and colleagues (1992), *evaluation* is a term that should be used when referring to the actual process used while arriving at a diagnosis. The term *assessment* is an "umbrella concept" that encompasses diagnosis, evaluation, and any measures used to determine a client's understanding of tasks, his or her progress toward accomplishing goals, and the effectiveness of intervention strategies. Assessment is an ongoing process that should be consistently practiced while we are engaged in intervention activities. Taylor and Payne (1983; Taylor, 1986, 1990) defined *culturally valid* or *nonbiased assessment* as a process of collecting data using instruments and procedures that discriminate only in those areas for which they were designed (i.e., normal versus pathological behavior) and do not discriminate unfairly either for or against a client for cultural linguistic and/or behavioral reasons. Furthermore, nonbiased assessment does not penalize clients because of social variations within a culture based on such factors as age, gender, language, socioeconomic class, and mores.

## CULTURAL BIAS IN TESTING

According to Taylor and Payne (1983), Vaughn-Cooke (1986), Bailey and Wolery (1989), and Wyatt (1995), bias can occur during assessment if a child's performance on tests is unfairly influenced by such factors as race, language, behavior, mores, sex, cultural background, or religious affiliation. Adler (1993) discussed two types of bias that may occur in tests: deliberate bias and nondeliberate bias. According to Adler, a *deliberate bias* involves inclusion of test items that are not representative of the examinee's language, learning style, behavioral set, community, or culture. A *nondeliberate and nondesirable bias* is reflected in tests that are normed on individuals who are representative of mainstream society, administered to nonmainstream individuals, and interpreted to suggest inferiority of individuals from culturally, linguistically, and behaviorally diverse backgrounds.

Taylor and Payne (1983), Chamberlain and Medeiros-Landurand (1991), and Wyatt (1995) elaborated on four principal forms of bias that can exist in assessment procedures: situational bias, bias in directions or format, value bias, and linguistic bias. In their discussion of *situational bias,* Taylor and Payne (1983; Taylor, 1986, 1990) reported that mismatches can occur between clients and clinicians with respect to the social rules of learning, behavioral, and language interaction. Some of the major areas of mismatching they identified include rules of who may speak to whom and appropriate elicitation procedures. Wyatt (1995) points out that culturally specific learning styles and appropriate language behaviors among nonmainstream children may serve different communicative purposes; therefore, the rules of production and interpretation will need to be different in the assessment process. When mismatches occur between clients' rules and clinicians' rules, clinicians may interpret the mismatch as a sign of a disorder.

*Directions* or *format bias* can occur when individuals being tested are unfamiliar with the framework of the procedures used during the assessment or when directions are presented that are inconsistent with clients' everyday lives and/or do not consider different behavioral cognitive or learning styles. Grossman (1995) stated that the format of an assessment procedure refers to how the tasks and questions are presented to the child and to how the child is expected to respond to them. Some examples of directions or format bias are (1) when the child is asked to recognize the correct picture, answer, or solution to a problem or to produce it themselves; (2) whether the child is expected to respond orally, in writing, or by performing a task; and (3) whether there are time constraints. Since different cultural, behavioral, and linguistic factors could influence task analyses and performance, "fair assessments" must address how these differences might have an impact upon performance.

Taylor and Payne (1983; Taylor, 1986, 1990) reported that *value bias* might occur when the examinee is required to indicate a preference for one set of stimuli over another or when he or she is expected to make a judgment about what a person should do in a given situation. Other examples of this type of bias include timed tests that do not allow time for contemplation and tasks that are contemplative in nature. According to Taylor and Payne (1983; Taylor, 1986, 1990), test items are discriminatory when a correct response requires individuals being tested to show knowledge or acceptance of a value that may be unfamiliar or unacceptable to them.

*Linguistic bias* can be manifested in two ways. The most obvious manifestation of this bias is the child whose first or preferred language or dialect is not English or is a variety of English that is different from General American English Dialect (GAED). When a child is tested using a test that is based on proficiency in General American English, practitioners must ensure that the examinee is fully proficient in GAED. One can easily think of problems inherent in the assessment process when monolingual/monodialected English-speaking service providers try to conduct assessment of students whose English is limited and/or bidialectual. The most typical adjustment made in this type of situation is to request the assistance of a translator or interpreter. Linguistic bias can also occur when a diagnostician assumes that the client speaks a particular dialect because of his or her racial/ethnic group or native geographic region. Bias is manifested if the examiner alters the assessment procedure based on that presumption. Not all people belonging to an identifiable ethnic and/or cultural group speak dialects. Even when dialects are spoken by those individuals, the dialects may vary significantly due to several economic, educational, political, behavioral, and/or historical factors.

Grossman (1995) and Wyatt (1995) discuss content and gender bias. *Content bias* tends to occur in testing situations where all children are assumed to have had exposure to certain "basic" concepts. Obviously, not all children are exposed to the same things in the same way in their home and community environments. Additionally, parents, teachers, schools, and communities do not offer content or learning experiences in the same way.

According to Grossman, each gender is likely to respond correctly to test items with which they are more familiar and/or more interested, and those that use same-gender pronouns. This could result in *gender bias*. Grossman cited studies conducted in the 1970s and early 1980s that indicate test items generally include more male pronouns and more material that fits what are considered "male interests."

Losardo and Coleman (1996) discussed limitations and cultural biases of traditional assessment models and tools as follows:

- Standardized tests often do not take into account contextual learning or behavioral and cultural influences on the measurement of language.
- Many standardized instruments measure skills in restricted nondiverse settings.
- Normative samples frequently do not include various racial/ethnic/ cultural groups. When representatives of those groups are included, it is usually not in proportion to the groups' representation in the general population.
- The content of most standardized tests typically reflects formal language used in white middle-class school settings. Obviously this precludes accurate assessment of many segments of our community.
- Pictures and materials are not always culturally appropriate. Consequently, children/clients do not respond well to stimuli that may appear "foreign" to them.
- Standardized measures frequently do not take into account cultural differences in values, beliefs, and attitudes.

In an attempt to make standardized tests "fairer" to children whose linguistic, behavioral, and/or learning styles are nonmainstream, some test developers have produced adaptations of traditional tests. According to Losardo and Coleman (1996), problems with these tests include the fact that there is inadequate knowledge of language, learning, and behavior development across and within different ethnic groups. Secondly, test translations are usually based upon a mainstream or Eurocentric view. That view assumes that the language learning and behavioral development of minority children is the same as the development of majority culture children. It does not account for unique multicultural language, learning, and/or behavioral characteristics (e.g., code switching and language borrowing). Another problem associated with test adaptations is nonspecific multicultural scorings that in some cases may lead to lower standards and expectations.

The use of translated tests also may negate the norms established by the mainstream culture. In addition, there are many aspects of language that cannot be easily translated. Another problem is that, generally, only selected linguistic structures/concepts and behaviors considered important by majority culture are included in the tests. Also, the content assessed by the test might not be something the child is exposed to on a regular basis, if at all. Items that are considered to be "common objects" within mainstream culture may not be that common in other cultures. Additionally, if the concept exists in another language, culture, or behavioral set, test developers may not be able to translate it from the mainstream cultural repertoire using a one-word label (Erickson & Iglesias, 1986a).

## NONBIASED ASSESSMENT

Recognizing that there are many potential problems that could occur during the assessment of individuals from culturally, behaviorally, and linguistically diverse backgrounds, speech-language pathologists and other special service providers need to make adjustments in traditional assessment procedures in order to make the process as nonbiased as possible. Bogatz, Hisama, Manni, and Wurtz (1986) and Tucker (1993) offered four characteristics of nonbiased assessment. According to Tucker (1993), nonbiased assessment

1. Is ongoing.
2. Results from a team effort.
3. Involves the child's parents as active participants.
4. Investigates all relevant data sources such as observations, historical data, language dominance, educational achievement, sensorimotor development, adaptive behavior, medical or developmental history, personality, and intellectual development.

Erickson and Iglesias (1986a) stated that it is the responsibility of communication specialists, educators, and other healthcare practitioners to determine what are the most appropriate and fair assessment materials and procedures to use when working with diverse populations of individuals. They pointed out that culture, behavior, and language use varies depending on the people who are interacting with each other, topics being discussed, situations in which conversations take place, cultures involved, and the language learning environment to which children are exposed while they are acquiring language learning skills.

Some general strategies for overcoming bias in assessment of culturally, linguistically, and behaviorally different children were offered by Chamberlain and Medeiros-Landurand (1991). They include the following:

1. Increasing knowledge and awareness of the child's cultural, behavioral, learning and linguistic background.
2. Determining the child's level of acculturation.
3. Controlling for cultural variables.
   a. Recognize and identify the specific cultural variables that may affect the assessment results.
   b. Analyze formal tests for the specific cultural content and style(s) they require of students.
   c. Change testing procedures so as not to interfere with the testing outcomes.
   d. Teach majority or Eurocentric test-taking strategies.
4. Determining the languages and learning styles used in testing and matching the language and learning styles used for assessment with the child's skills and purposes.
5. Using interpreters/translators.

According to Bailey and Wolery (1989) and Wyatt (1994), it is not likely that a completely unbiased test will ever be developed. Scholars suggest that we use the following strategies to make the assessment process more culturally, linguistically, and behaviorally valid:

1. Use multiple culturally sensitive measures and gather data in naturalistic contexts.
2. Use a multidisciplinary, multicultural team approach to evaluation.
3. Involve parents as significant partners in the assessment process and focus intervention goals and objectives on those things considered important to parents.
4. Focus on describing skills rather than on labeling the child.
5. Provide services in mainstreamed culturally sensitive environments instead of self-contained programs.

6. Examine test manuals to ensure that they are not biased against children of a certain gender or culture.
7. Examine test manuals to determine evidence of fair use of the test with both boys and girls and in nonmainstream backgrounds.

Erickson and Iglesias (1986a) presented several options for nondiscriminatory assessment procedures. They include the following:

1. Before using a test, examine each item to determine if the child would have had access to the information being tested.
   a. Reword instructions from a culturally sensitive perspective.
   b. Provide additional time for the child to respond. Utilize learning and behavioral time parameters that appear to be consistent to the child's background.
4. Continue testing beyond the ceiling.
5. Record all responses, particularly when the child changes an answer, explains, comments, or demonstrates. Analyze responses from a culturally sensitive perspective.
6. Compare the child's answers to features of his or her dialect, first language behavioral and learning style. Rescore phonology and language tests, giving credit for variation due to culture/language.
7. If the test does not have practice items, develop several to ensure that the child understands what is expected during the assessment task.
8. In addition to pointing to stimulus items on picture vocabulary recognition tasks, have the child name the picture to determine the appropriateness of the label for the pictorial representation.
9. Have the child explain why the "incorrect" response was made.
10. Have the child identify the actual objects, actions, body parts, and so on, especially if he or she has had limited experience with books, line drawings, or the testing process.
11. For those items found to be incorrect according to the test manual, compare the child's answers with reported features of the child's language or dialect and rescore when appropriate.
12. Score the test results in two ways. First, record scores as indicated in by the examiner's manual. Next, rescore each item, allowing credit for those items that are considered correct in the child's language system and/or experience.
13. Compare both sets of scores with the norms. Typically, the adjusted scores are higher than the unadjusted scores for normal children. Children with communication disorders will achieve low scores no matter how the test is scored.
14. When reporting results of such testing, indicate that adjustments have been made. The evaluator should describe which items were

modified, what was done to modify test procedures, and the differences in the child's responses after such modification.

## DISTINGUISHING BETWEEN COMMUNICATION DIFFERENCES AND COMMUNICATION DISORDERS

Van Riper (1978) defined a communication disorder as a speech difference that (1) calls attention to itself, (2) interferes with communication, and (3) places an emotional burden on the speaker. This definition needs to be revisited in light of what we now know about the social, cultural, and political aspects of communication acquisition and use. Speakers of regional dialects are likely to call attention to themselves when they are outside their home region. Use of certain words and phrases with people who are not native to the speaker's home region may cause breakdowns in communication. If the regional dialect is often ridiculed, the speaker may experience some emotional distress. Most researchers would probably agree that these individuals should not, however, be considered to have a communication disorder.

The American Speech-Language-Hearing Association (1983) issued a position paper on social dialects that states that a dialect is not a disorder of communication. A speaker with a communication *difference* can also have a communication disorder. That person should receive intervention services for the communication *disorder*. Speech-language professionals must be able to accurately distinguish between differences and disorders in order to appropriately serve clients from culturally and/or linguistically diverse backgrounds. Stockman (1986) addressed this concern. According to Stockman, decisions about what is and is not normal communication influence every clinical decision made about speakers who exhibit language impairment. In order to make sound clinical judgments, clinicians must have some definition of what constitutes normal behavior. Furthermore, according to Stockman, the formulation of therapy goals and assessment of treatment progress are guided by what clinicians assume to be the requirements for normal language performance. Stockman views the lack of an adequate empirical definition of normal language behavior as the single most critical barrier to culturally valid assessment of nonmainstream speakers. She concluded that a determination of what is normal language should be framed in terms of the kind of linguistic behavior typically exhibited by most speakers in a given linguistic community.

Taylor (1986) addressed the issue of distinguishing between communication differences and communication disorders. According to Taylor, based on what is now known about language use by people around the world, a communication disorder can only be defined from the vantage point of the speech community of which a given speaker is a member. Taylor recommends a revision of the standard definition of a communication disorder, so that communication would have to meet certain social linguistic, behavioral, and acoustic criteria in order to be defective. It would

1. Be considered defective by the individual's indigenous culture or language group.
2. Operate outside the minimal norms of acceptability *of that culture* or language group.
3. Call attention to itself, *within the indigenous culture* or language group, or
4. Interfere with communication *within the indigenous culture* or language group.
5. Cause the speaker to be "maladjusted" *as defined by the indigenous group.*

Taylor (1986) offered several guidelines for distinguishing between language differences and language disorders. He suggested that clinicians should view clinical encounters as socially situated communicative events. Those events are subject to the cultural rules governing what is considered to be appropriate by clients and clinicians. Clinicians must also recognize that clients may perform differently under differing clinical conditions. That becomes especially significant when the client and clinician are representative of different cultural/linguistic backgrounds. Clinicians must also recognize that different modes or channels of communication may result in varying displays of linguistic or communicative performance. Taylor (1990) also stated that clinicians should utilize ethnographic techniques for evaluating communicative behavior and establish cultural norms for determining whether a communication disorder exists. Furthermore, Taylor (1990) asserted that clinicians should recognize possible sources of conflicts in cultural assumptions and communicative norms in clients prior to clinical encounters. If clinicians are aware of possible sources of conflict, they can take steps to prevent them from occurring during service delivery. Finally, Taylor (1990) suggested that speech-language professionals should recognize that learning about culture is an ongoing process. Such recognition should result in a constant reassessment and revision of ideas about people and "appropriate" communicative behaviors. The guidelines suggested by Taylor (1990), when implemented by diagnosticians, should result in professionals making accurate differentiation between communication differences and communication disorders.

## THE HUMAN FACTOR IN
## THE ASSESSMENT PROCESS

Assessment is a subjective process. It is highly influenced by a number of variables, including cultural, sociopolitical, and linguistic context (Chamberlain & Medeiros-Landurand, 1991). Holland and Forbes (1986) discussed the importance of clients' and clinicians' nonverbal behaviors during the assessment process, particularly when those individuals acquired their communication skills in different cultures. They reported that, unless the examiner is especially vigilant, he or she may miss nonverbal clues signaling discomfort, shyness, anger, and other emotions that the client is unable or unwilling to verbalize. They also suggested that the examiner must be aware of the potential impact of his or her nonverbal behavior on the performance of the client. For example, negative judgments or attitudes (coldness, condescension, disapproval, etc.) can be inadvertently communicated to clients nonverbally. According to Holland and Forbes (1986), a comfortable nonverbal rapport is as important as creating a comfortable physical setting for assessment purposes. Erickson and Iglesias (1986a) also commented on the importance of interpersonal variables in the clinical interactions. They suggested that establishing effective working relationships with our clients is a vital component in any type of effective clinical management. They believe differences in the verbal and nonverbal rules between clients and clinicians can result in unintentional episodes that could have an adverse impact on the ability to conduct effective clinical work.

According to Barrera (1994), when diagnosticians and clients and/or their families bring different world views, expectations, values, and behaviors to the assessment process, the already difficult task of diagnosis and evaluation is made even more complex. Barrera (1994) stated that it is the subjective aspect of the observation component of assessment that is particularly relevant to culturally valid assessment. In Barrera's (1994) opinion, competent assessment requires a sensitivity to the ways children and their families perceive, believe, evaluate, and behave.

## THE ASSESSMENT PROCESS

Barrera (1994) discussed steps in what she called "culturally responsive assessment." According to Barrera, the steps involved in culturally responsive assessment are not significantly different from those required by any assessment. She believes there are certain aspects of each step, however, that are especially critical when assessing children from nonmainstream backgrounds. The steps include (1) gathering background information, (2) formulating hypotheses, (3) engaging in active assessment, (4) analyzing and interpreting information, (5) reporting findings, and (6) developing program/intervention.

Cultural considerations for each of these steps are discussed below.

Step 1. *Gathering background information.* It is important to determine the child's background and how it is similar and different from that of the examiner. The examiner must learn as much as possible about the child's background before starting to observe and judge the child's behavior and development. According to Barrera, social groups reinforce, value, and reward some choices over others. She stated that, without knowing about the child's experience, it is not possible to understand whether a particular behavior demonstrated by the child indicates a need or a strength. A preassessment conference will help examiners gather valuable information to help make that determination.

Step 2. *Formulating hypotheses.* After gathering the necessary background information, hypotheses about modifications that should be made in the typical assessment procedures and materials should be formulated.

Step 3. *Conducting the assessment.* Barrera stated that the procedures used during this step should be aimed primarily at gathering two types of information: what the child knows and can do within his or her current environment and what the child's learning abilities, strengths, and needs are in relationship to new sociocultural environments. She emphasized the importance of *distinguishing observations from inferences* during this process.

Step 4. *Analyzing and interpreting information.* It is not enough to simply record the presence or absence of behaviors. It is also critical to determine what such presence or absence reflects. She suggests that the examiner should seek to determine whether the child is exhibiting age-expected behavior and skills for his or her cultural or linguistic community; whether those behaviors will serve the child well as he or she leaves home and enters new environments; and whether the child has had opportunity to learn the expected behaviors and skills.

Step 5. *Reporting findings.* According to Barrera, the greatest assessment bias often lies not in the actual assessment but in how the data are reported. For example, there may be no mention of correct responses obtained outside of the standardized procedures. She believes it is not only important to report what the child actually did, but we should also report how that performance was elicited and measured. Furthermore, it is important to include information about community behavioral expectations, because if a child is developmentally on par with peers in his or her community, the child should not be considered to have a language or learning disability.

Step 6. *Developing programs/intervention.* The final step of the assessment process is development of specific goals, objectives, and strategies. A discussion of how this can be accomplished in a culturally sensitive way follows later in this chapter.

## PREASSESSMENT

As has been discussed earlier in this text, in order to comply with various legal mandates and to provide appropriate services for our young clients, assessment and intervention procedures must be family-focused. One of the best ways to implement this goal is to have a preassessment conference. Crais and Cripe (1996) identified four goals for preassessment planning. Those goals are (1) to identify what the family wants and/or needs from assessment, (2) to identify family priorities and preferences for assessment activities, (3) to identify areas and activities of strength for the child, and (4) to determine the roles that family members will take in the assessment.

Moore and Beatty (1995) stated that a preevaluation conference should preferably be conducted in the client's home, if that is comfortable for the family. They suggested that service providers confirm the appointment the day before the conference. The confirmation may be done by phone, if the family has one. In some cases, the confirmation may have to be accomplished through a third party.

## A FRAMEWORK FOR ALTERNATIVE AND CULTURALLY APPROPRIATE ASSESSMENT MODELS

Losardo and Coleman (1996) presented four culturally appropriate assessment models. These models are discussed in the professional literature as strategies to be considered when trying to assess young children using naturalistic intervention. Losardo and Coleman believe they are particularly appropriate when examiners are assessing children from culturally different backgrounds. The models presented were: (1) embedded approaches, (2) alternative approaches, (3) dynamic approaches, and (4) comprehensive models. *Embedded approaches* are observational assessment activities that provide opportunities for children to demonstrate language and literacy abilities within the natural context. Examples of this type of activity include nonstandardized elicitations, play-based models, naturalistic or milieu approaches, and critical experiences. Advantages of these activities are that they measure language as used in daily routines, activities, and meaningful contexts and involve use of familiar tasks and culturally appropriate materials.

*Alternative approaches* include assessment activities that provide a profile of the literacy abilities of children through completion of real-life tasks. Examples of this kind of activity include performance assessment and authentic assessment. Advantages of using alternative approaches are that performance assessment allows children to demonstrate language skills in meaningful real-life situations and gives a more authentic view of the child's skills, and portfolio documentation of various forms of language use provides a concrete and meaningful picture of children's progress.

*Dynamic assessment approaches* use strategies that involve guided instruction to provide information on children's responsivity to training. Examples of dynamic approaches include curriculum-based language, learning and behavioral assessment, mediated learning approaches, and assessment of children's narratives. A dynamic assessment measures language, learning, and behavioral skills and children's responses to adult mediation. It allows for modifications such as rewording instructions, providing additional time or practice, and repeated presentation of a task. Dynamic assessment also allows children to provide an explanation for their responses.

*Comprehensive models* use a multidimensional approach and allow use of a variety of strategies, including ethnographic interviews and descriptive observations. Comprehensive models also allow for the collection of information from family members and other people familiar with the child. Finally, they provide the opportunity for description of language learning styles and behavior use across a variety of contexts (school, home, community, etc.).

Losardo and Coleman (1996) discussed necessary conditions for successful implementation of culturally sensitive assessment models. Among the conditions for successful initiation of multiculturally specific learning, language, and behavioral paradigms are:

I. Collaborative relationships with families
   - Relationships based on trust and mutual respect.
   - Respect for individual preferences for levels/degrees of involvement.
   - Appreciation of the importance of the family's role in development of the child's language.
   - Recognition that parents/primary caregivers are the experts on their own child.
II. Culturally appropriate materials and activities
   - Ethnic foods, dolls, utensils, etc.

- Books depicting different groups' manners, customs, clothing.
- Pictures depicting different skin tones, family compositions, neighborhoods, etc.

III. Awareness of cultural characteristics of individuals involved.
- Behavioral, language, and learning expectations in variety of settings and interactions.
- Child-rearing practices and family mores.
- Narrative styles and general communication expectations.
- Willingness to "perform" in the presence of adults and/or strangers.
- Types of activities likely to be ongoing and sanctioned in the home.
- Common play-based activities.

IV. Awareness of holidays/special days common to the culture.
- Events involved.
- Significant characters/heroes.
- Possible offensiveness of holidays celebrated by the dominate culture.

V. Awareness of culturally based learning, behavioral sets, styles, and how to make adjustments from European-based or mainstream culture models and interactions to accommodate the particular cultures involved.

There is no one way to assess the learning, behavioral, and linguistic styles of children with diverse backgrounds. A combination of interviewing, observation, testing, and sampling/probing offers a holistic approach that can incorporate not only the child but also significant others and familiar communication contexts. As you will see in the next section, several aspects of multicultural assessment are especially important when assessing the language, learning, and behavior of non-mainstream children.

## CULTURALLY DIFFERENT CHILDREN: ASSESSMENT CONCERNS

Within the multicultural population is a continuum of proficiency in English (ASHA Position Paper, 1985), including bilingual English proficient, limited English proficient (LEP), and limited in both English and their native language. Still, they may have a language impairment in English. It is important that the speech-language pathologist be able to distinguish between a disorder and a language difference. The speech-language pathologist must appreciate the rule-governed nature of the native language and know the contrastive features of the native language. Elective speech and language services may be provided to individuals who are bilingual English proficient and who desire more standard production of English. It is important for the speech-language pathologist to remember, however, that native dialects are not disorders. Individuals who are limited English proficient (LEP) are proficient in their native language but not in English. Assessment and intervention should be conducted in the native language as mandated by federal law (PL 94-142 and PL 95-561), legal decisions (*Diana v. Board of Education,* 1970; *Larry P. v. Riles,* 1972), and state educational regulations.

## Overcoming Bias in an Assessment

The goal of learning, behavior, and communication assessment with children is to differentiate difficulties that result from experimental and cultural factors from those that are related to language impairment (Damico, 1991). Both cultural and linguistic factors influence performance in an assessment (Chamberlain & Medeiros-Landurand, 1991). These may lead to misinterpretations and miscommunication. The speech-language pathologist must be careful not to stereotype behavior and draw incorrect and unfair conclusions. For example, Latin American children may seem uncooperative and inattentive, when, in fact, their behavior signifies different concepts of time, body language, and achievement.

The speech-language pathologist, healthcare practitioner, and educator can avoid biasing data interpretation by asking the following questions (Damico, 1991):

1. Are there other variables, such as limited exposure to English, infrequency of error, testing procedural mistakes, extreme test anxiety, or contextual factors, that might explain the difficulties exhibited with English?
2. Are similar problems exhibited in $L_1$?
3. Are the problems exhibited related to second language acquisition or dialectal differences?
4. Can the problems exhibited be explained by cross-cultural interference or related cultural phenomena?
5. Can the problems exhibited be explained by any bias effect related to personnel, materials, or procedures that occurred before, during, or after assessment?
6. Is there any systematicity or consistency to the linguistic problems exhibited that might suggest an underlying rule?

The speech-language pathologist, healthcare practitioner, and educator should interpret the child's performance in light of the intrinsic and extrinsic biases inherent in the assessment process (Miller, 1981). Intrinsic biases, such as knowledge needed and normative samples, are part of the test, while extrinsic biases, such as sociocultural values and attitude toward testing, reside in the child.

Language use patterns of both the child and the speech-language pathologist and the language learning history of the child also may influence the assessment. Communication and interactive style are culture bound.

Bias can be overcome by addressing cultural and linguistic influences in a four-step process (Chamberlain & Medeiros-Landurand, 1991):

1. Recognize and identify variables that might affect the assessment.
2. Analyze tests and procedures for content and style.
3. Take variables into account and change procedures.
4. Teach test-taking strategies.

The speech-language pathologist, healthcare practitioner, and educator should be mindful that each child's level of acculturation will differ with the age of the child and the extent of exposure to both cultures (Berry, 1980).

## Use of Interpreters

The accuracy of testing with children with LEP may be increased by using interpreters who speak the child's primary language (Watson, Grouell, Heller, & Omark, 1986). When an interpreter is not available, family members can aid the speech-language pathologist.

## Lack of Appropriate Assessment Tools

We can expect the performance of nonmainstream children to be affected by cultural divergences and the performance on formal tests to reflect these differences. Likewise, negative listener or tester attitude affects children, causing poor performance. The result is lower expectations and inappropriate referral or classification (Brophy, 1983; Cummins, 1986).

Few, if any, nonbiased standardized language tests are available for evaluating children who are bidialectal and bilingual (Bernstein, 1989). Tests are typically unique to one culture or language. In two judicial decisions regarding placement of Mexican American and African American children in classes for the retarded (*Diana v. State Board of Education,* 1969; *Larry P. v. Riles,* 1979), the courts ruled that judgments made on the basis of responses to tests whose norming populations are inappropriate for these children are discriminatory.

Many of the tests widely used in healthcare service delivery, education, and speech-language pathology (Carrow, 1974; Kirk, McCarthy, & Winfield, 1968; Lee, 1971; Mecham, Jex, & Jones, 1967) are normed on population samples with a disproportionately high number of middle-class white children. For example, older versions of the Peabody Picture Vocabulary Test (PPVT) have been shown to yield lower scores for lower socioeconomic groups and for middle-class African American children (Adler & Birdsong, 1983; Cazden, 1972; Wolfram, 1983). Error analysis suggests that some test items may be culturally biased against African American children. On the revised PPVT, African American children do more poorly than the norming population. Error patterns suggest that the children do not know the words and that the score spread is too narrow to be revealing (Washington & Craig, 1992).

In general, poor performance leads to lower expectations (Adler, 1990). It is inappropriate to compare children with LEP to native speakers of English. The use of chronological norms is especially questionable, given the great variety in developmental rate among minorities (Seymour, 1992). The nonmainstream child typically does not have language similar to a native speaker of English of a certain age. The problem is in deciding which standard to use (Lahey, 1992).

The following five guidelines should be considered prior to using standardized tests with minority children (Musselwhite, 1983):

1. What is the relationship of the norming population and the client? Are enough minority children included to give a fair representation? Are separate norms used for different minority groups?
2. What is the relationship of the child's experience and the content areas of the test? Items using farm content, for example, may have little relevance for children in the inner city.
3. What is the relationship of the language and/or dialect being tested and the child's language and/or dialect dominance? This issue is critical in determining language impairment. The determining factor should be the child's ability to function within her or his own linguistic or dialectal community (Erickson & Iglesias, 1986a).
4. Will the language of the test penalize a nonstandard child by use of idiomatic or metaphoric language?
5. Is the child penalized for a particular pattern of learning or style of problem solving?

American English standardized tests can be used with modified procedures to enhance performance. Modifications may aid the speech-language pathologist in describing the child's language and communication skills. Obviously, the scores from such testing would be invalid and should not be reported.

Dual sets of norms—those from the test and locally prepared ones—can be used to compare the performance of minority children to that of the standard group and of their peer group (Musselwhite, 1983), but they must be used cautiously (Seymour, 1992). The test, however, is still in Standard American English. It seems more appropriate to measure the child's performance in his or her dialect and compare this performance to that of other children also using that dialect (Seymour, 1992). Unfortunately, we have very little data on this development and even fewer tests.

Parents, who presumably speak the same dialect, may be used as referents when very few normative data are available (Terrell, Arensberg, & Rosa, 1992). A language test can be given to both the parent and the child. Once the speech-language pathologist has gathered enough data, he or she can compare the child's performance with that of the adult. Assuming the adult has no language impairment, child use that reflects parent use but that differs from Standard American English would represent a dialectal difference, not a disorder. For example, omission of final plosives would result in omission of the regular past tense marker *-ed*. Just testing the child, the speech-language pathologist might assume that the child does not have past tense, when in fact, this is a dialectal characteristic. Parental omission would confirm a dialectal difference.

Some tests, such as the Preschool Language Scale (PLS; Zimmerman, Steiner, & Evatt, 1979) and the Test of Auditory Comprehension of Language (TACL; Carrow-Woolfolk, 1985), have been normed on population samples from different languages, such as children speaking English and Spanish, by using English and a Spanish translation. Results of translated tests must be used very cautiously because they assess structures important for speakers of English and ignore those of the other language. For example, *hitting* something with a stick in English is *sticking* in Spanish, but that verb is not used when *hitting a ball*. In Spanish, one cannot *stick a ball*.

The standardized norms from such translated tests could be used to identify children with language differences. Children who exhibit language disorders relative to their peer group could be identified by use of the peer group norms.

Even this procedure may bias some results, given the diversity of some populations, such as Hispanics. Norms for all speakers of a language fail to consider dialectal variations in that language. Other variables, such as socioeconomic status, family grouping, length of time exposed to English, and quality of $L_1$ used at home, affect the child's performance. Locally prepared norms may be more appropriate.

The speech-language pathologist is encouraged to use language tests designed for and normed on a population that reflects the child's background. She or he should be proficient in $L_1$ and familiar with its variations or use the expertise of an interpreter.

## AN INTEGRATED MODEL FOR ASSESSMENT

Current methodology in language assessment has been described as a "discrete point approach" (Acevedo, 1986; Mattes & Omark, 1984) in which language is treated as an autonomous cognitive ability divided into many components (Damico, 1991). Language is not viewed as holistic; rather, it is separate from environmental variables and context.

It is not surprising that several special service providers have suggested an integrated approach similar to the one presented in this chapter, one that uses the child's natural environment and depends on descriptive analysis, rather than on normative test scores. Language and communication are not static, divisible, and autonomous, but dynamic, synergistic, and integrative (Damico, 1991). Such an assessment would focus on the functional or use aspects of language and on flexibility of use. The overall question would be: "Is this child an effective communicator in this context?" The criterion is not norm-referenced, but "communication-referenced" (Bloom & Lahey, 1978), with the speech-language pathologist determining the indices of proficiency. As mentioned earlier in the chapter, data would be collected in natural settings (Erickson & Iglesias, 1986b). The child would converse with his or her natural conversational partners, parents, teachers, and peers.

As in the integrated, functional approach mentioned earlier, assessment would begin with data gathering. This collection process might include screening all children for other than English and for nonstandard dialectal use. This step could be followed by referral information from classroom teachers on children experiencing academic difficulty (Chamberlain & Medeiros-Landurand, 1991). Early intervention may prevent difficulties or inappropriate classification later (Garcia & Ortiz, 1988). A teacher checklist of the child's language functions, a questionnaire, and/or caregiver interview might follow.

In addition to verifying demographic information, the speech-language pathologist should observe the child in the classroom and with peers and caregivers. Of interest is the child's language use, academic strengths and weaknesses, and learning style.

Data collection and observation would be followed by testing and language sampling. Sampling should include a wide variety of settings and activities to increase the accuracy of the language sample collected (Bernstein, 1989). Parents can be trained to listen to their child, to observe language use, and to discuss linguistic interactions (Erickson & Omark, 1981).

Family and community members can aid the speech-language pathologist in assessing performance, especially in the language sample (Bleile & Wallach, 1992). In one study, African American Head Start teachers were asked to judge children with poor speech and those with normally developing speech (Bleile & Wallach, 1992). The poor speech samples were analyzed and a set of community standards derived.

## FINAL NOTE

Despite the incredible difficulties inherent in assessing nonmainstream children, there is hope. The same integrated, functional methodology proposed for native speakers of English can be used with some modifications with these children as well. With sensitivity, unbiased administration of testing, and sampling within the everyday context of the child, a fair assessment can be accomplished. Too often, a battery of readily available tests, given to every child regardless of possible language impairment, passes for thorough assessment. As with intervention, assessment procedures must be designed for the individual client. Standardized tests are only a portion of this process. Standard tests are aids to the healthcare practitioner, educator, and/or speech language pathologist. They cannot substitute for informed clinical judgment.

A thorough assessment includes a variety of procedures designed to heighten awareness of the problem and delineate more clearly the abilities and impairments of the child. For training to be truly functional, a thorough description of the child and the child's language, learning styles, culture, and behavioral sets must be obtained. Then, and only then, does the culturally different child receive a chance for "fair" assessment and treatment.

Erickson and Iglesias (1986b) point out that specialists in communication, learning theory, and behavioral sciences are challenged to identify and evaluate elusive behavior such as human verbal and nonverbal interactions. In becoming a culturally competent clinician, Battle (1998) points out, it is important to develop an awareness of the beliefs and attitudes held by the clinician and his or her clients. Acquisition of critical multicultural assessment skills increases a clinician's power, energy, and professional integrity (Lynch & Hanson, 1992; Pedersen, 1988). Clinicians must become culturally aware of their own values and beliefs in order to effectively recognize and respect the value system(s) of persons who are unlike them. Practitioners must comprehend and value the differences that exist among children and their families if they are to acquire accurate information about the cultural, learning, and behavioral factors that influence the clinical situation. In order to develop cultural, behavioral, and learning style awareness, culturally sensitive clinicians must always strive to serve children and their families in an appropriate manner.

In conclusion, professionals who accept the important challenge of culturally sensitive assessment must develop skill in interacting with clients from a variety of cultures with a myriad of learning, behavioral, and language features (Battle, 1998, Lynch & Hanson, 1992). Competent clinicians must be able to generate, receive, and analyze language, learning, and behavioral stimuli across and within discrete culturally different contexts. The culturally competent clinician must solicit continuous self-assessment regarding cultural differences. Culturally competent clinicians must be knowledgeable about multicultural resources if they are to provide quality clinical services in an increasingly culturally diverse world (Battle, 1998).

## STUDY QUESTIONS AND ACTIVITIES

1. What are some of the concerns that have been raised regarding the validity of norm-referenced tests when they are used across different cultural groups?
2. Discuss the following types of bias that can occur during assessment if children's cultural backgrounds are not considered.
   - deliberate
   - nondeliberate and nondesirable
   - situational
   - directions or format
   - value
   - linguistic
   - content
   - gender
3. What are four characteristics of nonbiased assessment offered by Tucker (1986)?
4. Discuss Chamberlain and Medeiros-Landurand's (1991) general strategies for overcoming bias in assessment of culturally, linguistically, and behaviorally different children.
5. Explain how you might apply Erickson and Iglesias' (1986a) options for discriminatory assessment procedures when working with one of your culturally diverse clients.
6. Read the following case example and answer the questions at the end.

   Diane Jones is from a small rural area in the Appalachian mountains. Since she was a little girl she has wanted to be a teacher. After graduating from high school in 1997 she enrolled in the teacher education program at Smokey Hollow College. She has earned good grades and was placed on the Dean's List of Scholars for the last three semesters. Diane is now in the process of applying for official admission to the college's school of education. Part of that process involves passing a speech proficiency examination that is administered by the speech and hearing clinic at a nearby university. Diane had to obtain verification from the university clinic that she had no speech problems in order for her to continue in the education major.

Diane failed the speech proficiency screening and was referred for a complete speech-language evaluation. She was administered a standard diagnostic protocol. She passed a pure-tone hearing screening test and an examination of the oral speech mechanism. Her voice and fluency characteristics were judged to be normal. She exhibited problems on the norm-referenced articulation and language measures. Specifically, there were problems with the pronunciation of some vowels, deletions of some consonants, and mispronunciation of a few words. The primary problem with the language test was with the sentence imitation task. The sentences had to be repeated back to the examiner exactly as they had been said. On some items Diane deleted final consonants, did not indicate the /s/ marker on the third person present tense, and did not add suffixes to show possessiveness. In conversational speech, Diane expressed herself well but one of the clinicians described Diane as sounding like "somebody from the backwoods." The clinicians recommended that Diane should be enrolled in speech therapy. Diane filed an appeal with the clinic director. You are the clinic director.

- How would you handle this situation?
- What advice might you give to the examiners regarding interpretation of the test data?
- What would you say to Diane about her communication skills and her chosen profession?
- Would you recommend further assessment? If so, what would you suggest that the examiners do?

# REFERENCES

Acevedo, M. A. (1986). Assessment instruments for minorities. In F. H. Bess, B. S. Clark, & H. R. Mitchell (Eds.), *Concerns for minority groups in communication disorders* (pp. 46–51). Rockville, MD: American Speech-Language-Hearing Association.

Adler, S. (1990). Multicultural clients: Implications for the SLP. *Language, Speech, and Hearing Services in Schools, 21,* 135–139.

Adler, S. (1993). Nonstandard language: Its assessment. In S. Adler, *Muticultural communication skills in the classroom.* Boston: Allyn & Bacon.

Adler, S. L., & Birdsong, S. (1983). Reliability and validity of standardized testing tools used with poor children. *Topics in Language Disorders, 3*(3), 76–87

American Speech-Language-Hearing Association (1983). Social dialects: A position paper. *Asha, 25*(9), 23–24.

American Speech-Language-Hearing Association (1985). Clinical management of communicatively handicapped minority language populations. *Asha, 27,* 29–32.

Anderson, N. B., & Battle, D. E. (1993). Cultural diversity in the development of language. In D. E. Battle (Ed.), *Communication disorders in multicultural populations* (pp. 158–186). Boston: Butterworth-Heinemann.

Bailey, D., & Wolery, M. (1989). *Assessing infants and preschoolers with handicaps.* Columbus, OH: Merrill.

Barrera, I. (1994). Thoughts on the assessment of young children whose sociocultural background is unfamiliar to the Assessor. *Zero to Three, 15,*

Battle, D. (1998). Communication disorders in a multicultural society. In D. E. Battle (Ed.), *Communication disorders in multicultural populations* (pp. 3–39). Boston, MA: Butterworth-Heinemann.

Bernstein, D. K. (1989). Assessing children with limited English proficiency: Current perspectives. *Topics in Language Disorders, 9,* 15–20.

Berry, J. W. (1980). *Acculturation* as varieties of adaptation. In A. M. Padilla (Ed.), *Acculturation: Theoretical models and some new findings* (pp. 9–26). Boulder, CO: Westview.

Bleile, K. M., & Wallach, H. (1992). A sociolinguistic investigation of the speech of African American preschoolers. *American Journal of Speech-Language Pathology, 1,* 54–62.

Bloom, L., & Lahey, M. (1978). *Language development and language disorders.* New York: John Wiley & Sons.

Bogatz, B. E., Hisama, T., Manni, J. L. & Wurtz, R. G. (1986). Cognitive assessment of nonwhite children. In O. L. Taylor (Ed.), *Treatment of communication disorder in culturally and linguistically diverse populations.* Austin, TX: Pro-Ed.

Brophy, J. (1983). Research on the self-fulfilling prophecy and teacher expectations. *Journal of Educational Psychology, 75,* 631–661.

Carrow, E. (1974). *Carrow Elicited Language Inventory.* Austin, TX: Learning Concepts.

Carrow-Woolfolk, E. (1985). *Test of Auditory Comprehension of Language, Revised Edition.* Allen, TX: DLM Teaching Resources.

Cazden, C. B. (1972). Preface. In C. Cazden, V. John, & D. Hymes (Eds.), *Functions of language in the classroom.* New York: Teachers College Press, Columbia University.

Chamberlain, P., & Medeiros-Landurand, P. (1991). Practical considerations for the assessment of LEP students with special needs. In E. V. Damico & J. S. Damico (Eds.), *Limiting bias in the assessment of bilingual students* (pp. 111–156). Austin, TX: Pro-Ed.

Crais, B., & Cripe, J. (1996). *Child assessment.* Flat Rock, NC: SIFT-OUT Workshop.

Cummins, J. (1986). *Schooling and language minority students: A theoretical framework.* Los Angeles: California Association for Bilingual Education.

Damico, J. S. (1991). Descriptive assessment of communicative ability in limited English proficient students. In E. V. Hamayan & J. S. Damico (Eds.), *Limiting bias in the assessment of bilingual students* (pp. 157–217). Austin, TX: Pro-Ed.

Damico, J. S., Smith, M. D., & Augustine, L. E. (1996). Multicultural populations and language disorders (pp. 272–299). In M. D. Smith & J. S. Damico (Eds.), *Childhood language disorders.* New York: Thieme Medical Publishers.

Diana v. California State Board of Education. United States District Court, Northern District of California, C-7037, RFP, 1969.

Erickson, J. G., & Iglesias, A. (1986a). Assessment of communication disorders in non-English proficient children. In O. L. Taylor (Ed.), *Nature of communication disorders in culturally diverse populations*. San Diego: College Hill Press.

Erickson, J., & Iglesias, A. (1986b). Speech and language disorders in Hispanics. In O. L. Taylor (Ed.), *Nature of communication disorders in culturally and linguistically diverse populations*. San Diego, CA: College Hill Press.

Erickson, J. G., & Omark, D. R. (Eds.) (1981). *Communication assessment of the bilingual bicultural child*. Baltimore: University Park Press.

Garcia, S. B., & Ortiz, A. A. (1988). Preventing inappropriate referrals of language minority students to special education. *New Focus: Occasional Papers in Bilingual Education, 5*, 1–12.

Grossman, H. (1995). *Teaching in a diverse society*. Boston: Allyn & Bacon.

Haynes, W. O., Pindzola, R. H., & Emerick, L. L. (1992). *Diagnosis and evaluation in speech pathology* (4th ed.). Englewood Cliffs, NJ: Prentice-Hall.

Holland, A. L. (1983). Nonbiased assessment and treatment of adults who have neurologic speech and language problems. *Topics in Language Disorders, 3*, 67–75.

Holland, A. L., & Forbes, M. (1986). Nonstandard approaches to speech and language assessment. In O. L. Taylor (Ed.), *Treatment of communication disorders in culturally and linguistically diverse populations*. Austin, TX: Pro-Ed.

Juarez, M. (1983). Assessment and treatment of minority-language-handicapped children: The role of the monolingual speech-language pathologist. *Topics in Language Disorders, 3*(3), 57–66.

Kirk, S. A., McCarthy, J. J., & Winfred, K. (1968). *The Illinois Test of Psycholinguistic Abilities*. Urbana, IL: University of Illinois Press.

Lahey, M. (1992). Linguistics and cultural diversity: Further problems for determining who shall be called language disordered. *Journal of Speech and Hearing Research, 35*, 638–639.

Larry P. v. Riles, No. C-71-2270RFP, U.S. District Court, Northern District of California (1979).

Lee, L. (1971). *Northwestern Syntax Screening Test*. Evanston, IL: Northwestern University Press.

Leonard, L. B., & Weiss, A. L. (1983). Application of nonstandardized assessment procedures to diverse linguistic populations. *Topics in Language Disorders, 3*(3), 35–45.

Lewis, R. B. (1997). Assessment of student learning. In A. I. Morey & M. K. Kitano (Eds.), *Multicultural course transformation in higher education: A broader truth* (pp. 71–88). Boston: Allyn & Bacon.

Losardo, A., & Coleman, T. J. (1996). A framework for alternative and culturally appropriate assessment models. South Carolina Speech-Language-Hearing Association Convention, Hilton Head.

Lynch, E. W., & Hanson, M. J. (1992). Steps in the right direction: Implications for interventionists. In E. W. Lynch & M. J. Hanson, *Developing cross-cultural competence: A guide for working with young children and their families* (pp. 355–377). Baltimore, MD: Paul H. Brookes.

Mattes, L. J., & Omark, D. R. (1984). *Speech and language assessment for the bilingual handicapped*. San Diego, CA: College Hill Press.

Mecham, M., Jex, J., & Jones, J. (1967). *Utah Test of Language Development.* Salt Lake City: Communication Research Associates.

Miller, J. (1981). *Assessing language production in children.* Baltimore, MD: University Park Press.

Moore, S. M., & Beatty, J. (1995). *Developing cultural competence in early childhood assessment.* Boulder, CO: University of Colorado-Boulder.

Musselwhite, C. R. (1983). Pluralistic assessment in speech-language pathology: Use of dual norms in the placement process. *Language, Speech, and Hearing Services in Schools, 14,* 29–37.

Paul, R. (1995). Child language disorders in a pluralistic society. In R. Paul, *Language disorders from infancy through adolescence: Assessment and intervention.* St. Louis, MO: Mosby-Yearbook.

Pederson, P. (1988). *A handbook for developing multicultural awareness.* Alexandria, VA: American Association for Counseling and Development.

Secord, W. A., & Wiig, E. H. (1990). *Best practices in school speech-language pathology: Collaborative programs in the schools—concepts, models, and procedures.* San Antonio, TX: Psychological Corp.

Seymour, H. N. (1992). The invisible children: A reply to Lahey's perspective. *Journal of Speech and Hearing Research, 35,* 638–639.

Stockman, I. (1986). Language acquisition in culturally diverse populations: The black child as a case study. In O. L. Taylor (Ed.), *Nature of communication disorders in culturally and linguistically diverse populations* (pp. 117–155). San Diego: College Hill.

Taylor, O. L. (1986). *Treatment of communication disorders in culturally and linguistically diverse populations.* Austin, TX: Pro-Ed.

Taylor, O. L. (1990). Language and communication differences. In G. H. Shames & E. H. Wiig (Eds.), *Human communication disorders* (3rd ed.; pp. 126–158). Columbus, OH: Merrill Publishing Company.

Taylor, O. L., & Payne, K. (1983). Culturally valid testing: A proactive approach. *Topics in Language Disorders, 3,* 8–20.

Terrell, S. L., Arensberg, K., & Rosa, M. (1992). Parent-child comparative analysis: A criterion-referenced method for the nondiscriminatory assessment of a child who spoke a relatively uncommon dialect of English. *Language, Speech, and Hearing in Schools, 23*(1), 34–42.

Tucker, G. R. (1993). *Policy and practice in the education of culturally and linguistically diverse students.* Alexandria, VA: TESOL.

Van Riper, C. (1978). *Speech correction.* Englewood Cliffs, NJ: Prentice Hall.

Vaughn-Cooke, F. B. (1986). The challenge of assessing the language of non-mainstream speakers. In O. L. Taylor (Ed.), *Treatment of communication disorders in culturally and linguistically diverse populations* (pp. 23–48). San Diego: College Hill.

Washington, J. A., & Craig, H. K. (1992). Articulation test performances of low-income, African-American preschoolers with communication impairments. *Language, Speech, and Hearing Services in Schools, 23,* 203–207.

Watson, D. L., Grouell, S. L., Heller, B., & Omark, D. R. (1987). *Nondiscriminatory assessment test matrix, vol. 2.* San Diego, CA: Los Amigos Research Associates.

Wolfram, W. (1983). Test interpretation and sociolinguistic differences. *Topics in Language Disorders, 3*(3), 21–34

Wyatt, T. (1994). Nonbiased assessment of the African American child (videotape). Layton, UT: Info-Link Bulletin.

Wyatt, T. A. (1995). Language development in African American English child speech. *Linguistics and Education, 7*(l), 7–22.

Zimmerman, I. L., Steiner, V. G., & Evatt, R. L. (1979). *Preschool Language Scale Manual,* Columbus, OH: Merrill Publishing Co.

# 7

# SERVICE DELIVERY IN RURAL AREAS

## LORI STEWART-GONZALEZ

As we begin to consider service delivery in rural areas, let us understand that the unique characteristics of rural America must, in many cases, drive how we approach the development, organization, and implementation of service. Wendell Berry, a native Kentucky writer, speaks frequently of understanding the endemic needs of rural areas first, if we are to provide equal opportunities for service delivery in rural areas while not ignoring the cultural differences that remain influential in those areas. Berry wrote:

> My feeling is that if improvement is going to begin anywhere, it will have to begin out in the country and in the country towns. This is not because of any intrinsic virtue that can be ascribed to rural people, but because of their circumstances. Rural people are living and have lived for a long time at the site of the trouble. They see all around them, every day the marks and scars of an exploitive national economy. They have much reason, by now, to know how little real help is to be expected from somewhere else. They still have, moreover, the remnants of local memory and local community (Berry, 1990, p. 168).

We might easily apply Berry's argument to the issue of service delivery in rural areas. That is, we must seek solutions that are cooperatively determined and focused on the individual needs of a community. No

**129**

text alone could possibly provide the answers to the problems of service delivery in these areas. Without acceptance and cooperation from within the rural areas, material such as this fails to be relevant. The need for local involvement shows us why many efforts, including government programs, have been unsuccessful. It is not completely possible to effect change from without; the change must also come from within those rural areas. To that end, the focus of this chapter will be on those ideas, programs, and models that empower the citizens of rural areas to help effect change for themselves.

The purpose of this chapter is to describe the challenges to service delivery in rural areas and to present innovative programs seeking to address the needs of rural America. The programs described in this chapter were not all developed for delivery of speech-language pathology services. It seemed appropriate to investigate a range of practices, regardless of discipline, in order to identify the most positive aspects of the programs and develop eclectic approaches for individuals with communicative disorders who live in rural areas. Additionally, the author's approach to the presentation of this information is grounded in her own personal and professional experiences in rural areas of Kentucky and Florida. Several programs offered as examples are current Kentucky programs in the fields of health care and education. Also, the impressions and insights of several practitioners with experience in rural areas are included.

## WHAT ARE RURAL AREAS?

About 24 percent of the population in the United States (61.7 million people) reside in rural or nonmetropolitan areas (Parker, 1993). According to the Census Bureau, a rural community has "fewer than 2,500 inhabitants or fewer than 1,000 inhabitants per square mile" (Herzog & Pittman, 1995, p. 114).

Rural communities are complex social, economic, and political entities. Although some communities are vital and growing, others show little or no growth—in fact, they show stagnation and are suffering from an out-migration or exodus of adults of working age (Herzog & Pittman, 1995). Some rural areas are made up of thriving family-owned farms, while others may consist of scattered communities loosely connected by county designations. There is no one type of program in rural areas; there may be hospitals or schools that provide services for a small number of individuals in a remote area or for a larger number in closer proximity to services (Gold, Russell, & Williams, 1993).

Because of the population shifts and economic stagnation that exist in many rural areas, the profile of rural communities is changing. Older adults (age 65 and over), a population traditionally in need of services, is increasing in proportion to other segments of rural society (Herzog & Pittman, 1995). This demographic shift is occurring in part because of the movement of adults of working age out of these communities and into more expansive urban areas where a greater variety of higher paying, professional-level jobs exist (Herzog & Pittman, 1995). Rural communities face many of the same problems found in urban areas with one of the primary problems being poverty. For example, children make up 30 percent of the rural population living in poverty (Lahr, 1993) and these children are at risk for many problems (i.e., communication disorders, educational difficulties, and health problems). It must be emphasized that regardless of the specific profile of any one rural area, many of the difficulties encountered in the provision of services are the same for much of rural America.

In the United States 4.8 million students attend schools in rural districts (Herzog & Pittman, 1995), and in many of these areas, it is difficult to find sufficient personnel to provide the full range of services in the schools (Dopheide, Ellis, & Duncan, 1988; Farmer, 1996; Foster & Harvey, 1996; Joyce & Wienke, 1990; Lemke, 1995; Luft, 1992–1993; Thompson-Smith, 1996). Consequently, these nearly five million children do not receive adequate services. Furthermore, the American Speech-Language-Hearing Association (ASHA) has identified rural and remote populations as one of the six underserved communicatively disabled populations (ASHA, 1985a, 1985b). With these factors taken into account, service delivery in rural areas presents numerous challenges to the communication disorders profession. However, it must also be noted that service to this specific population offers countless opportunities to make positive differences and to build rewarding professional careers.

Service delivery in rural areas cannot always follow the traditional models presented in our academic training programs. One area may require the services of an itinerant professional flown into a remote area of Alaska (Olmstead & Bergeron, 1993) while another area may have access to both center- and home-based services for children and their families. Thus, no single model of service delivery is appropriate for all rural areas (RECSETF, 1990). To place these models in a relevant context, it is important to understand why traditional methods and models must be modified or adapted to meet the needs of a rural environment.

## BARRIERS TO SERVICE DELIVERY

Current literature dealing with rural issues in general is an excellent source for further detail about barriers to service delivery in rural areas

(ASHA, 1985a, 1985b; Fox, 1996; Helge, 1981, 1991; Wheeler & Hall, 1995). Cultural, geographical, social, and economic factors impede service delivery in rural areas. Many rural areas are isolated and impacted significantly by weather-related problems due to poor roads and rugged terrain (Sarachan-Deily, 1992).

Furthermore, transportation alone is an important challenge even in good weather conditions. We are familiar with the phrase "as the crow flies" as a way of noting that in a rural setting the actual distance between two locations can be significantly different from the distance as defined by the time it takes to travel that distance. An individual may report that she lives only 6 miles from the town, but it takes her as long to get to work as the individual who lives 20 miles from the same town but near a major highway. Because of this disparity between distance and travel time, most individuals in rural areas tend to talk about the time it takes to get somewhere rather than the number of miles between two places.

The emphasis of this chapter is not placed on the details of those barriers that cannot be readily changed (i.e., geographical, climate, or poverty rates), although some attention to these conditions and the challenges they present to service delivery is necessary. Rather than focus only on those factors that make service delivery difficult in rural areas, the challenge becomes to determine what approaches are effective in dealing with these obstacles and to identify those barriers that may be positively affected by new policies or programs. Also, we should attempt to identify the characteristics of service delivery in rural areas that might facilitate improved practice and positively impact our professional efforts. In this way, rural areas might receive services equal to those of other areas of society.

For example, one barrier to service delivery is isolation, which can be positively impacted if considerable attention is devoted to reducing its effects. Isolation may come in the form of social and professional isolation for service providers or isolation of client from needed services. For the service provider, social and professional isolation are among the most serious problems in rural areas and significantly impact the recruitment and retention of providers in all arenas of service delivery (Bornfield, Hall, & Hoover, 1997; Green, Roebuck, & Futrell, 1994). Approximately 15 percent of all teachers (including speech-language pathologists) will leave after their first year, and as many as 50 percent of first-time teachers will leave after seven years (Green et al., 1994), thereby creating a shortage of educators with a significant degree of experience. Thus, it is important that ways be developed to recruit and retain these professionals for work in health care and educational settings.

# ADVANTAGES OF RURAL WORK SETTINGS

The barriers to service delivery in rural areas are paradoxically viewed as advantages by many living and working in these areas (Collins, 1992; Herzog & Pittman, 1995). Given the typically negative stereotypes of rural life, the advantages found in service delivery in rural areas are often ignored by those outside the rural community. Based on descriptions from graduate students who were also employed as special educators in rural areas, Collins (1992) identified several factors—including community, family, and social support—that were classified as advantages to service delivery in rural areas of Kentucky. To these professionals, having knowledge of the students and their families provided a connection that enhanced services. Collins (1992) identified advantages in the administrative support provided to professionals in rural areas. The rural educators indicated that the lack of bureaucracy allowed for ease in obtaining materials and allowed professionals the freedom to set their own schedules. Geography, long identified as a barrier to service delivery, was actually viewed as advantageous by these rural educators. They were knowledgeable of community-based services and were able to make home visits to the families of their students, which would have been problematic without knowledge of the rural area (Collins, 1992).

Lemke (1995) detailed factors positively impacting service delivery in rural schools. These included more autonomy regarding curriculum, smaller classes with fewer behavior problems, increased family involvement in school activities and daily activities, and fewer differences among "classes" and "cultures" of students. In addition, teachers living and working in rural areas reported greater job satisfaction than teachers in urban areas (Lemke, 1995).

# INNOVATIVE SOLUTIONS

Many states have innovative programs in place to help improve the quality of services delivered to individuals in rural areas. The intention of these programs is to increase the number of professionals capable of providing quality services. Additionally, there are smaller, creative programs being implemented across the United States. It is the challenge to professionals working in rural areas to utilize applicable components of these innovative and creative programs. While many of these programs focus on services other than communication disorders, many of their features can be adapted or modified. Therefore, the information about innovative solutions will not be limited to only those programs that are providing services for the communicatively impaired. Other programs have much to offer and may spark creativity in some professional working in a rural area. Along with adapting programs used elsewhere, it is also crucial to seek the input and involvement of the rural community themselves when determining solutions for problems in service delivery to those areas (Herzog & Pittman, 1995).

## Kentucky Educational Reform Act Early Start Program

In 1990, the Kentucky legislature passed the Kentucky Educational Reform Act (KERA) in response to a court ruling mandating the equalization of educational funding and opportunities for all children in the Commonwealth. An important component of this landmark reform was the Kentucky Preschool Program (KPP). This initiative created a free statewide preschool program for children at-risk and the provision of services for three- and four-year-old children with disabilities was mandated in 1991.

In addition, Kentucky is using federal money to provide additional funding for before and after school care. More than 220 new programs for child care with a focus on rural areas have been initiated in the years between 1995 and 1996 (Holcomb, Cartwright, Dreisbach, & Fritz, 1996). In a recent report on the status of child care programs nationwide, child-friendly programs from other states including Colorado, Georgia, Illinois, and West Virginia were summarized. These states have also initiated programs that improve service delivery for prekindergarten children including many living in rural and remote areas (Holcomb et al., 1996). For example, Colorado has in place a program called First Impressions that networks with state and private agencies to enhance preschool services and in Georgia, more than $157 million has been used to expand the preschool program for four-year-olds (Holcomb et al., 1996).

## Kentucky Homeplace: Empowerment Not Dependence

Kentucky Homeplace, a state-funded grant program, was piloted in 1995 and 1996 to help individuals in twenty-three Kentucky counties seek appropriate heath care, as well as other basic needs (UK Center for Rural Health, 1996). The strength of this program is the use of Family Health Care Advisors, local members of the community who are trained to provide or seek the necessary services. These advisors also serve as facilitators to help clients access health care by making appointments, providing transportation, seeking services, and serving as liaisons between agencies and providers and clients. In short, the advisors help the members of the rural communities in any way possible (UK Center for Rural Health, 1995). Two of the primary reasons this program works are that (1) the advisors are trained as generic health advisors, enabling them to deal with clients of all ages with a variety of health care needs, and (2) there is a careful process for the selection of the advisors. Individuals are chosen from the communities where they will be working, and they are selected because they have "status" within the community. These individuals are usually active in social and service groups within the community and are respected by large segments of the population (UK Center for Rural Health, 1996).

Programs such as this offer cyclical empowerment by allowing citizens from within the communities to fuel the process of getting those in need of services to the appropriate source. Ideas such as empowering the individuals needing services could be applied to all areas of service delivery including communication disorders. Local volunteers could be trained to provide basic information about prevention of communication disorders or about how to access the service delivery system through local school districts, home health agencies, or hospitals.

## ASHA's REACH Program

The REACH, or remote/rural education, access, consultation, and habilitation, model was developed in 1991 by the Ad Hoc Committee on Services to Remote/Rural Populations (ASHA, 1991). The committee was formed following the ASHA-sponsored National Colloquium on Underserved Populations and was charged with the mission of determining alternate forms of service delivery in rural areas and developing recommendations for service delivery, education, and research. Six target areas were identified including "data, grant funding, training programs, continuing education, professional resource development and consumer resources" (ASHA, 1991, p. 282).

Recommendations about needed data collection and analysis were made and the Research Division of ASHA was identified as the entity that should compile the data. The REACH model identified some innovative continuing education programs that were actively engaged in the dissemination of information regarding service delivery to rural populations, and they recommended that ASHA take a leading role in making information available to its membership. In terms of professional resource development, ASHA was urged to assist in the development of networks in rural areas through identification of members willing to serve in their communities. Funding sources were to be identified and modifications in current Clinical Fellowship Year regulations were to be developed. Finally, it was recommended that ASHA develop a resource guide with national, regional, and local information for dissemination to members in rural areas (ASHA, 1991). Although an ambitious project, REACH provided a framework for addressing the needs of service providers and clients in rural and remote areas.

## Special Education Cooperatives and Consortia: Making the Most of Limited Resources

The old adage, "there is strength in numbers," certainly applies to cooperatives. A cooperative is developed when several smaller school districts pool money to hire specialized personnel, purchase materials, and provide specialized or technical support. In many rural areas, several school districts have contributed money to develop a centralized cooperative that serves the needs of all the participating districts. These cooperatives are not meant to replace standard services provided (and mandated) within each district. Rather, they allow for enhanced service at a lower cost to each district. A cooperative may hire a director who serves as the point of contact for all special education providers in the area. Furthermore, a cooperative may use funds to purchase necessary, but infrequently used, assessment or treatment materials. These cooperatives may also provide specialized training for educators beyond the standard in-service programs offered through individual districts.

Smaller school districts may also form consortia in order to maximize recruitment efforts. Advertisements can be funded by all districts, allowing for an expanded audience. Administrators can rotate attendance at career fairs and other state or regional meetings in order to maximize participation without draining resources at the local level (Lemke, 1994). The cost-sharing aspect of cooperatives and consortia has considerable appeal for educators and administrators in rural areas.

Practitioners may develop more informal groups through local associations or networks. This networking, done on a much more informal basis than the cooperatives or consortia mentioned above, allows practitioners to contact professionals at other schools to discuss service delivery issues. Such activity will provide a support network for rural practitioners and also allow for the sharing of materials, accessing the state organization with more clout, and development of workshops in a region or county. Case Example 7.1 provides an illustration of networking. Networks of speech-language pathologists can seek local sources, such as the Lion's Club or Sertoma organizations, for assistance with purchase of specialized equipment.

## ALTERNATIVE FORMS OF SERVICE DELIVERY

When personnel and resources are limited, alternative solutions to providing services—such as use of paraprofessionals or collaboration—must be developed. These alternatives are not to be considered replacement of service provision by trained professionals, but may, in many instances, be

---

### Case Example 7.1: Local School District Network

Suzanne recently moved to a rural area to begin working in the Monroe County school district. Her job requires travel between several small schools located in remote areas. She is the only speech-language pathologist serving these schools and her only opportunities for interaction with other speech-language pathologists are at the initial inservice meetings and her state convention. To deal with the professional isolation, Suzanne initiates an informal network to increase the contact between the speech-language pathologists in Monroe County.

She begins by locating the names and addresses of all the speech-language pathologists in Monroe County. She contacts each professional by phone with an invitation for an informal dinner at a local site. At the dinner, she outlines her plans and polls the professionals for interest; all of the speech-language pathologists are eager to participate. The rest of the evening is spent brainstorming possible actions that would increase communication and interaction. The suggestions included: (1) circulation of e-mail addresses for the members of the group, (2) development of a listserv for discussion of professional topics related to school practice, (3) implementation of quarterly dinner meetings or brown bag lunches, (4) presentation of treatment programs at these dinner or luncheon meetings (the presentations will be rotated among all members and may be from the literature or the professionals' practices), and (5) solicitation of funding from the state association to provide an evening workshop each year.

*Discussion Exercises:*

1. What other suggestions could be implemented to increase communication among the speech-language pathologists in Monroe County?
2. What are some other possibilities for funding?
3. How might the network track the success of their activities?
4. What are some suggestions to increase their strength?

---

the single source of service delivery. Thus, it is important to maximize and enhance services to the greatest degree possible while continuously monitoring overall program effectiveness. Use of paraprofessionals, parents, or community members allows practitioners to stretch their resources by indirectly impacting the lives of more children. In addition, the establishment of regional-community linkages also enhances service delivery.

## Use of Paraprofessionals

In many rural areas, paraprofessionals or speech-language pathology assistants (SLPAs) are used in order to provide services to more clients when few professionals are available. A paraprofessional should receive some specialized training in the discipline (e.g., speech-language pathology, physical therapy, respiratory therapy), but must work under the direct supervision of a certified professional (ASHA, 1996). The use of SLPAs has been a controversial topic in the field of communication disorders. Proponents for the use of SLPAs see their use as providing added access to care and extending the resources of the certified professionals (Spar, 1995). However, those who oppose the use of SLPAs fear that service quality will be reduced and that the value of services provided by certified clinicians will be questioned (Spar, 1995).

Many states (30 as of 1995) are currently using paraprofessionals in some way and have laws or regulations controlling their use (Paul-Brown, 1995). In Kentucky, individuals holding a bachelor's degree in communication disorders may be employed as speech assistants in the schools under the supervision of a certified or licensed speech-language pathologist. There is some concern that SLPAs with bachelor's degrees will be used without concern for the need for supervision—that they will be viewed as autonomous practitioners (Paul-Brown, 1995). Given the limited resources in rural areas, it is easy to understand the temptation for administrators to misuse paraprofessionals in order to provide more less expensive services. Thus, it is the responsibility of professionals in these areas to provide the needed oversight to insure that this does not occur. This can be accomplished by keeping all speech-language pathologists and SLPAs aware of scope of practice for both as well as legal and ethical responsibilities for each practitioner.

In 1996, in response to the need for a more formalized approach to training and use of paraprofessionals, ASHA issued guidelines including training levels, job duties, and supervisory requirements. The guidelines provided a scope of practice for the paraprofessionals as well as a listing of activities that are outside of the recommended practices for these individuals (ASHA, 1996). The ASHA guidelines for paraprofessionals require training culminating in an associate degree, as well as a clinical practicum experience during the two-year program. Because the guidelines have only recently been published, few training programs are implementing them.

## Collaborative and Consultative Models

The collaboration and consultation model is another service delivery alternative to maximize the impact of the practitioner. The speech-language pathologist can serve more children through collaboration and consultation with the classroom teacher (Sarachan-Deily, 1992). This widely used models allows the speech language pathologist to work closely with the classroom teacher to develop appropriate teaching or intervention strategies for use with the children identified with communication problems (Owens, 1995). In this way, the speech-language pathologist and teacher can develop appropriate goals and implement effective remediation programs that meet the needs of all children in the classroom. The speech-language pathologist may also team teach with the classroom teacher so that the classroom (rather than the therapy room) becomes the primary context for learning, and the children are allowed to interact with all their peers. In most school districts, regardless of geographical setting, this model is being used to some degree. (For detailed information regarding specific implementation of collaborative consultation programs in the school setting, the interested reader is directed to the following resources: Borsch & Oaks, 1992; Brandel, 1992; Ferguson, 1992a; 1992b; Montgomery, 1992; Roller, Rodriquez, Warner, & Lindahl, 1992).

Olson and Bostick (1988) described a successful collaboration with medical professionals in a rural Idaho community to develop and implement a procedure for medical screening and referral for infants at risk. The authors reported that the initial implementation was only partially successful because a little more than half of the infants in need of referral were actually referred. At the end of the first year, the screening instrument was revised and the project staff reestablished the collaborative relationship with the medical community and continued regular contact with these individuals. Following the program modifications, the screening and referral programs were deemed successful by all participants (Olson & Bostick, 1988).

## Use of Parents and Other Community Members

As previously stated, an often reported advantage to working in rural areas is parent involvement in school programs and activities (Collins, 1992; Lemke, 1995). The involvement of parents in the schools has historically been in the form of participation in parent-teacher organizations or as "homeroom mothers." Since the implementation of PL 94-142 and 99-457, parents have become an integral and important resource for the educational community. Parental involvement provides an excellent opportunity to enhance and extend service delivery. Inservice training programs detailing techniques for language stimulation for children with communication disorders presented in easily understood language would be a first step in educating parents in order to maximize service delivery. Parent groups could be formed to provide a vehicle for dissemination of information regarding wellness and prevention of communication disorders (Donahue-Kilburg, 1993). Such groups allow the speech-language pathologist to reach several families at one time and stretch already over-burdened resources. Further, prevention information, as well as techniques for early language stimulation, may reduce the number of children who need direct services at a later date.

Rather than simply involving parents in the programming for a child with communication problems, the entire family should be viewed as a valuable resource (Gallegos & Medina, 1995). Using family members as guest speakers for other families, sponsoring social events or health fairs for families, or developing newsletters and calendars of important events have all been used effectively in rural communities to increase family involvement (Gallegos & Medina, 1995). Among other successfully implemented ideas, Gallegos and Medina (1995) suggested the use of translators when necessary during the family activities and all programmatic interactions. Further, they stressed the importance of developing resources for the family such as toy or book libraries or directories of services in the surrounding area.

Parents or community members are particularly important for situations where more direct services are required and where resources are extremely limited, or in some cases, nonexistent. A program involving community members was used to provide direct services to individuals on one of the remote islands of the Bahamas (Thompson-Smith, 1996). Family members or other members of the remote community were trained to provide basic services for children with communication problems. The program, initially piloted on the most remote island of the Bahamas, trained eighteen facilitators to provide these services. Participants (including parents, family members, community members) agreed to participate for one year so training time could be used to the fullest extent. The program was recently extended to another island and plans are in place to extend to other islands within the next five years (Thompson-Smith, 1996).

In areas where many of the residents are non-native English speakers, it is necessary to use interpreters during assessment and treatment. In 1985, ASHA presented recommendations for the use of interpreters that included their use when the practitioner is not fluent in the client's native language and no other professionals are available. Professional interpreters or individuals in the health care or education fields should be sought as interpreters initially. If no such individuals are available, community members become important resources as interpreters or advocates for service delivery. These individuals can transfer information between the clinician and families. It is important that these individuals receive sufficient training about communication development and disorders in children, the assessment and treatment process, and the procedures for serving as an appropriate interpreter (ASHA, 1985a). An informed parent or community member will enhance services for the underserved population of children.

## *Regional-Community Linkage*

One of the primary weaknesses in programs that "come into" rural areas to offer services is that they are often based on perceived rather than actual need. Consequently, the services are not accessed by those living in rural areas because they are often not needed. An innovative program in Missouri called Project LINCS used a five-phase process for developing linkage between regional and local services and targeted expansion of services to developmentally delayed infants (Gautt, 1988). An initial analysis determined what individuals in the local area felt were the true needs of residents. After this analysis, a program was established in the local communities reflecting these local needs. However, at each stage, the linkage was evaluated in terms of the "best fit" for a given community and changes were made as needed. A strength of this model is that it recognized how ineffective it can be to simply provide a service because it is assumed to be "good" for the area. This program moved away from the notion of helping those "poor rural folks," an alternate system of service delivery that is doomed to failure (Gautt, 1988). Similar to Kentucky Homeplace, this innovative program recognized the need for establishing community linkages before initiating the program. Further, this community linkage model could be readily applied to programs providing services for individuals with communication disorders.

Of the several program models described, there exist components that can be replicated or modified to develop a program tailored to the unique needs of residents a given rural area. However, practitioners must take into account numerous factors such as geographic barriers and the availability of services. In some areas, center-based models will not be feasible. Furthermore, if there are few professionals serving an area, it may not be a good use of limited resources to have those professionals traveling great distances between clients, thus losing valuable time that could be used for service delivery (RECSETF, 1990). It cannot be overstated how important knowledge about specific needs and existing resources is to appropriate decision making regarding center- or home-based programs, collaborative/consultative programs, or programs that offer a combination of several models. It is also important to remember that flexibility is key to the planning and implementation of effective programs (RECSETF, 1990).

## PERSONNEL ISSUES

### *Avoiding Burnout and Isolation*

As previously stated, one of the primary complaints from speech-language pathologists is the isolation found in rural areas (Foster & Harvey, 1996). In many cases, speech-language pathologists are itinerant and may feel that they do not have a true association with any one school or agency. Additionally, because only one practitioner may provide services for a large geographic area, there is little opportunity for professional collaboration among speech-language pathologists in rural areas (Bell, Bull, Barrett, Montgomery, & Hyle, 1993). Administrators can develop programs or activities that can reduce these feelings of isolation. Regular staff meetings of all speech-language pathologists (or related staff, such as physical and occupational therapists) would provide opportunities for discussion of issues related to service delivery in the specific community or surrounding areas (Gold et al., 1993). District administrators committed to retaining their staff could provide activities that lead to personal and professional growth and address the problems of service providers in a very specific area (Bainer, 1993). For example, the district could provide payment of professional dues, monetary support for continuing education programs, or release time for attendance at professional meetings (Lemke, 1995). Such policies would go far in the retention of employees. Other solutions to isolation may be found in the effective use of technology. Listservs (mailing lists and electronic discussion groups) and e-mail make it possible for professionals to be in constant contact with colleagues in the profession.

### *Orientation Programs*

In order for a new employee to be satisfied in the rural setting, the process of orientation or induction should be started as soon as the contract is signed (Lemke, 1995). Through this process, the employee is informed of all policies and procedures of the given work setting as well of the mission and strategic plan of the agency. Further, for professionals in the school setting, the culture of the district, the curriculum, and the goals for service delivery are presented (Lemke, 1995). It is also crucial that information about the community be presented. Itinerant service providers should be given detailed maps of the area, including the official highway or road names as well as the local names. Information about the closest gas stations, grocery/drug stores, and hospitals should also be included. Policies that relieve some of the hassles for the itinerant professional should be developed and explained to all involved parties. For example, the itinerant service provider should be asked to leave a weekly schedule with all designated individuals so the professional may be contacted if roads are closed because of inclement weather or if clients have canceled appointments. These efforts can allow the professional to know of schedule changes before traveling 50 miles to a child's home only to find that the family is away.

Many may question the need for this induction of new employees. It involves advance preparation and a departure from the "sink or swim" mentality seen in some school districts. However, the process of induction has some very definite benefits. In one study of school induction programs, 85 percent of the teachers who were oriented to the district continued to teach in the area compared with the usual 50 percent of new teachers who were not exposed to such a program (Lemke, 1995). The induction process has been shown to "reduce job stress, increase feelings of effectiveness, and improve retention" (Lemke, 1995, p. 28). The professional that is made to feel an integral part of the professional and social environment will be more likely to remain on the job (Lemke, 1995). Case Example 7.2 illustrates an orientation program.

## Growing Your Own

The idea of "growing your own" is particularly powerful for programs in rural areas. Individuals who live in these areas tend to have more positive perceptions of the areas, see many advantages to living and working in the area, and are more likely to return to these areas for their first employment (Bell et al., 1993; Collins, 1992). Thus, administrators should seek individuals from the community as potential service providers (Gold et al., 1993; Lemke, 1995). Scholarships or stipends should be made available to interested individuals for educational programs. Using funds as seed money will pay off in terms of allegiance to the rural area and can guarantee that a service provider will work for a district for a specified period of time in order to fulfill the scholarship obligations (Gold et al., 1993; Lemke, 1995).

Further, the literature about training programs emphasizes the importance of teaching students about the rural experience (Helge, 1983, 1991; Joyce & Wienke, 1990; Marrs, 1984; McIntosh & Raymond, 1990; Sarachan-Deily, 1988). In some programs, students are currently being instructed in cultural differences and the need to develop sensitivity in dealing with other cultural groups. By training professionals from rural

## Case Example 7.2: Orientation Program

Linda has lived and worked in a rural area for her entire life, with the exception of six years spend at the state university. She has worked for a rural hospital for six years and the hospital was recently purchased by a larger hospital corporation. The hospital will be expanding its services to include inpatient, out-patient, and home health assessment and treatment. Because of her knowledge of the area and experience working with the population, she has been asked to develop and implement an orientation program for all the rehabilitation professionals that will be hired by the corporation for employment in a six-county area.

Linda has observed the importance of orientation or induction and knows that it will pay off in terms of personnel stability. She developed an orientation module for new employees hired for the Rehabilitation Department, which includes speech-language pathologists, occupational therapists, and physical therapists. The module covers the following topics: (1) mission and goals of the corporation and the individual hospitals or agencies; (2) duties and responsibilities of rehabilitation personnel; (3) regional highlights including recreational, shopping, and cultural information; and (4) demographic profile of each of the counties served by the corporation. Linda also prepared an information packet for each participant. The packets include: (1) brochures about sites of local and regional interest, (2) maps of the area, (3) housing information, (4) social services catalog, and (5) directory of schools and churches.

During the modules, Linda takes each group on a tour of the facility and provides time for presentations from corporate and hospital administration. She has placed local crafts on a table in the back of the presentation room and serves regional foods at the luncheon.

### *Discussion Exercises:*

1. What other information could be presented in the module? Think about presentations from hospital personnel.
2. What other information should be presented in the information packet?
3. Linda has been asked to report on the success of the orientation program. List some methods of evaluation for the program.

areas to return to rural areas, the problems with cultural differences may be reduced because these professionals are aware of many of the customs and practices of rural areas.

## Mentoring Programs

The use of mentors for beginning professionals is one way to reduce professional isolation and increase retention (Wei, Shapero, & Boggess, 1993). Mentoring programs offer benefits to both participants. The mentor can assume a challenging role that will rejuvenate attitudes toward the job and lessen the chance of burnout, and the beginning professional is offered a nonthreatening, experienced source of information (Wei et al., 1993). Thus, morale is improved for all participants and in turn, service delivery is enhanced. Because mentoring may be one of the keys to job satisfaction and retention, administrators would be well advised to develop a formal plan for a mentoring program. Green and colleagues (1994) outlined an innovative program that utilized a mentor teamed with university personnel to provide support to beginning teachers in Arkansas. One of the program goals was to assist the first-year teacher in the changing role of student to teacher. Roles and duties for all participants were outlined and the program was viewed as successful for all participants because of the combination of theory and practice.

## Continuing Education

Beginning in 1993, ASHA received grant funding from the U.S. Department of Education to provide practitioners with information to enhance service delivery to diverse populations through the development of a program called Building Bridges. This program was "one piece of a societal effort to achieve optimal outcomes by attempting to bridge the relationship between communication development and school success" (ASHA, 1993, p. 4). One of the six modules of this program was called Special Populations: Economically Disadvantaged and Geographically Remote. The topics covered in the module included demographics of the population, barriers to services, approaches to service delivery, and prevention (ASHA, 1993).

Local districts or cooperatives could pool resources to bring appropriate speakers to the rural area. Those specialists who are able to discuss a specific disorder or treatment program in a rural context would be particularly welcomed. Practitioners in rural areas could also lobby state associations to include presentations dealing with rural/remote service delivery at the state convention and area workshops.

## RESPONSIBILITIES OF TRAINING PROGRAMS

There have been many attempts to develop creative training programs for meeting the personnel shortages and special needs in rural areas (Andrew & Jaussi, 1993; Dopheide et al., 1988; Farmer, 1996; Joyce & Weinke, 1990; McIntosh & Raymond, 1990; Prater, Miller, & Minner, 1996). Some have been successful and others less so. Few university programs offer course work specifically geared toward service delivery in rural areas. In fact, there is little understanding of the cultural differences that will be encountered when the working professional moves to the rural area (Marrs, 1984). Since "culture clash" has been identified as a primary problem associated with retention, it seems that some effort should be made to address these problems. Programs should attempt to teach those necessary "survival skills" for life and work in rural areas (Marrs, 1984). Some training programs are making efforts at increasing the students' exposure to rural issues and some programs have developed specialized programs to educate rural professionals. It is important to look at those programs that have had a positive impact on the training of professionals who are later employed in rural areas. A few of those exemplary programs that target training professionals for rural service delivery are summarized below.

## Speech-Language Pathology Rural Project

The Communication Disorders Program at West Virginia University was the 1989 national award winner for exemplary rural special education programs in the area of preservice/inservice training (Chezik, Pratt, Stewart, & Deal, 1989; Lipinski, 1991). With funding from the federal and state departments of education, the Communication Disorders Program initiated the project designed to deal with the recruitment, training, and retention of speech-language pathologists in rural areas. The recruitment efforts began by identifying students at the junior, senior, and graduate level who indicated interest in serving in rural areas. Student participants received financial assistance and tuition waivers in exchange for participation in a program geared toward rural service delivery. Participants completed two courses in rural issues and a one-semester externship at a rural site. Further, all participants agreed to work in a rural area following completion of the program (Chezik et al., 1989).

## Three-Year Summers-Only Program

Farmer (1996) outlined an innovative program that provided training for bachelor's-level practitioners so they could receive their master's degrees while continuing employment in the rural school setting. Programs that allow these practitioners to increase their knowledge and clinical skills while remaining on the job would be very beneficial. The program discussed by Farmer (1996) provided a curriculum presented across three consecutive summers. The academic program was the same as that of other full-time students. No formal training in rural/remote issues was provided. However, all participants were currently employed in rural/ remote areas. The participants were able to remain in full-time employment while upgrading their skills in the summer. Participants in the program were allowed to complete a field study and gain clinical clock hours at their rural employment site, provided they did not receive compensation for the clinical work. Farmer (1996) reported that this Three-Year Summers-Only project allowed the reduction of barriers such as distance, employment commitments, and scheduling. Similar programs have been implemented in other states. In Ohio, a group of universities joined together to provide a master's program for speech-language pathology assistants. Each program was responsible for teaching a set number of courses and the teaching was presented via distance learning avenues.

## Rural Behavior Disorders Project

Educators at West Virginia University developed a program to enhance service delivery to students with behavior disorders (BD) who resided in rural areas (Joyce & Wienke, 1990). Program participants were chosen from those educators who were providing services to BD students in rural areas but who did not hold the appropriate state certification. Individualized instruction was then developed that guided the student to meet all competencies. In terms of rural issues, students were required to demonstrate: (1) knowledge of alternative service delivery models in rural areas, (2) skills for working with families in rural areas, and (3) knowledge of rural culture. Some of the competencies related to rural service delivery included the ability to (1) identify alternative service delivery, team building, and collaboration models suited for rural areas; (2) interact successfully with parents in rural areas; (3) recognize cultural characteristics of rural areas; and (4) deal effectively with the remote aspects of rural employment (Joyce & Wienke, 1990). All students were given reading assignments for each seminar and were required to develop questions to be used by the student facilitators during class discussions. Further, each student was observed in his or her classroom by project staff and the sessions were videotaped for review and discussion by the entire class. This program allowed students to develop needed competencies for work with BD students in rural areas (Joyce & Wienke, 1990).

## The School Extension Agent Program

For most individuals employed in rural areas, all information about rural issues takes place in the workplace (Helge, 1983). In order to address the rural training that is learned on the job, a "school extension agent" program was established in South Carolina using the Agriculture Cooperative Extension Service Agent model (McIntosh & Raymond, 1990). The school extension agents were university-trained to provide direct consultation and demonstrations to large groups regarding services for children with mild-to-moderate handicaps. The courses were infused with information dealing with service provision in rural areas. Through use of network information services, the school extension agents were taught to provide materials and information and, if necessary, access direct services from specialists in the field. The program was based on the assumptions that (1) the university campus is not the best environment for training rural service providers, (2) many rural providers do not remain on the job, and (3) rural communities tend to be reluctant to interact with unfamiliar service providers. So instead of recruiting "outsiders," elementary teachers employed in rural areas were selected and retrained to serve as these school extension agents. Following training, the teachers were available for immediate consultation (for groups and individuals) and provided demonstrations and referral information when needed. This program allowed for long-term service continuity for children with mild-to-moderate handicaps and decreased the need for moving these children to different schools further from home (McIntosh & Raymond, 1990). Similar programs are being implemented in Arizona and Michigan (Thompson-Smith, 1996). Special educators are being trained as support facilitators to provide consultative services. This idea of school extension agents could be readily adapted to provide district-based extension agents specialized training in areas such as augmentative communication or autism.

## Teacher Preparation Program for Deaf Education

Andrew and Jaussi (1993) incorporated knowledge of Appalachian culture into a teacher preparation program for deaf education. In addition to specific training in deaf education and the deaf culture, students were presented with information about Appalachia. Dialectal differences were studied, and the history of the Appalachian dialect was presented. Students studied arts and crafts from the region and many participated in cultural activities (e.g., clogging) from Appalachia. Student self-reports indicated increased knowledge of Appalachian culture and language. Further, 67 percent of the students trained in the project were initially employed in rural areas (Andrews & Jaussi, 1993).

## Appropriate Clinical Experience: Kentucky's Area Health Education Centers Program

One of the recommendations made repeatedly is that training programs provide appropriate clinical experiences that place students in rural or remote areas. The urban clinical experience cannot be generalized to this very different setting. One such program that attempts to create a realistic and appropriate clinical experience is the Kentucky Area Health

Education Centers (AHEC) program. The AHEC program provides personnel and services to enhance health care to medically underserved populations throughout Kentucky. The program, run through the Universities of Kentucky and Louisville, has seven AHEC centers, one urban and six rural (Hughes & Todini, 1996). Over 1700 students in the disciplines of medicine, dentistry, pharmacy, nursing, physical therapy, physician's assistants, and speech-language pathology were placed in 89 counties throughout the state (Hughes & Todini, 1996).

The graduate students in communication disorders at the University of Kentucky are placed in a semester-long rotation in a rural area. During the rotation, housing is provided at no cost and a modest food stipend is provided. The AHEC program allows students to live and work in a rural setting and allows first-hand experience of the rural life. Such experience may assist the non-rural professional in identifying positive aspects of the setting and in dispelling many of the stereotypes about rural life.

The literature describing exemplary programs for the training of rural practitioners emphasizes the need for course content dealing with specific rural issues (Joyce & Weinke, 1990; Marrs, 1984). Courses in rural culture, characteristics of rural communities, and the unique requirements of rural employment must be offered in order to realistically train service providers (Andrews & Jaussi, 1993; Helge, 1983, 1991; McIntosh & Raymond, 1990; Sarachan-Deily, 1988). In addition, in order for students to be exposed to the rural experience, programs should include a rural rotation or externship (Sarachan-Deily, 1988). The challenges are many for training programs, but the impact on those with communication handicaps is considerable.

## A LOOK TO THE FUTURE

### Use of the Internet: Closing the Gap

The use of the Internet in the profession of communication disorders is gaining wide acceptance and understanding. *Asha* magazine now has a regular feature on the use of the Internet in the field (for examples, see Kuster, 1995, 1996, 1997). In these *Asha* magazines, Kuster provides web sites and listservs dealing with communication disorders and related areas for the readership. These features are an excellent source for the beginning net-surfer, because of basic instructions are provided and the content is all related to communication disorders. Web sites and listserv addresses are continually changing, thus it is not feasible or practical to list them in this text.

Kuster and Kuster (1995) provided an excellent overview of Internet resources for communication disorders specialists. They described the various services and information available through the Internet including e-mail, listservs, and the world-wide web. All these electronic resources are available for use in the place of employment or the practitioner's home, if these areas are "wired." As rural districts begin to see the benefits of this information highway, and as more funds are made available for hardware and software products, service delivery will change significantly. The speech-language pathologist will be able to access information from databases across the United States or the world in order to learn more about a rare genetic syndrome. Conversations between professionals working in rural areas can occur at any time with practitioners from across the nation being involved. Thus, the barriers of isolation and distance prevalent in rural areas can be somewhat overcome (Sarachan-Deily, 1992)

One often-asked question is how this new technology will be received by those practicing in rural areas. In 1996, Howley and Howley studied the computing and telecommunication skills of teachers in rural areas as well as potential use of telecommunication services. Results indicated that teachers in rural areas were familiar with word processing and instructional use of computers. Additionally, although receptive to the use of other telecommunication systems, very few teachers had access to the Internet either in their homes or classrooms. These same teachers indicated the need for such access and the potential such access would bring. How well such technology would be used, when available, is still open to speculation (Howley & Howley, 1996). It is the responsibility of training programs to show preservice teachers and other preprofessionals the power inherent in such technology. For those professionals currently in the field, staff development should focus on the use of telecommunications for classroom and professional use in order to take advantage of the wealth of information available online (Howley & Howley, 1996). These individuals must be taught to access this technology and to negotiate this new superhighway of information.

## Use of Distance Learning

The term *distance learning* has made its way into the mainstream of education. It is no longer the technology of the future, but is being used successfully to bring information to remote locations (Barker & Taylor, 1995). Barker and Taylor (1993) defined distance learning in terms of time and distance sensitivity and presented two types of distance learning as examples. Classroom-focused distance learning is the "live, simultaneous transmission of a teacher's lessons from a host classroom or studio to multiple receive site classrooms in distant locations" (Barker & Taylor, 1993, p. 2). Thus, the communication occurs in real-time and simultaneous interactions between sites is possible. The second type of distance learning, network-focused, involves the use of technology at a time and place convenient to the user. Use of electronic databases, e-mail, and the Internet are all examples of the network-focused distance learning. Students, practitioners, teachers, and parents can access information at any time in order to enhance learning or to add information to existing knowledge (Barker & Taylor, 1993).

## CONCLUSIONS

The professional living and working in a rural area has chosen a challenging path. There are challenges in keeping current with technology and service delivery and staying motivated to keep on the chosen path. As proposed here, many successful initiatives are being implemented across the United States. The rural professional could adapt any of the initiatives and use only those aspects that "fit" into a given job setting and geographic location. Many have responsibility for making service delivery in rural areas successful. University educators, special education directors, hospital administrators, and the working professionals all have a role in making rural service delivery work. Much is at stake in improving service delivery. All professionals must work together to enhance the communicative abilities of a large segment of our population and provide quality services to these individuals. The time for positive change is now.

## STUDY QUESTIONS AND ACTIVITIES

1. Stereotypes exist for every segment of society. What are some of the stereotypes you know about rural areas and individuals from rural areas? List these stereotypes and identify possible sources of the stereotypes.
2. If you were hired to work in a rural area, what benefits, equipment, and services would you want to request at the time of the job negotiations? Provide a listing of each and a brief rationale for how each would enhance service delivery.
3. You have been chosen to serve as a recruiter for a county school district. You have been asked to interview potential speech-language pathologists at the state convention. What information would you provide for the interviewees and how would you present information about your rural work setting?
4. One of the difficulties faced by speech-language pathologists in rural and remote areas is the time involved in travel. School-based professionals often have more than one school assigned and there is some problem establishing a presence in these schools. What are some ways an itinerant speech-language

pathologist could increase visibility at schools he or she serves only one or two days weekly?

5. Orientation programs are important to acquaint a new employee to the job setting and the community. Assume you are the Director of Speech Services in a rural county. Develop an outline for a series of three inservice presentations to orient new speech-language pathologists to the schools and to the community.

6. List some ways technology may be used to enhance service delivery for professionals serving rural areas. How might a speech-language pathologist gain access to such technology?

## REFERENCES

American Speech-Language-Hearing Association. (1985a, June). Clinical management of communicatively handicapped minority language populations. *Asha, 27,* 29–32.

American Speech-Language-Hearing Association. (1985b). 1985 National Colloquium on Underserved Populations report. *Asha, 27,* 31–35.

American Speech-Language-Hearing Association. (1991). REACH: A model for service delivery and professional development within remote/rural regions of the United States and U.S. territories, *Asha, 33* (Suppl. 6), 5–14.

American Speech-Language-Hearing Association. (1993). *Building Bridges: Special populations: Economically disadvantaged and geographically remote.* Rockville, MD: Author.

American Speech-Language-Hearing Association. (1996, Spring). Guidelines for training, credentialing, use, and supervision of speech-language pathology assistants. *Asha, 38* (Suppl. 16.), 21–34.

Andrews, J. F., & Jaussi, K. (1993). Teacher education in deafness in Appalachian Kentucky. *Rural Special Education Quarterly, 12*(4), 8–21.

Bainer, D. L. (1993). Problems of rural elementary school teachers. *Rural Educator, 14*(2), 1–3.

Barker, B., & Taylor, D. (1993). *An overview of distance learning and telecommunications in rural schools.* Paper presented at the annual meeting of the National Association of Counties, Chicago. ERIC ED 365 502.

Barker, B., & Taylor, D. (1995). Case studies in the current use of technology in education. *Rural Research Report, 6*(10), 1–5, ERIC ED 391 619.

Bell, T. L., Bull, K. S., Barrett, J. M., Montgomery, D., & Hyle, A. E. (1993). Future special education teachers perceptions of rural teaching environments. *Rural Special Education Quarterly, 12*(4), 31–38.

Berry, W. (1990). *What are people for?* San Francisco: North Point Press.

Bornfield, G., Hall, N., Hall, P., & Hoover, J. H. (1997). Leaving rural special education positions: It's a matter of roots. *Rural Special Education Quarterly, 16*(1), 30–37.

Borsch, J. C., & Oaks, R. (1992). Effective collaboration at Central Elementary School. *Language, Speech, and Hearing Services in Schools, 23*(4), 367–368.

Brandel, D. (1992). Collaboration: Full steam ahead with no prior experience! *Language, Speech, and Hearing Services in Schools, 23*(4), 369–370.

Chezik, K. H., Pratt, J. E., Stewart, J. L., & Deal, V. R. (1989). Addressing service delivery in remote/rural areas. *Asha, 31*, 52–55.

Collins, B. C. (1992). Identification of the advantages and disadvantages of special education service delivery in rural Kentucky as a basis for generating solutions to problems. *Rural Special Education Quarterly, 11*(3), 30–34.

Donahue-Kilburg, G. (1993). Family-centered approach to promoting communication wellness. *Asha, 35*, 45–46.

Dopheide, B., Ellis, L., & Duncan, R. (1988). An accelerated education program for speech-language clinicians for serving rural and remote schools. *Rural Special Education Quarterly, 7*(3), 10–13.

Farmer, S. (1996). Speech-language pathology education and training for rural areas: A state and university "goodness of fit" model. *Rural Special Education Quarterly, 15*(1), 13–17.

Ferguson, M. L. (1992a). Implementing collaborative consultation: An introduction. *Language, Speech, and Hearing Services in Schools, 23*(4), 361–362.

Ferguson, M. L. (1992b). The transition to collaborative teaching. *Language, Speech, and Hearing Services in Schools, 23*(4), 371–372.

Foster, F., & Harvey, B. (1996). Retention of rural speech pathologists. *Rural Special Education Quarterly, 15*(3), 10–19.

Fox, M. (1996). Rural school transportation as a daily constraint in students' lives. *Rural Educator, 17*(2), 22–27.

Gallegos, A. Y., & Medina, C. (1995). Twenty-one ways to involve families: A practical approach. *Rural Special Education Quarterly, 14*(3), 3–6.

Gautt, S. W. (1988). Community linkage development: Expanding services to developmentally delayed infants in rural areas. *Rural Special Education Quarterly, 7*(1), 17–19.

Gold, V., Russell, S. C., & Williams, E. U. (1993). Special education in northwest Ohio: A case study of rural service delivery problems. *Rural Special Education Quarterly, 12*(3), 42–46.

Green, C., Roebuck, J., & Futrell, A. (1994). Combating isolation: A first year teacher support program. *Rural Educator, 15*(3), 5–8.

Helge, D. I. (1981). Problems in implementing comprehensive special education programming in rural areas. *Exceptional Children, 47*, 514–520.

Helge, D. I. (1983). Increasing preservice curriculum accountability to rural handicapped populations. *Teacher Education and Special Education, 6*(2), 137–142.

Helge, D. (1991). At risk students: A national view of problems and service delivery strategies. *Rural Special Education Quarterly, 10*, 42–52.

Herzog, M. J. R., & Pittman, R. B. (1995, October). Home, family, and community: Ingredients in the rural education equation. *Phi Delta Kappan*, 113–118.

Holcomb, B., Cartwright, C., Dreisbach, S., & Fritz, A. L. (1996, June). Child care: How does your state rate? *Working Mother*, 18–39.

Howley, A. A., & Howley, C. B. (1996). Receptivity to telecommunications among K–12 teachers in a rural state: Results of a West Virginia survey. *Rural Educator, 17*(1), 7–14.

Hughes, S., & Todini, C. (1996). *Annual report of the Kentucky Area Health Education Centers program.* Lexington, KY: University of Kentucky.

Joyce, B., & Wienke, W. (1990). Preparing teachers in behavior disorders through an innovative teacher training program. *Rural Special Education Quarterly, 9*(2), 4–9.

Kuster, J. M. (1995). Internet: The Internet—providing important links for practicing professionals. *Asha, 37*(4), 29–30.

Kuster, J. M. (1996). Internet: Electronic publications. *Asha, 38*(3), 47.

Kuster, J. M. (1997). Internet: Ethics and the Internet. *Asha, 39*(1), 33.

Kuster, J. M., & Kuster, T. A. (1995, February). Finding treasures on the Internet: Gopher the gold! *Asha, 37*(2), 43–47.

Lahr, M. (1993). Families with children and headed by women fare worst. *Rural Conditions and Trends, 4*(3), 50–53.

Lemke, J. (1994). How to keep qualified teachers in rural and small towns: Why administrators need to know! *Small Towns, 25,* 22–25.

Lemke, J. C. (1995). Attracting and retaining special educators in rural and small schools: Issues and solutions. *Rural Special Education Quarterly, 14*(2), 25–30.

Lipinski, T. A. (1991). Preservice/inservice training: Speech-Language Pathology Rural Project. *Rural Special Education Quarterly, 10*(2), 39–40.

Luft, V. D. (1992-1993). Teacher recruitment and retention practices in rural school districts. *Rural Educator, 14*(2), 20–24.

Marrs, L. W. (1984). A bandwagon without music: Preparing rural special educators. *Exceptional Children, 50*(4), 334–342.

McIntosh, D. K., & Raymond, G. I. (1990). Training special education teachers in rural areas: A viable model. *Rural Special Education Quarterly, 9*(1), 2–5.

Montgomery, J. K. (1992). Perspectives from the field: Language, speech, and hearing services in schools. *Language, Speech, and Hearing Services in Schools, 23*(4), 363–364.

Olmstead, P. J., & Bergeron, L. (1993). A rural/remote perspective: Alaska. *Asha, 35,* 43–45.

Olson, J., & Bostick, M. (1988). Developing at-risk referral procedures for rural areas. *Rural Special Education Quarterly, 7*(1), 9–10.

Owens, R. E. (1995). *Language disorders: A functional approach to assessment and intervention* (2nd ed.). Boston: Allyn & Bacon.

Parker, T. (1993). Nonmetro college completion rates fall further behind metro. *Rural Conditions and Trends, 4*(3), 32–33.

Paul-Brown, D. (1995). Speech-language pathology assistants: A discussion of the proposed guidelines. *Asha, 37*(9), 4(3), 39–42.

Prater, G., Miller, S. A., & Minner, S. (1996). The rural special education project: A school-based program that prepares special educators to teach Native American students. *Rural Special Education Quarterly, 15*(1), 3–12.

Roller, E., Rodriquez, T., Warner, J., & Lindahl, P. (1992). Integration of self-contained children with severe speech-language needs into the regular education classroom. *Language, Speech, and Hearing Services in Schools, 23*(4), 365–366.

Rural Early Childhood Special Education Task Force (RECSETF). (1990). Response to PL 99-457, Titles I and II: Issues concerning families residing in rural and remote areas of the United States. *Rural Special Education Quarterly, 9*(1), 24–27.

Sarachan-Deily, A. B. (1988). Preparation of teachers to work with communicatively handicapped students in rural schools. *Rural Special Education Quarterly, 7*(3), 6–9.

Sarachan-Deily, A. B. (1992, April). Beyond the one-room schoolhouse. *Asha, 34,* 34–37.

Spar, F. T. (1995). Speech-language pathology assistants. *Asha, 37*(9), 39.

Thompson-Smith, T. (1996). *Speech-language-hearing service delivery: Rural and remote.* Paper presented at the annual meeting of the American Speech-Language-Hearing Association, Seattle, WA.

UK Center for Rural Health. (1995). *Kentucky Homeplace Fourth Quarterly Report.* Hazard, KY: UK Center for Rural Health.

Wei, S. B., Shapero, S., & Boggess, B. W. (1993). Training and retaining rural special educators. *Rural Special Education Quarterly, 12*(4), 52–59.

Wheeler, J. J., & Hall, P. S. (1995). Supported employment in rural areas: The demographics of job development in South Dakota. *Rural Special Education Quarterly, 14*(1), 20–23.

# 8

# LANGUAGE DISORDERS IN CULTURALLY DIVERSE POPULATIONS: INTERVENTION ISSUES AND STRATEGIES

## LEMMIETTA G. MCNEILLY and THALIA J. COLEMAN

Many spoken languages and dialects are found in the United States. Those languages and dialects are inherent characteristics of the cultural heritages of individuals who live in this country. Most of those people want to preserve the language differences of their cultural heritages. According to the principles of the American way of life, they have a right to do that. This country consists largely of individuals who immigrated here, bringing with them cultural diversity that permeates all aspects of their lives. It would not be appropriate to welcome people to our country while at the same time insisting that they leave their heritages behind. People's languages are as much a part of their cultural heritages as their religions and feelings of nationalism (Hulit & Howard, 1997).

Children with cultural differences come to school with varying degrees of skill in their first language and in English. They also differ in the amount of exposure they have had to the mainstream culture, their learning skills, and their social skills (Kuder, 1997). Consequently, children from culturally and linguistically different backgrounds are often erroneously labeled as language disordered. One of the responsibilities of speech-language pathologists is to make a determination about which children are simply exhibiting language differences and which ones actually have language disorders that require special intervention. Many teachers, speech-language pathologists, and other service providers are from the majority culture and may perceive linguistic differences as "problems." For example, a dialect or accent may be mistaken for a speech or language disability (Ratner & Harris, 1994).

Speech-language professionals must be prepared to take on many roles as they work in settings that serve culturally diverse clients. First of all, they must be able to conduct thorough and appropriate assessments to determine if there are deficits in both the primary language and in English. Second, they must serve as educators/mentors for professional colleagues regarding the nature of communication differences versus communication disorders and the appropriate actions to take in either case. Third, they must collaborate with classroom teachers regarding appropriate strategies for ensuring that all students are able to *code switch*—use formal or informal English as required or expected in given situations. Finally, they must ensure that they *themselves* have come to terms with the issues of cultural diversity in this country and are able to articulately and convincingly serve as advocates for unbiased and culturally valid services for all children. Part of that advocacy would involve encouraging decisions based on children's needs and program effectiveness rather than on factors such as prejudice, fear, and cost (Kuder, 1997). Additionally, the Individuals with Disabilities Act (IDEA) requires that disorders be determined based on the child's individual needs.

## LANGUAGE DIFFERENCE OR LANGUAGE DISORDER?

### Language Disorder

There has been much debate about what constitutes a language disorder. This debate has yielded many attempts to define this aspect of communication impairment. The Committee on Language, Speech, and Hearing Services in Schools of the American Speech-Language-Hearing Association, as cited in Paul (1995), defined language disorder as the impairment or deviant development of comprehension and/or use of spoken, written, and/or other symbol system. The disorder may involve (1) the form of language (phonologic, morphologic, and syntactic systems), (2) the content of language (semantic system), and/or (3) the function of language in communication (pragmatic system) in any combination (Committee on Language, Speech, and Hearing Services in Schools, 1982, p. 949). Our discussion of language disorders will be based on the description offered by Paul (1995). According to Paul, children with language disorders have a significant deficit in learning to talk, understand, or use any aspect of language appropriately as determined by results obtained by informal and standardized measures.

## Language Difference

The issue of distinguishing between language difference and language disorder was discussed in chapter 6. As was mentioned there, many children from culturally and linguistically different backgrounds who are referred for language assessment do not have disorders. However, some children from culturally/linguistically different backgrounds do have language disorders. When they do, it is the responsibility of the speech-language pathologist to provide intervention in a culturally sensitive way (Paul, 1995).

Harris (1994) summarized key aspects of the American Speech-Language-Hearing Association's (1985) position paper on providing clinical services for individuals from culturally and linguistically diverse backgrounds who have communication impairments. The position paper states that children with limited English proficiency (LEP) are considered to have a communication disability when there is limited competence in both the English language and the one spoken most frequently by the child. According to the position statement, assessment of children who have limited proficiency in English should be conducted in the client's primary language with a proficient bilingual examiner. ASHA's position papers on social dialects (1983, 1987) declared that no English dialect can be considered a language disorder and should not be treated as such. Harris (1994) believes children speaking dialects should be treated in a manner similar to that of children who are bilingual or have limited proficiency in English. She believes teachers and other service providers must study, respect, and value each child's cultural and linguistic differences.

There are several morphological, syntactical, and pragmatic components of English that vary across the various vernacular forms of English present in America. The dialectal variations and vernacular usage of English spoken in different regions of the country and by members of various ethnically diverse populations need to be validated for the community in which the child resides. An examiner who is not familiar with the specific features of the dialects spoken might misinterpret communication behaviors as disorders when they are merely differences. The reader is referred to the list of suggested readings at the end of this chapter for more information about the specific features of several common dialects of American English.

Stockman (1986) stated that it is complicated to separate the child with a linguistic difference from one with a language disorder. One reason for this difficulty, according to Stockman, is the lack of an adequate empirical definition of what is normal language behavior for nonmainstream speakers. Stockman believes this lack of an adequate definition of normalcy results in inaccurate language assessment. Each speech language pathologist has the responsibility of quantifying and qualitatively describing normal language for speakers of vernacular American English for the communities in which they are providing services.

## ASSESSMENT AND INTERVENTION

### Assessment Considerations

All good intervention programs should begin with unbiased accurate assessments. Many of the issues regarding culturally valid assessment were discussed in chapter 6. Given that assessment serves as the foundation for program development, additional comments specific to assessment of language skills of children from culturally diverse groups will be offered in this chapter.

Harris (1994) pointed out that no one test can account for all of the variables that may have an impact on language competence and performance. She asserts that, even if there were one test that encompassed all critical considerations, that test would not be standardized with children using every dialect of every language from every culture in this country. Harris concluded that standardized tests are extremely limited as to what aspects of language they can effectively test and on whom.

Nelson (1989, as cited in Langdon & Cheng, 1992) noted that the focus of assessments of speech and language disorders has shifted from diagnosing the cause of a problem to determining strategies to help students cope more efficiently with the demands of appropriate language for classroom environments and to become better communicators. Kayser (1989, as cited in Harris, 1994) reported several items to consider when assessing language skills of children from culturally/linguistically different backgrounds, particularly clients whose first language is not English. The responses to these items will result in decisions regarding disorder versus difference diagnosis as well as make an impact upon the intervention choices for the child and family. They are:

- Language used by the family
- Child's length of stay in this country
- Educational level of parents

- Work experience of parents
- Use of language outside of the home by the family
- Language used in newspapers and other media by the family
- Attitude of the family toward the dominant language and culture
- Attitude of the community towards the dominant culture

If the language used by the family is not English and the child has lived in this country for a very short time, it is safe to assume that the child has not had adequate opportunities for learning to speak English.

## Intervention Considerations

It is very important for the examiner to understand the family attitudes toward the dominant language when making intervention recommendations to the family. The speech language pathologist will be more successful when he or she utilizes intervention strategies that are congruent with the family's values and beliefs regarding language usage in the community. Other considerations, such as child-rearing practices, self-concept, learning styles, reactions to examiners, and so on, were discussed earlier in this book. These factors will also have an impact on the nature of intervention with children who present with language disorders. We believe valid and appropriate assessment is an absolute prerequisite to effective intervention. In fact, we consider assessment to be the foundation of all other intervention activities. As we seek to improve the efficacy of language intervention with children who are from nonmainstream backgrounds, it is important that we have based our goals and the strategies for obtaining those goals on results obtained using culturally valid assessment strategies.

## BEST PRACTICES IN LANGUAGE INTERVENTION: CHILD-CENTERED, INTERACTIVE, AND NATURALISTIC STRATEGIES

Many speech-language pathologists are now using language intervention approaches that emphasize the communicative or functional aspects of language rather than focusing on discrete parts or language form alone. What has been learned about the nature of language and the normal acquisition of language over the past decades has had a tremendous impact on how speech-language professionals engage in the intervention process. In some settings, language is now being taught in the context of daily routines and conversational interactions. Professionals tend to use methods and procedures that are child-centered, interactive, and naturalistic (McCormick, 1997). Most of those strategies are especially appropriate and effective when used with children who have cultural and/or linguistic differences. Some of the approaches that could be used with children from most (perhaps all) backgrounds and strategies that may be especially effective when working with children who have different behavioral and learning styles are described in this chapter.

Beaumont (1992) summarized some of the child-centered, naturalistic considerations for language intervention. They include:

1. Using authentic, purposeful communication interactions as part of teaching strategies.
2. Planning activities that use themes, events, and experiences.
3. Incorporating communication events from children's home and community into activities.
4. Connecting intervention activities to things children experience as part of their larger curriculum context.
5. Creating an environment that facilitates and encourages a wide range of language uses.
6. Integrating form, content, and use in all intervention/educational activities.
7. Planning intervention around what is considered to be *effective communication and learning* instead of around deficits.

McCormick (1997) also described several naturalistic methods that are currently being used with children to improve their language skills. They are as follows:

1. **Milieu Language Teaching.** This umbrella term covers several naturalistic language teaching procedures. It is based on observations that have been made of how parents and other caregivers interact with their children who are developing language skills normally. Parents and professionals using this approach talk about objects, events, and relations that have attracted the child's attention. They follow the child's lead rather than making a decision on their own regarding the conversational topic. Trainers model, imitate, and expand desired and actual communication efforts by the child. They repeat and clarify words, statements, and requests as appropriate. Additionally, they use higher frequencies and stress to call the child's attention to important sentence elements. According to McCormick, the difference between milieu teaching and other naturalistic approaches is that milieu teaching uses *explicit* prompts.
2. **Scaffolding.** This approach helps children understand and use language at a more complex level. The difficulty of requests made to the

child is gradually increased. As that happens, the instructor provides the child with just enough support to enable him or her to be successful at completing the task. Beaumont (1992) presents the following characteristics of effective scaffolding:

- Connecting the task to something the child already knows.
- Directing the child's attention to the most important aspects of the task.
- Questioning the child in a way that will lead to problem-solving strategies.
- Demonstrating strategies that are effective.
- Modeling devices to aid memorization.
- Following cues from the child to determine when to intervene.
- Providing the proper balance between success and error to allow the child to grow without becoming discouraged.
- Appropriately withdrawing intervention as the child becomes more successful at communication tasks.
- Relinquishing control of the task to the child.

The reader is referred to the list of recommended readings at the end of this chapter for additional resources describing the scaffolding approach.

3. **Routines and Script Training.** McCormick (1997) discussed routines as activities that are repeated frequently and always in the same way. Social routines include activities such as games, rhymes, jokes, songs, stories, and courtesies. Maintenance routines include classroom activities such as collecting lunch money, taking attendance, cleaning up, and distributing materials. McCormick suggested that professionals consider the type of materials involved, time requirements, and the number and repetitiveness of the actions and subroutines involved when deciding which routines are more suitable for promoting communication skills than others.

   Nelson and Gruendel (1986) described *scripts* as generalized representations of familiar events and routines that show an established pattern of behavior. According to McCormick, the goal of script training is to create interactive, systematic repetitions of events where each child plays his or her predictable role. This is done in such a way as to (a) provide children with opportunities to practice social roles, (b) observe and model other children's communication skills, and (c) increase understanding of how to solve interpersonal conflicts.

4. **Interactive Modeling.** According to McCormick, this procedure is sometimes called *recasting, interactive language instruction,* or *focused stimulation.* The procedure gives children more deliberate and focused practice, more time, more repetitions, and intensified focus on new words and concepts. Target forms or operations are embedded in play

or curriculum activities and routines. The trainer uses the target forms/operations repeatedly in contexts where they are appropriate. Children are not requested nor required to respond.

5. **Situated Pragmatics.** Dunchan (1995) described situated pragmatics as an instructional approach that assists children with communication disorders to understand and be included in the normal flow of interactions in daily situations. According to McCormick, supports are provided in several contexts such as playground, classroom, telephone, which are tailored to fit the child's difficulties or build upon his or her strengths.

Several excellent sources exist that provide information about child-centered, interactive, and naturalistic strategies for language intervention. An extensive review of all of those strategies is beyond the scope of this chapter. For more information the reader is referred to the list of suggested readings at the end of this chapter.

## LANGUAGE INTERVENTION WITH CHILDREN WHO ARE BILINGUAL OR LIMITED IN ENGLISH PROFICIENCY

### *Determining Language for Intervention*

According to Beaumont (1992), one of the most important and most difficult decisions that the speech-language pathologist must make when working with children who are bilingual or limited in their use of English is determining the language to be used for intervention. Beaumont discusses several variables that must be taken into account to arrive at a decision about what best suits the needs of the student and about what resources are available in the school. Intervention should be conducted in the first language if all following circumstances exist:

1. The first language continues to be the child's dominant language for several aspects of communication. In addition, the student is familiar with more concepts in the first language.
2. The student's background knowledge and prior experiences have been developed and coded linguistically in the first language.
3. The first language reflects the cultural environment in which the student was raised.
4. The student may potentially lose the ability to communicate with family members who speak only in that language if the first language is not enhanced (Beaumont, 1992, pp. 349-350).

Beaumont (1992) suggested that there should be a thorough assessment of the student's language preference and proficiency levels in each language he or she speaks. This testing should be comprehensive and done using general language proficiency testing. Furthermore, the languages in which students have received instruction and the amount or length of time that they have received instruction in each language should be determined. Since some children's school experiences may have been inconsistent due to frequent moves, erratic attendance, or changes in the language of instruction from one year to another, those children may need special attention to ensure that their programs are integrated appropriately.

Speech-language pathologists might consider determining whether students will have opportunities to interact with peers in along a continuum from formal to informal situations using both languages. Observing students in several situations and consulting with the classroom teacher can do this. Some children may be highly motivated to acquire the second language due to the desire to belong to a particular social group. According to Beaumont (1992), the attitude of teachers and service providers toward the student's primary language is also very important. It may be difficult for students to sustain the motivation to use second language if school personnel ignore or merely tolerate it. Additionally, Beaumont contends that the attitudes and proficiency of parents and other family members are also important. As natural communication partners are family members and generally children are concerned about the way their communication is perceived by others that they interact with regularly and respect. These variables may impact expected outcomes from intervention.

Finally, Beaumont (1992) suggests that the speech-language pathologist should have at least minimal linguistic competence in the student's first language. Minimal linguistic competence would allow the speech language pathologist to support the child's primary language and engage in basic conversations. If, however, the clinician is going to instruct the student using a foreign language, she or he "should be at least a strong intermediate level speaker of the language and should have near-fluent pronunciation skills" (Beaumont, 1992, p. 351).

## Intervention Issues

Harris (1994) contends that the first steps to effective intervention for children from culturally and linguistically diverse backgrounds must include knowledge and respect for each child's culture and language. She discussed several issues with regard to teaching children who are bilingual or limited in their proficiency in English. Several excellent resources are available that provide *comprehensive* information about language intervention with children who are bilingual or have limited proficiency in English. The reader is referred to the suggested readings at the end of this chapter.

Cummins (1989) and Ruiz (1989) offer some suggestions that would be helpful for speech language pathologists who are working with language disordered individuals who have a primary language other than English. These suggestions are especially helpful for professionals who are attempting to help students gain facility in both languages instead of just in English. The suggestions include

- Signs in school written in the "minority" language(s).
- Tutors who speak the "minority" language.
- Displays of pictures of various cultures represented at the school.
- Newspaper articles written in the "minority" student's primary language(s).
- "Minority" language integration into content areas.
- Collaborative learning to provide opportunities for natural language practice.

## Increasing Communicative Opportunities

A child who exhibits a different speaking pattern, limited English proficiency, or vernacular form of English may not engage in communicative interactions in classrooms as readily or as frequently as do other children. Additionally, children who present with language disorders and who have difficulty expressing their needs to others within and across culturally familiar situations tend to communicate less frequently than children who present with age appropriate language skills. Bunce (1997) suggested several ways to help those children. They include:

1. Setting up a buddy system. This would allow all students to have a peer resource who would be available to check their work and discuss their ideas.
2. Using gestures and demonstrations liberally while avoiding overly complex syntax when talking.
3. Using role-playing as a mechanism to provide contextual support. Activities could include dramatic play, and acting out stories or historical events. Care should be taken to ensure that the themes are appropriate for the child's background or culture.
4. Using peer teaching and modeling of responses. Some students may understand instruction from peers better than that from the teacher.
5. Using some group work and cooperative learning.

6. Recording instructions on audiotape. This allows students to replay instructions until they have a clear understanding of what they mean. The taped instructions can also be paired with written instructions to provide additional opportunities to learn language.
7. Allowing additional time for students to make responses.
8. Describing what students are observing.
9. Using small-group activities and one-on-one interactions with the teacher in order to help students feel more comfortable about speaking.
10. Making corrections indirectly by expanding or recasting utterances.
11. Using activities that enable the child to work from a global or holistic perspective before dealing with discrete parts of the whole.
12. Using *whole-language* activities such as language-experience stories, choral reading and/or poetry activities, predictable books or stories, puppets reading and retelling stories, and other writing activities.
13. Using tutors, when available, who speak the child's first language.
14. Using content area books that are available in the child's first language.
15. Using reading materials where the "star" of the story is from the student's linguistic or cultural group.

## SUMMARY AND CONCLUSIONS

The language assessment and intervention approaches presented in this chapter represent an array of options for the clinician. It should be clear that there is no single best clinical practice for all children from any culture. However, we have presented a number of clinical considerations that should be addressed so that you are capable of eliciting information that is truly representative of the child's best language skills. We need to analyze the results of assessment tools with knowledge of the child's culture. We need to be knowledgeable about the dialects and languages primarily spoken in the home. We must ask questions regarding rules for children to communicate with adults. We should analyze the errors obtained and ask if any cultural barriers exist that would prevent the child from being able to provide the desired response. We need to clearly distinguish between "errors" based on cultural or environmental opportunities versus disordered language. Families can help us make that decision, if we ask the right questions.

Families have a major role to play in accurate assessment verification as well as therapeutic strategies that are culturally appropriate for the family. The clinician should bring good observational and listening skills to the clinical environment, be flexible, and make appropriate changes that include cultural values and practices that are adhered to by the family. We are trained professionals, and parents and family members are the experts in their family practices and cultural beliefs. They are also excellent reporters of the behaviors presented by the child involved in clinical intervention. They also can provide the clinician with information regarding communication skills in the home and community outside of the therapy room. We will get the answers if we ask questions in culturally appropriate and respectful ways.

There are few articles documented in the literature regarding language intervention for culturally diverse populations, therefore this is an area in which treatment efficacy studies are desperately needed. Studies that systematically study specific treatment protocols for culturally diverse populations are indicated for the future. However, the information presented in this chapter serves as a framework upon which language intervention can be developed so that speech language pathologists can achieve expected outcomes for children from culturally and linguistically diverse populations. English-only-speaking speech-language pathologists often feel unsure about their options, therefore it was our intent to present some specific choices and considerations that one should employ as a part of planning therapy programs.

## STUDY QUESTIONS AND ACTIVITIES

1. What cultural considerations should I take into account when planning a therapy program for a language-disordered child from a culture that is different from mine?

2. The family speaks Spanish only, but they want 3-year-old Juan to learn to speak English primarily and they want him to receive speech therapy because he has lived in the United States for six months and has not picked up any English. Describe the approach you would take regarding interviewing parents, assessment and intervention strategies, or recommendations.

3. One child is a 3-year-old boy who speaks in single English word utterances, is the only child of two university professors, lives in Illinois, and is Caucasian. The second child is a 3-year-old boy who speaks in single English word utterances and is the son of bilingual migrant farmers. The family recently moved to Illinois from Florida and will be leaving in six months for another state. Would the intervention materials and strategies and goals recommended be the same for the two children described above? Explain why or why not.

4. Write a lesson plan for the first week of therapy with a 7-year-old African American girl from a rural community in the south who recently moved to Washington, DC with her family. She has documented expressive and receptive vocabulary skills two years below age level. Explain why you selected

the materials utilized and the rationale for the short-term goals identified for the week.

5. The following case studies may be used to stimulate discussions for interactive learning activities in the classroom. Some questions that might be suggested for discussion include:

   • How would you seek to modify traditional intervention strategies when working with this child?

   • What challenges might there be to the intervention process?

   • What intervention goals and strategies would you develop?

**Case Example 8.1**

Mary, a 3-year-old child adopted from China by a mother who is Caucasian, has lived in America with her single mother for twelve months. Mary's mother is very concerned about Mary's communication skills. She wants to maintain ties with her Chinese heritage and therefore attends a parent-child playgroup weekly with other children who have been adopted from China.

Mary smiles and is a happy friendly little girl. She enjoys books and manipulative toys. She plays well alone and next to other children. She is generally quiet while playing. She uses some single words including "ma," "juice," "no," "go," and "bye-bye." Her pragmatic skills consist of greetings, protests, requesting objects/actions, and responses to requests. Her expressive language is characterized by few spontaneous initiations with peers or adults. She tends to be a passive communicator, she responds nonverbally and maintains good eye contact with communication partners. Her mother wants Mary to receive speech therapy to help increase her language skills. She is eager to receive information about ways that she can facilitate language in the home environment. She spends several hours each day just sitting and talking or playing with Mary. They also go on field trips monthly.

After two months of therapy in the home, Mary's communication skills have increased significantly. She plays with other children and talks while playing. Her mother is very pleased and feels equipped to handle further development of Mary's communication skills.

**Case Example 8.2**

Adam is a three-and-half-year-old Caucasian child living with his family in a suburban community. His father is the sole family provider and the mother does not work outside of the home. Adam has a brother who is one year older and a sister who is two years younger. He presents with some interesting language skills. He is unable to answer questions about objects or pictures within his environment. He can spontaneously label items within his environment. He can name all of his letters and can spell some simple words. He has difficulty retrieving words to express his needs and has difficulty making choices when his mother offers two or more items. He has temper tantrums that last for several minutes. His spontaneous speech is characterized by phonological processes and is quite unintelligible to the unfamiliar listener. He speaks in primarily two- to three-word utterances.

His mother is concerned about his speech, the family history is positive for stuttering, and the child's pediatrician stated that he will be fine if they just give him some more time and let his language improve. Adam's mother wants a speech language assessment for Adam and therapy. She doesn't feel that Adam's problems will go away with age.

**Case Example 8.3**

Ricardo is a 30-month-old child of bilingual parents who live in a rural southern community. He watches some children's television programs in English such as "Barney" and "Arthur." His Spanish language skills are age appropriate; however, his parents are concerned about the development of his English language skills. They have avoided teaching colors or shapes because they aren't sure about which language they should use to teach these pre-academic skills. They don't want to confuse the child. Ninety percent of the time Spanish is spoken in the home. There are no Spanish-speaking speech-language pathologists in the community. He is presently at home but will attend an English-only preschool next year. They are interested in strategies for facilitating his success in school. He uses some English words and understands some simple directions presented in English with pictures or objects.

## REFERENCES

American Speech-Language-Hearing Association. (1983). Social dialects—a position paper. *Asha, 25*(9), 23–24.

American Speech-Language-Hearing Association. (1985). Clinical management of communicatively handicapped minority language populations. *Asha, 27*(6), 29–32.

American Speech-Language-Hearing Association Committee on the Status of Racial Minorities. (1987). Social dialects position paper. *Asha, 45.*

Beaumont, C. (1992). Language intervention strategies for Hispanic LLD students. In H. W. Langdon & L. L. Cheng (Eds.). *Hispanic children and adults with communication disorders: Assessment and intervention.* Gaithersburg, MD: Aspen Publishers.

Bunce, B. H. (1990). Bilingual/bicultural children and education. In L. McCormick & R. L. Schiefelbusch (Eds.), *Early language intervention: An introduction* (2nd ed.). Boston: Allyn & Bacon.

Committee on Language, Speech, and Hearing Services in Schools. (1982). Definitions: Communicative disorders and variations. *Asha, 24,* 949–950.

Cummins, J. (1989). A theoretical framework for bilingual special education. *Exceptional Children, 56,* 111–119.

Dunchan, J. F. (1994). *Supporting language in everyday situations.* San Diego, CA: Singular.

Harris, L. (1994). Looking at cultural and linguistic diversity. In V. Ratner & L. Harris (Eds.), *Understanding language disorders: The impact on learning* (pp. 105–132). Eau Claire, WI: Thinking Publications.

Hulit, L. M., & Howard, M. R. (1997). Language diversity: Regional social/cultural, and gender differences. In *Born to talk: An introduction to speech and language development* (pp. 301–331). Boston: Allyn & Bacon.

Kuder, S. J. (1997). *Teaching students with language and communication disabilities.* Boston: Allyn & Bacon.

Langdon, H. W., & Cheng, L. R. L. (1992). *Hispanic children and adults with communication disorders: Assessment and prevention.* Rockville, MD: Aspen Publishers.

McCormick, L. (1997). Language intervention and support. In L. McCormick, D. F. Loeb, & R. L. Schiefelbusch (Eds.). *Supporting children with communication difficulties in inclusive settings: School-based language intervention.* Boston: Allyn & Bacon.

Nelson, K., & Gruendel, J. (1986). Children's scripts. In K. Nelson (Ed.), *Event knowledge: Structure and function in development.* Hillsdale, NJ: Erlbaum.

Paul, R. (1995). *Language disorders from infancy through adolescence: Assessment and intervention.* St. Louis: Mosby Year Book.

Ratner, V., & Harris, L. (1994). *Understanding language disorders: The impact on learning.* Eau Claire, WI: Thinking Publications.

Ruiz, R. (1988). Bilingualism and bilingual education in the United States. In C. Paulston (Ed.), *International handbook of bilingualism and bilingual education* (pp. 539–560). New York: Greenwood Press.

Stockman, I. J. (1986). Language acquisition in culturally diverse populations: The Black child as a case study. In O. L. Taylor (Ed.), *Nature of communication disorders in culturally and linguistically diverse populations* (pp. 117–155). San Diego, CA: College-Hill Press.

## SUGGESTED READINGS

Cheng, L. L. (1991). *Assessing Asian language performance: Guidelines for evaluating limited English proficient students* (2nd ed.). Oceanside, CA. Academic Communication Associates.

Gutierrer-Clellan, V. F., & Quinn, R. (1993). Assessing narratives of children from diverse cultural/linguistic groups. *Language, Speech and Hearing Services in Schools, 24*(1), 2–9.

Hamayan, E. V., & Damico, J. S. (1991). *Limiting bias in the assessment of bilingual students.* Austin, TX: Pro-Ed.

Fradd, S., & Weismantel, M. (1989). *Meeting the needs of culturally and linguistically different students: A handbook for educators.* Boston: Little, Brown and Co.

Langdon, H. W., & Cheng, L. L. (1992). *Hispanic children and adults with communication disorders: Assessment and intervention.* Gaithersburg, MD: Aspen Publishers.

Luterman, D. (1991). *Counseling the communicatively disordered and their families.* Austin: Pro-Ed.

McCardle, P., Kim, J., Grube, C., & Randall, V. (1995). An approach to bilingualism in early intervention. *Infants and Young Children, 7*(3), 63–73.

Perozzi, J. A., & Sanchez, M. L. C. (1992). The effect of instruction in L1 on receptive acquisition of L2 for bilingual children with language delay. *Language, Speech, and Hearing Services in Schools, 23*(4), 348–352.

Taylor, O. L. (1986). *Treatment of communication disorders in culturally and linguistically diverse populations.* Austin: Pro-Ed.

van Kleeck, A. (1994). Potential cultural bias in training parents as conversational partners with their children who have delays in language development. *American Journal of Speech-Language Pathology, 3*(1), 67–68.

# 9

# PHONOLOGICAL DISORDERS IN CULTURALLY DIVERSE POPULATIONS: INTERVENTION ISSUES AND STRATEGIES

## CORINE C. MYERS-JENNINGS

The ability to speak is one of our most precious gifts (Secord, 1989). Speech is the most frequently used vehicle for communication and the most efficient. Speech production is a vehicle for carrying language. Not all of us, however, use this gift in the same way. In the United States today, linguistic and cultural diversity is a major topic in our field. Many professionals who are presently serving individuals with communication disorders are now learning how to assess and treat phonological problems and how to address articulation problems. With the challenge of learning about child phonology, clinicians are faced with decisions of determining if what they have examined is a disorder or a difference. When examining phonology in various cultural groups, a further challenge is to determine if an observed pattern is a part of the individual's dialect or if it is a phonological deviation. The aim of this chapter is to focus on assessment and treatment issues as they apply to various cultural groups.

## CHILD PHONOLOGY

Much has changed over the years in child phonology. Our knowledge of the linguistic aspects of language has opened our understanding to the role of phonology as a component of language . All human beings have substantially the same speech apparatus, so the total repertoire of human sounds is effectively the same for the whole species, but the selection made from this total repertoire varies quite considerably from community to community (Grunwell, 1987). The study of the linguistic rules governing the sound system of the language, including speech sounds, speech sound production, and the combination of sounds in meaningful utterances is *phonology* (Creaghead & Newman, 1989). The study of the total range of speech sounds that can be made by human beings is the concern of *general phonetics* (Grunwell, 1987). *Articulation* refers to the actions of the organs of speech in producing the sounds of speech (Creaghead & Newman, 1989). Each language has specific sounds, or *phonemes,* that are characteristic of that language. Phonemes are combined in specific ways to form linguistic units known as words.

A phoneme is the smallest linguistic unit of speech that signals a difference in meaning (Bernstein & Tiegerman-Farber, 1997). The words *hat* and *bat* differ from each other in only one way—their initial sound. Because this initial sound difference produces two different words, the difference is a meaningful one. Therefore, /h/ and /b/ are, by definition, two different phonemes.

Phonemes are classified by their acoustic properties (the pattern of their sound waves), their articulatory properties (where in the oral cavity they are produced or place of articulation), and their production properties (manner of articulation) (Bernstein & Tiegerman-Farber, 1997). The use of phonemes is governed by two sets of rules. One set describes how sounds can be used in various word positions. These are called *distributional rules.* In English, for example, the *ng* sound as in the word *long* is a single phoneme that never appears at the beginning of a word. The second set of rules determines which sounds may be combined. They are called *sequencing rules.* In English, for example, the sound sequence *rs* may not appear in the same syllable (Bernstein & Tiegerman-Farber, 1997). Phonological rules govern sounds and their distribution and sequencing within a language. Children must learn the phonological rules of the language, and they must develop the motor skills to produce not only individual speech sounds but the movements necessary for their rapid combination. Most often children learn the phonological system used in their immediate environment and community. In order to understand disordered phonology and phonological differences, one must also have information regarding normal development.

## Vocal Development

Most studies of language acquisition and vocal development have involved Standard American English (SAE) speakers (Bloom & Lahey, 1978; Brown,

1973; Ingram, 1976). For most children, the acquisition of the sounds of their language takes place during the first four years. By age 4 children know a great deal about the phonological system of the language, with later development to occur primarily in the areas of morphophonology of complex word forms and metalinguistic knowledge (Ingram, 1976). Some children produce nearly all phonemes correctly in sentences by $2^{1}/_{2}$ to 3 years, whereas others continue to have a few phonetic errors at age 6. Most children can be understood by strangers by $3^{1}/_{2}$ years or earlier and exhibit adult-like articulation (Creaghead, 1989).

Just as for other behaviors, children's imperfect productions of spoken language are patterned and not random. A major portion of the acquisition of the phonological system of the language occurs during the first year. At birth, reflexive crying is the only type of sound that infants emit. The sounds of crying are primarily nasalized vowels. Within the first few months, however, children begin to gain control over the vocal mechanism. Sounds continue to be reflexive, but they become more varied (Creaghead, 1989).

From 4 to 6 months, alternations of resonances and constrictions will become consonant-vowel (CV) or vowel-consonant (VC) syllables. Vocalizations are more fully resonated, but they are not yet distinguishable as specific vowels. In the same way, specific consonants will not generally be identified. During this stage, almost total constrictions that resemble /k/ or /g/, /p/ or /b/ may be heard. These will become stops. Raspberries appear, precursors of fricative sounds (Oller, 1980).

At 6 to 10 months reduplicated babbling occurs. Babbling, unlike the sounds of crying, shrieking, cooing, yelling, and fussing, is defined by the production of well-formed or canonical syllables that have many of the acoustic characteristics of adult speech. Canonical syllables are defined in specific physical terms relating to duration, as well as to frequency, amplitude, and their changes over time (Oller, 1986). Variations in the specific phonemes are evident but the phonemes will be stops, nasal, glides, and fricatives.

From 10 to 14 months the productions are still primarily CV sequences, as in the previous stage, but now the reduplicative nature of the utterances is no longer present, and a variety of consonants and vowels can co-occur, for example [bawidu] (Oller, 1980). This type of utterance is referred to by Oller as variegated babbling. During this stage the consonantal repertoire increases substantially. A second characteristic of this stage is the presence of adult-like intonation patterns. Parents often believe their children are producing whole sentences—statements, questions, exclamations—but in their own language. It is during this time that variations in the phonetic inventory are very evident. Consonants resemble the productions of those in the child's environment. Myers-Jennings (1994) examined the vocal development of African American and Caucasian infants from 6 to 14 months who lived in rural areas in Florida and South Carolina. Fifteen infants were observed from the canonical babbling period through variegated babbling period. Infants were observed to produce basically the same CV combination during the canonical babbling period and started to resemble the CV combinations in their immediate environment when they stated to use different consonants in a single combination. Mothers were observed saying combinations such as "gubudu" and the infants matched and reproduced these combinations with the same intonational, inflectional, and pitch patterns. As the infants were observed during a free vocal play period without a model, they produced the CVCVCV combinations similar to those normally produced in their environment.

## Phonological Development in Normally Developing African American Children

Because General American English (GAE) and African American English (AAE) are dialects of the same language, several features, such as initial consonants (except /v/), are noncontrastive. The early phoneme development of speakers of AAE does not differ from that of speakers of GAE. At 36 months, the conversational speech of African American children contains the same minimal core of initial consonants expected of speakers of standard English (e.g., /n,m,b,p,d,t,g,k,f,s,h,w,j/) (Seymour & Ralabate, 1985; Seymour & Seymour, 1981; Steffersen, 1974). The features that contrast between AAE and GAE in the medial and final positions of words—final consonant deletion, final consonant cluster reduction, unstressed syllable deletion, and interdental fricative substitution (e.g.,/th/ and /v/)—normally develop after age 5 (Haynes & Moran, 1989; Moran, 1993; Seymour & Seymour, 1981; Stockman, 1991, 1995; Stockman & Settle, 1991; Vaughn-Cooke, 1986; Wolfram & Fasold, 1974).

## Phonological Development in Normally Developing Spanish-Speaking Children

Oller and Eilers (1982) examined babbling in normally developing Spanish-speaking infants. These infants produced CV syllables containing oral and nasal stops with front vowels. Normative data presented by Goldstein (1995) indicates similar information. Researchers have reported that the determination of the normalcy of the development of phonology in children learning Spanish is difficult because of the number of dialects within the Spanish language and the differences in criteria used to determine the normal developmental stages (Goldstein & Iglesias, 1996b). However, researchers (Anderson & Smith, 1987; Pandolfi & Herrera, 1990) agree that it is likely that, by the time normally developing Spanish-speaking children reach 3 years of age, they will use the dialectal features of the community and will have mastered the vowel system and most of the consonant system (Iglesias & Goldstein, 1998). By completion of preschool, normally developing children will exhibit some difficulty with consonant clusters and a few phones, specifically, [c], [th voiced], [s], [t°], [flap], [r], [h], [j], and [l] (Acevedo, 1991; Eblen, 1982; Jimenez, 1987; Linares, 1982). These children, to some degree, will still occasionally exhibit specific phonological processes—cluster reduction, unstressed syllable deletion, stridency deletion, and tap/trill /r/ deviation—but will likely have suppressed velar and palatal fronting, prevocalic singleton omission, stopping, and assimilation (Goldstein & Iglesias, 1996a; Stepanof, 1990).

   Iglesias and Goldstein (1998, p. 158) cited research showing that children's acquisition and development of vowels have received more attention recently (e.g., Clement & Wijnen, 1994; Pollock & Keiser, 1990), although few studies have examined the production of vowels in Spanish-speaking children. Oller and Eilers (1982) found that the mean proportion occurrence of vowel-like productions in 12- to 14-month-old English and Spanish-speaking children was remarkably similar. They noted that, in general, the children were likely to produce more anterior-like than posterior-like vowels. Maez (1981) indicated that by 18 months the three subjects in the study had mastered (i.e., produced correctly at least 90 percent of the time) the five basic Spanish vowels, [Á], [e],[µ], [o], and [a]. Maez's study, however, focused on consonant development and did not indicate if vowel errors occurred.

## Phonological Development in Speakers of Asian Languages

Few studies have investigated phonological development in children who speak Asian languages. Limited information is available, but researchers have examined phonological development in specific language/dialect groups. So and Dodd (1994) investigated phonological development in Cantonese-speaking children with phonological disorders and also provided data on development in normally developing Cantonese-speaking children (Iglesias & Goldstein, 1998, p. 161). In the normally developing Cantonese-speaking children So and Dodd noted phoneme acquisition similar to English but at a more rapid rate. In general, anterior consonants were acquired before posterior consonants, and oral and nasal stops and glides were acquired before fricatives and affricates. They also noted the exhibition of phonological processes and found that by age 4;0 no process was exhibited more than 15% of the time. Between the ages of 2;0 and 4;0, these children showed processes similar in quantity (greater than 15 percent) and kind to English-speaking children: assimilation, cluster reduction, stopping, fronting affrication, and final consonant deletion.

## PHONOLOGICAL DISORDER OR A VARIATION (DIALECT)?

A phonological disorder can be defined as a significant deficit in speech production or perception or in the organization of phonology in comparison to a child's peers (Howell & Dean, 1991). Children who are learning to talk have to master two main tasks. They have to learn how to articulate a number of different speech sounds (phonetic) and they also have to learn how to contrast and combine these sounds to produce meaningful pronunciation patterns (phonemic). In other words, they have to know how to integrate features of voice, place, and manner to physically produce phonetic segments, and they have to acquire the rules of adult language that determine how these segments are organized to form words (Howell & Dean, 1991).

A dialect is a variation or a mutually intelligible form of a language associated with a particular region, social class, or ethnicity. Several varieties of American English are spoken in the United States, some of which depend on context and interlocutors (register). Registral varieties are dependent on participants, settings, and topics (Iglesias & Anderson, 1993, p.147 ). We may use one register when talking to our friends and another when speaking to an individual when we are trying to give directions to a particular location. To determine if a phonological disorder exists, Fey (1992, p. 228) suggested that the following basic questions may be answered:

1. *What sounds does the child produce and are they used correctly or not?* This question of the child's phonetic repertoire really involves the child's articulatory skills and may require not only careful analysis of spontaneous speech samples, but also traditional articulation testing and subsequent stimulability testing.
2. *What syllable shapes does the child produce?* An analysis of the syllabic and lexical shapes found in the child's speech may indicate that the child is using a particular acquisition strategy such as focusing on sound contrasts at the end of the word while erring on sound at the beginning. It will also help identify any strong phonotactic constraints that seem to be limiting the child's production. Phonotactic constraints are restrictions that a child may develop on where certain sounds can occur in a syllable or word and on the sequences

of sounds. This affects the position of occurrence of sounds as well as on combinations and possible orders.

3. *What phonological contrasts are present in the child's spontaneous speech output?* For this assessment of the child's phonemic repertoire, emphasis is on contrast, not on correctness.

4. *When the child has failed to preserve contrasts in his or her speech output, what factors seem to be involved?* The information gleaned from answering the questions above may give some indication as to the level at which the child's problems are occurring, that is, perceptual, organizational, or articulatory.

5. *What phonological rules are active in the child's system?*

Information on the characteristics of particular languages and dialects, together with data on normal phonological development, can be extremely useful in conducting less biased phonological assessments and in differentiating children with dialectal differences from those with phonological disorders (Iglesias & Goldstein, 1998). Sensitivity and knowledge of the linguistic influences on a child's speech, as well as the social characteristics of the child's community, are required for clinicians who serve children with phonological disorders from culturally diverse backgrounds (Iglesias & Goldstein, 1998). Wolfram (in press) explains many variables across languages. Phonological variation is a very natural development in language, as all living languages undergo continual change. One source of variation comes from within the language itself as languages naturally adjust and readjust their phonological systems over time. Today's General American English is much different from that spoken centuries ago, as some sounds have been lost and others changed. For example, the current spelling *gh* in *thought* once represented a sound (pronounced something like the German ch [X]) that has since been lost.

Other sound differences come from outside the language, as English has adopted sounds from other languages with which it has come into contact. The introduction of the phoneme /Z/ into English (e.g., azure, leisure) is attributable to the influence of French borrowings into English (Wolfram, in press).

Other differences in current English varieties reflect the peculiar language contact history of a group of speakers (Wolfram, in press). For example, the pronunciation of standard English /sh/ as /ch/ in some Hispanic-English dialects is a reflection of Spanish language background, where the /ch/ is not contrasted with /sh/ (typically only /ch/ is found). Similarly, a Vietnamese English speaker may pronounce this /ch/ as /s/ (e.g., wish as wis), reflecting influence from the Vietnamese language, which does not differentiate either /sh/ or /ch/ from /s/. Again, these changes from outside are really no different from those that have affected English historically, but the particular language of influence (e.g.,

Spanish or Vietnamese) and the acceptance of such variation into the mainstream system set these changes apart from the historical influence on English phonology. In some cases, variation from outside is transitional, occurring simply as a function of learning English as a second language. In other cases, changes from outside may be incorporated into a more stable, community variety of English that is passed on to successive generations of speakers who learn English as a first language. It is important to separate native speaker phonological variation from second language variation, although both types of situations characterize the language communities (Wolfram, in press).

## CHARACTERISTICS OF AFRICAN AMERICAN VERNACULAR ENGLISH (AAVE)

AAVE is spoken by some, but not all, African Americans. AAVE is generally considered a dialect of American English. Like all American English dialects, AAVE is systematic, complete with rule-governed phonological, semantic, syntactic, pragmatic, and proxemic systems. Some of the major phonological features that distinguish AAVE and GAE as reported by Iglesias and Anderson (1993, p. 149) are as follows:

1. Word-final consonant cluster reduction, particularly when one of the two consonants is an alveolar (e.g., *test* /test/—-> /tes/).
2. Stopping of word-initial interdentals (e.g., *they* /(voiced th)e/ ——> [de], *thought* /θat/—-> [tat] ).
3. Substitution of f/θ and v/th (voiced) in intervocalic position (e.g., *nothing* /n θIh/—> [n fIh], *bathing* /be ih/—->[bevih]).
4. Substitution of f/θ in word-final position (e.g., *south* /saμθ/→ saμf]).
5. Deletion of /r/ (e.g., *sister* /sIster/—->[sist \], *Carol* /kærəl/-→[kæəl]).
6. Deletion of /l/ in word-final abutting consonants (e.g., *help* /help/ —>[hep]).
7. Substitution of [I] for /e/ before nasals (e.g., *pin* /pIn/ and *pen* /pen/ pronounced as [pIn]).
8. Deletion of nasal consonant in word-final position with nasalization of preceding vowel (e.g., *moon* /mun/—-> [mu]).

## CHARACTERISTICS OF SPANISH PHONOLOGY

A brief overview of the Spanish consonant and vowel system is presented here (for a more complete analysis, see Goldstein, 1995). Spanish phonology has 18 consonants and 5 primary vowels (compared to 24 consonants,

*Spanish phonetic repetoire*

3 semivowels, and 12 to 14 vowels in English). The 5 primary vowels are two front vowels /i/ and /e/ and the three back vowels /u/, /o/, and /a/. The 18 phonemes are the unaspirated stops, /p/,/t/, and /k/; the voiced stops, /b/,/d/, and /g/; the voiceless fricatives, /f/,/c/, and /s/; the affricate, /t°/; the glides, /w/ and /j/; the lateral, /l/; the flap /rr/ and trill /r/; nasals /m/,/n/ (nasalized), and /h/.

Children who speak Spanish have some difficulty learning English as a second language and may produce some English sounds differently from monolingual English speakers because of the similarities and contrasts of the two languages (Battle, 1997, p. 391). For example, since there is no /th/ or /v/ in Spanish, these sounds are difficult for many children learning to speak English. Also, although many consonant sounds are similar, the consonants are not all produced in the same way. The /t/, for example, is aspirated in English, but it is unaspirated in Spanish. Moreover, in Spanish, /t/ is dental, while in English it is alveolar. While these differences are subtle, they add to the perception of language difference when Spanish speakers produce English words and may be mistakenly classified as a disorders (Battle, 1997).

## CHARACTERISTICS OF ASIAN PHONOLOGY

*Tones*

Many, but not all, Asian languages are tone languages; for example, Cantonese is a tone language but Japanese is not (Iglesias & Goldstein, 1998). In tone languages, differences in word meanings are signified by differences in pitch. Tone languages are generally composed of register tones (typically two or three in a language) and contour tones (also usually two or three per language) (O'Grady, Dobrovolsky, & Aranoff, 1993). Register tones are level tones, usually signaled by high, mid, and low tones; contour tones are a combination of register tones over a single syllable. An example of Mandarin Chinese is H——>[ma] *mother* high tone; LH——>[ma] *hemp* low rise; MLH——> [ma] *horse* fall rise (O'Grady et al., 1993).

There are few syllable-final segments and few consonant clusters in Asian languages (Iglesias & Goldstein, 1998). For example, (1) the only syllable final consonants in Mandarin Chinese are /n/ and /h/; (2) there are no labiodental, interdental, or palatal fricatives in Korean; and (3) Hawaiian contains only 5 vowels and 8 consonants (Iglesias & Goldstein, 1998). Given the differences between Asian language and English, Cheng (1987) notes possible phonetic "interference" by speakers of Asian language learning English. Syllable structure varies greatly in the Asian language. Laotian contains three syllable types (CVC, CVVC, and CVV), Khmer exhibits eight (CVC, CCVC, CCCVC, CVVC, CCVVC, CC-CVVC, CVV, CCVV) yet contains few polysyllabic words (Cheng, 1987).

Vietnamese has a limited number of final consonants (voiceless stops and nasals); the only final consonant in Hmong is /h/; Korean contains no fricatives or affricates in words-final position. For more information on Asian phonology, it is suggested that the reader consult Cheng (1987, 1993) and Wang (1989).

## CHARACTERISTICS OF NATIVE AMERICAN PHONOLOGY

Native American languages include sounds in their segmental inventories that do not appear in English (Ladefoged, 1993). Many contain ejectives, sounds made with a glottalic egressive airstream. These phonemes include /p',t',k',ts,/; for example, [p'o] (*foggy*) (Iglesias & Goldstein, 1998). They may also show voiceless stops in combination with the velar fricative, /p,t,k/); for example [p a] (*bitter* in Lakhota). Implosives—stops made with an ingressive glottalic airstream—may be part of the segmental inventories of these languages. Ejective and nonejective stops and ejective affricates may be produced with a lateral release, /tl'/, /tl/, and /ts'/, respectively (Iglesias & Goldstein, 1998). Examples from Navajo include [tl'`e`e?] (*night*), [tl`ah] (*oil*), and [ts'`aal] (*cradle*). These languages may contain nasalized vowels (Welker, 1995).

## ASSESSMENT

The assessment of phonological patterns in children from culturally and linguistically diverse populations requires determination of whether children's phonological systems are within the norm of acceptable speech for their linguistic communities. The assessment must be approached with an understanding of the social, cultural, and linguistic characteristics of the community from which a given child comes. The concept of "speech community" means that speech patterns of a given group of people will vary by age, length of time in the United States, frequency with which English is spoken in the home, sound systems of the first language, frequency of contact with the homeland, the geographical region in which people live, and their social status within the community (Proctor, 1994). It is vital that such information be obtained to guard against cultural stereotyping (Taylor, Payne, & Anderson, 1987). For example, it is inappropriate to assume that all African Americans speak AAVE. Members of the same race need not share the same speech community or culture. While one African American's production of /f/θ/ in the word *bath* may be regarded as a dialectal feature of AAVE, it would be inappropriate to make the same clinical judgment for another African American who also produced /f/θ/ without further investigation. The first speaker may be an AAVE speaker, the second speaker may not, and therefore his or her production would be considered a phonological error.

A very common situation occurs regularly in clinics, schools, and training institutions when clinicians make decisions about clinical needs based solely on race. Consider the following true story as an example. An African American family brought their 4-year-old son for an evaluation. The parents were well educated individuals. Effective communication skills were important to them. They did not speak AAVE in formal or casual situations. The clinician interviewed the family so this allowed her to hear the speaking patterns of the parents, which should have given her a small view of some of the speech patterns used in the child's immediate environment. The clinician gave a standardized test, and the child scored within the 4th percentile. The clinician made a decision that because this was an African American child she would subtract all error sounds that are dialectal features of AAVE from the total number of errors. The child's percentile rank changed and instead of a severe phonological problem, he just seemed to have some minor errors. The clinician did not consider the child's speech environment nor the child's patterns presented in his misarticulations. She based her decision on a standard score that was based on inaccurate assumptions. With the multicultural society that we live in today, we can no longer continue with practices like the ones reported in the example above. We must do thorough examinations of all aspects of an individual's speaking pattern and have knowledge of the speaking patterns of individuals in the various communities that we serve.

*[handwritten margin note: Case Study]*

*[handwritten note in text: Things to keep in mind:]*

Iglesias and Anderson (1993, p. 157) cite several issues that must be considered when assessing an individual whose language or dialect differs from that of the examiner. First, examiners must be aware of their own dialects and their effects on the assessment process. Seymour and Seymour (1981) noted that the client's perception of the formality of the situation affects linguistic phonological usage. Casual speaking settings may encourage the use of a particular dialect, while formal settings may inhibit and stigmatize speech forms other than Standard English.

*[handwritten margin note: Setting can effect phonological use]*

*[handwritten circled: 1]*

Second, examiners must be aware of the limitations of existing assessment tools. Few test makers have specifically addressed the issue of linguistic diversity in the construction of phonological assessment instruments or procedures. It is imperative for speech-language pathologists to review items to determine which have the potential for eliciting nonstandard responses. With prior identification of such items, and with knowledge of the phonological features of both standard and

*[handwritten circled: 2]*

nonstandard dialects, the clinician will be able to conduct culturally appropriate phonological assessments.

Iglesias and Anderson (1993, p. 158) also suggested an informal approach for determining acceptable responses. According to Iglesias and Anderson, the examiner should ask a member of the client's speech community, preferably an adult family member, to say the word. The clinician should then compare the adult's production with the client's production. However, as Eblen (1982) noted, children may use a casual speech form they have heard, while the adult in the interview setting would more likely use a formal variant. Another approach suggested by Hodson (1986) is to obtain normative data for clients in their respective communities by administering a test to normal peers in order to identify those dialectal patterns that may be unique for that particular speech community.

Many phonological examinations are performed to determine eligibility of children for services. In those situations standardized tests may be required. Regardless of the circumstances for the examination, procedures for assessment should include a spontaneous sample of the individual's utterances. Phonological assessment is often done in the context of a communication evaluation that also includes assessment of voice quality, fluency of speech, and aspects of language including syntax, semantics, pragmatics, and discourse. In addition, such related measures as hearing testing and oral cavity examination are usually included in a comprehensive communication evaluation. Auditory perception and speech sound discrimination are essential for the development of speech and should be examined during a phonological examination.

The spontaneous sample should be transcribed using narrow phonetic transcription that is sensitive to sound variations within a phoneme class by the usage of diacritics. Moran (1993) conducted a study on final consonant deletion in African American children. He noted that in the initial transcription of ten African American children, three transcribers scored the speech sample for final consonant deletion with 86 percent agreement. The three listeners were trained to do narrow phonetic transcription using diacritics to denote allophonic variation in consonants. After training, the agreement index fell to 61 percent. This reduced agreement is not surprising because, following training, there were more options available to the listeners when the presence of a final consonant was not entirely clear. A more precise description of the production of the phonemes was recorded.

Once the utterances or words have been transcribed, the productions can be analyzed. If a standardized test is used, the clinician should follow the procedures for scoring the test as recommended. Most tests will not account for dialectal features and typically score these features as errors. Researchers agree that accounting for dialectal features is a prime consideration in the assessment of children from culturally and linguistically diverse populations (Iglesias & Goldstein, 1998). Analysis of phonological information must take the child's dialect into account. Not accounting for dialectal features may result in misdiagnosis of the phonological disorder or escalate the child's severity rating.

A few studies have specifically examined the effect of dialect on the diagnosis of phonological disorders in children. Cole and Taylor (1990) found that not taking dialectal variations into account resulted in the misdiagnosis of phonological disorder for 5 of 10 children speaking African American English. Another study, using normally developing Spanish-speaking preschoolers as subjects, found that not taking dialect features into account resulted in 25 of 54 (46%) subjects incorrectly being labeled as phonologically disordered (Goldstein & Iglesias, in preparation). The results of this study indicated that certain phonological processes (e.g., final consonant deletion, weak syllable deletion, and liquid simplification) might be targeted unnecessarily for intervention if dialectal features were not taken into account. Washington and Craig (1992) noted that in the group of children with "impaired speech," taking dialect features into account resulted in a shift in diagnostic category for 3 of 8 children (from severe to moderate) on the Arizona Articulation Proficiency Scale–Revised and for 2 of 8 children (from mild to normal) on the Arizona Articulation Proficiency Scale–Second Edition. These studies indicated that children may be mislabeled as having a phonological disorder when, in fact, they do not and/or receive intervention for targets that are dialect features rather than disordered forms. Subsequently, the children might be enrolled inappropriately for intervention. Thus, the authors of these studies advocated that speech-language pathologists account for dialect features in all phonological analyses.

The clinician should do an independent and relational analysis from conversational speech or from single word tasks. An *independent analysis* describes the child's production without reference to the adult model. The independent analysis includes: (1) an inventory of phonemes classified by word position and articulatory features (e.g., stops fricative, affricative, nasal, glides); (2) an inventory of syllable and word shapes produced (e.g., V, CVC, CV, CVCV); (3) sequential constraints on the occurrence of phonemes (Stoel-Gammon & Dunn, 1985). A *relational analysis* compares the child's pronunciation to the adult forms or pronunciations. Patterns or systematic differences are then described in terms of sound segments, features, rules, phonological processes, or combination of these (Stoel-Gammon & Dunn, 1985). In the case of the relational analysis, the adult pronunciations or forms refer to General American English pronunciations. An independent and relational analysis allows the clinician to obtain the necessary data to determine

Independent vs. Relational Analysis

if a significant deficiency in speech production or in the organization of phonology has occurred. Any patterns or dialectal features can readily be identified from the results of the analysis.

ASHA's position paper on social dialects (American Speech-Language-Hearing Association, 1983) officially acknowledges the distinction between a speech-language difference and a speech-language disorder. The differentiation between linguistic difference and phonological disorder requires at least one more step in addition to traditional procedures (Proctor, 1994). Instead of completing a single contrastive analysis where the child's speech is compared to the standard dialect (GAE), the SLP will complete a second contrastive analysis to determine if productions are consistent with expectations set for the first dialect or language. To achieve the latter, the SLP will elicit and record the speaker's sample via audio or video tape. The contrastive analysis should be completed to (1) describe the vowels and consonants and/or processes produced by the speaker, (2) determine if the phonemes and/or the processes are consistent with GAE, and, if not, (3) determine if the phonemes and/or processes are consistent with another dialect or language. If the phonemes and/or processes are consistent with what is expected in the first dialect or first language, but different from GAE, there is a phonological difference present. Once these procedures are followed, an appropriate differentiation between a difference and a disorder can be accomplished.

The assessment of speakers of languages other than English presents a challenge to the speech-language pathologist. As with complete phonological assessments for monolingual speakers, a detailed phonological assessment for bilingual speakers typically would include both formal measures (i.e., usually standardized assessments, of which there are few available in languages other than English) and informal measures (e.g., connected speech sample). The speech-language pathologist would use formal and informal measures to perform both independent and relational analyses, examining both consonants and vowels and phonological patterns/phonological processes (Bernthal & Bankson, 1998; Stoel-Gammon & Dunn, 1985). These analyses would ensure an adequate representation of phonological information (Bernthal & Bankson, 1998; Stoel-Gammon & Dunn, 1985). Opportunities to produce all consonants in syllable-initial and syllable-final position (if appropriate), all singleton consonants, all clusters (syllable-initial and syllable-final), and vowels (see Proctor, 1994 for more details regarding the assessment of vowels) should be included (Yavas & Goldstein, 1998). Ideally, the assessment tools used should be designed specifically to assess phonological patterns in the child's native language. However, not only are such tools often unavailable, but the normative data necessary is often also unavailable (Iglesias & Goldstein, 1998). In such cases, it is recommended that speech-language pathologists familiarize themselves with the phonological rules of the language and develop, in cooperation with native speakers of the language, informal assessments that provide the examiner with a measure of the child's ability to produce the phonemes of the child's native language. In cases where non-English tests are available, primarily Spanish, dialectal features of the speaker must be taken into consideration. Assuming a given individual speaks both English and a language other than English, the clinician should assess, whenever possible, both languages being conscious of possible interference errors and dialectal variations (Iglesias & Goldstein, 1998).

## TREATMENT

Once the results of an assessment are obtained, clinicians must decide from the assessment data and observations whether a disorder or difference exists. If a disorder exists, the unique characteristics of the child's system should be characterized in order to design the most appropriate treatment plan for the child. A phonological disorder is diagnosed after the speech-language pathologist (SLP) has accounted for the presence/absence of nondialect structural and neurological problems (e.g., dysarthria or apraxia) and has considered dialectal variations and/or the influence of another language (Proctor, 1994). A disorder is present when the client (Proctor, 1994, p. 216)

Diagnosing a disorder:

1. Is unintelligible or displays reduced intelligibility to the native speakers of the same speech community.
2. Misarticulates phonemes that are pronounced the same in both GAE and the first dialect or first language.
3. Produces idiosyncratic patterns that are not representative of the processes normally found in the first dialect/language, GAE, or as a function of borrowing or code switching.

The information from the assessment provides the basis for developing intervention goals and objectives. Assessment data also guides the clinician in selecting appropriate stimulus materials for use with the client. Finally, assessment provides a baseline from which to measure progress during the intervention program.

Successful intervention is a process that considers the communicative situations of a speaker. Normal phonological use involves both the production of sounds at a motor level and their use in accordance with the rules of the language. Two skills are intertwined and often it is difficult for clinicians to determine whether a client's errors reflect a lack of motor skills, a lack of linguistic knowledge, or deficiencies in both. It may be that in a given client, some errors relate to one factor, some to another, and some to both. Two broad categories are considered for phonological remediation: the motor approaches to phonological treatment and the cognitive-linguistic approaches to phonological treatment.

The *motor approaches to phonological treatment* focus primarily on the motor skills involved in producing target sounds and frequently include perceptual tasks as part of the treatment procedures (Bernthal & Bankson, 1993). Most of the motor approaches represent variations of the "traditional approach" to remediation. Remediation based on a motor perspective views phonological errors as motor based, with treatment focused on the placement and movement of the articulators so that segmental productions no longer violate adult standard pronunciations (Bernthal & Bankson, 1993). The usual remediation approach involves the selection of a to-be-corrected target speech sound or sounds, with instruction proceeding through a sequence of increasingly complex linguistic units (e.g., isolation, syllables, words, phrases, sentences) until target sounds are used appropriately in spontaneous conversation. Thus, speech production is viewed as a learned motor skill, with remediation requiring repetitive practice at increasingly complex motor levels until the targeted articulatory gesture becomes automatic (Bernthal & Bankson, 1993).

The *cognitive-linguistic approaches to phonological treatment* involve the establishment of phonological rules in a client's repertoire (Bernthal & Bankson, 1993). Instruction is oriented toward relationships among sounds (contrasts and other rules), as opposed to the individual sound focus of motor-oriented approaches to remediation. Treatment programs are designed to facilitate acquisition of linguistic rules and are not associated with single units of speech. There are two primary characteristics that are frequently associated with cognitive-linguistic-oriented treatment approaches. The first characteristic relates to the targeting of behaviors for treatment, and the second relates to instructional procedures. The treatment involves selecting for instruction certain target behaviors (sounds), called *exemplars,* that are likely to facilitate generalization to an entire class of sounds or sound-positions (e.g., other sounds containing a certain feature; other sounds in the same word-position). Exemplars can be selected that are designed to facilitate the acquisition of appropriate sound contrasts and/or sequences. Most treatment protocols that are based on a cognitive-linguistic model employ minimal contrast word-pairs, which in turn often involve minimal or maximal feature contrasts (Gierut, 1989; Weiner, 1981).

ASHA's (1983) position paper on social dialects provides guidelines to be followed if the client is a speaker of a dialect other than GAE. As reflected in this paper, the traditional role of a speech-language pathologist is to provide clinical services for communication disorders but not to treat dialectal differences. The position paper, however, identifies the following expanded role for the speech-language pathologist:

> Aside from the traditionally recognized role, the speech-language pathologist may also be available to provide **elective** clinical services to nonstandard English speakers who do not present a disorder. The role of the speech-language pathologist for these individuals is to prepare the desired competency in Standard English without jeopardizing the integrity of the individual's first dialect. The approach must be functional and based on context-specific appropriateness of the given dialect. (ASHA, 1983, p. 24)

For individuals with phonological differences, options can be offered. To offer the options, the SLP must develop awareness among speakers of the variation, discuss options with parents/guardians, obtain family permission to develop a culturally sensitive program, and request active participation on the part of the family. The availability of computers and home videotape equipment makes family participation more feasible. After the initial family conference, active family participation may occur via disk switching or exchanges of videotape. Children enjoy seeing themselves on television by route of videotape.

There is a scarcity of guidelines for the clinical management of children with phonological problems in which English is not the first language or for whom the dialect spoken is very different from the standard dialect. There are, however, intervention questions that should be addressed. Iglesias and Anderson (1993, p. 159) suggested the following question: Is the treatment objective for the client to use the appropriate speech sounds of his or her speech community? If so, then remediation should preferably be in the language(s) spoken in the child's environment. Such a decision requires the clinician to have a degree of competency in the client's first language or dialect. In spite of this, the decision is often made to provide remediation in English, a language that may not be spoken in the child's speech community. It is not uncommon for clinicians in this situation to suggest to parents that they speak English to their children, but they may later express concern that the English dialect spoken by the parents is not a "good model." While solutions to this problem are difficult to arrive at, it is clearly helpful if the clinician is bilingual.

To develop remediation goals when phonological differences are involved, Proctor (1994, p. 226) recommended the following:

1. Depending on degree, consistency, and frequency of occurrence of production of the dialectal difference, you may plan individual, small group, or classroom "Communication Time." Emphasize the fact that people speak differently in different countries; discuss positive values of being able to speak in more than one way. Focus on the fact that people speak differently in different situations and role play the possibilities. Have students develop scripts for different types of social situations. Have students develop narratives of different ways of talking. Talk about how we listen and what are conversational roles in different cultures; role play some of these situations. All of this serves to establish the importance of individual differences and that we can adjust how we speak at different times and in different places. Build in the fact that listening is important—we should listen to ourselves (self-monitor) and listen to others.

2. If you serve as a consultant to a classroom teacher, you can also develop bulletin boards. Have children bring information from home, for example, photos of grandparents who are from (name country) and speak (name language). Discuss the importance of being able to communicate in more than one way in more than one language.

3. Drill work may be incorporated into a particular child's program or into small groups with the same dialect (Berger, 1990; Kupfer & Kissel, 1990). Motoric drills may pose several difficulties unless the SLP is a speaker of the clients' native/home languages and is able to code switch between GAE and the variation. Perceptual training necessitates the ability to produce an auditory model and the clinician must know the segments that comprise a given client's native language and repertoire, the order of acquisition and ease of production of sounds, the frequency of occurrence of each phone in the language, and phonetic contexts that may facilitate production of the target sound (Bernthal & Bankson, 1993).

Children from the nondominant cultures are likely to produce either variations of American English or language that is influenced by family members who are non-native English. These children may be referred to as bicultural, bidialectal, or bilingual, suggesting the coexistence of two dialects or at least two languages that the same child understands and speaks.

The DeKalb Bidialectal Communication Program (DBCP) (Harris-Wright, 1987) has been used to make regular education students aware of the need for "functional flexibility" in verbal communication; to impart knowledge of the educational, social, and economic ramifications associated with the stigma of nonmainstream English; and to provide opportunities for students to develop and practice mainstream English skills. The instructional model is summarized as:

1. Preinstructional oral communication skills are videotaped for each student during reading and conversation with teacher.
2. Student communication skills are evaluated in relation to standard English skills by the teacher. These skills are profiled by degree of organization/content of expressive language, enunciation, grammar usage, vocal tone/intonation usage, and nonverbal communication.
3. Students view videotapes of various styles of communication that have been scripted and role played through monologues and dialogues. From this activity and detailed discussions about the role plays, students develop an awareness of ineffective and effective communication skills for various situations. The concept of "home communication" (dialectal skills) and "school communication" (General American English skills) are introduced in phase three. Students then view their preinstructional oral communication videotapes and the teacher to set goals for their communication skills on their Communication Checklist. This phase is called Awareness Training.
4. Activities from the specifically developed curriculum help students practice appropriately "choosing" and "using" dialectal or General American English communication skills in functional situations. The curriculum has five major teaching modules: (a) organization/content of expressive language, (b) enunciation, (c) General American English grammar usage, (d) vocal tone/intonation usage, and (e) nonverbal communication .
5. Student communication skills are again evaluated by the teacher according to the criteria defined in number two and students will view their pre- to post-communication videotapes to be made aware of their additional General American English oral communication skills. (Adler, 1993, p. 173)

We must keep in mind that each student enters school with a well-developed language system that should be respected and utilized, where appropriate, by the classroom teacher in planning and implementing General American English instruction. Effective communication is a basic skill to be mastered by all students. Speech-language pathologists should be knowledgeable about the dialect or differences of their clients. Clinicians must be aware that not all speakers of a particular dialect will show or use every characteristic of it. It is common knowledge that the future will bring an increasing number of immigrants to the United States. Many of these immigrants will exhibit non- or limited English proficiency. The clinician must be prepared to assess and treat all individuals who have a disorder and make recommendations to clients who exhibit differences. Regardless of whether services are provided in the individual speakers' first or second language or dialect, clinicians must know the phonological rules of the first language and its dialectal variations.

## STUDY QUESTIONS AND ACTIVITIES

1. What are some of the research findings regarding phonological development in normally developing African American children?
2. What are some of the research findings regarding phonological development in speakers of Asian languages?
3. Discuss issues related to determining whether a client is exhibiting a phonological disorder, a culturally related speech sound difference, or both.
4. List characteristics of each of the following
   • African American Vernacular English
   • Spanish phonology
   • Asian phonology
   • Native American phonology
5. Discuss information provided by Iglesias and Anderson (1993) and Proctor (1994) that may be used as guidelines for the clinical management of children with phonological problems in which English is not the first language or for whom the dialect spoken is very different from the standard dialect.
6. Read the following case example and answer the questions at the end.

   Kelly Mayes is from northern Massachusetts. She earned her master's degree in communication disorders from a well-respected university in the South and has decided to live in Savannah, Georgia. Kelly started her Clinical Fellowship Year last August in a small rural school in South Carolina.

   The people who live in the town are mainly working class families who have lived there for generations. They do not travel much outside of the state and have few interactions with people outside of their community. The citizens are generally honest, hardworking people who take pride in their little town and believe in being good to their neighbors.

   Kelly and her supervising therapist have an excellent relationship and Kelly is doing a good job with most of the students on her caseload. She has had some difficulty identifying children who have speech-sound disorders. Kelly failed nearly all of the children during routine speech screening. During follow-up diagnostic sessions Kelly continued to find a lot of children she thought needed to be in speech therapy for speech-sound disorders. When Kelly's supervisor made her next visit to the school, she questioned the large number of articulation/phonology failures. Kelly explained that she really did not know what to do with all of the children because "they talk so funny." According to Kelly, the sound errors were not errors in the traditional sense but that the children certainly were not producing the sounds the way they should be pronounced. She did not feel that she could allow them to "pass" the assessments "talking that way."

- If you were Kelly's supervisor, how would you handle this situation?
- What specific advise would you give to Kelly?
- What resources might you provide for Kelly to guide her in making future decisions about these children?

## REFERENCES

Acevedo, M. (1991, November) *Spanish consonants among two groups of Head Start children.* Paper presented at the convention of the American Speech-Language Hearing Association. Atlanta, Georgia.

Adler, S. (1993). *Multicultural communication skills in the classroom.* Boston: Allyn & Bacon.

American Speech-Language-Hearing Association. (1983). Social dialect position paper. *Asha, 25,* 23–25.

Anderson, R., & Smith, B. (1987). Phonological development of two-year-old monolingual Puerto Rican Spanish-speaking children. *Journal of Child Language, 14,* 57–78.

Battle, D. (1997). Language and communication disorders in culturally and linguistically diverse children. In D. Bernstein & E. Tiegerman-Farber (Eds.), *Language and communication disorders in children* (4th ed.; pp. 382–409), Boston: Allyn & Bacon.

Berger, M. I., (1990). *Speak standard, too.* Chicago, IL: Orchard Brooks.

Bernthal, J., & Bankson, N. (1993). *Articulation and phonological disorders* (3rd ed.). Englewood Cliffs, NJ: Prentice Hall.

Bernthal, J., & Bankson, N. (1998) *Articulation and phonological disorders* (4th ed.). Boston: Allyn & Bacon.

Bernstein, D., & Tiegerman-Farber, E. (1997). *Language and communication disorders in children.* Boston: Allyn & Bacon.

Bloom, M., & Lahey, M. (1978). *Language development and disorders.* New York: Wiley.

Brown, R. (1973). *A first language, the early stages.* Cambridge, MA: Harvard University Press.

Cheng, L. R. L., (1987). *Assessing Asian language performance: Guidelines for evaluating limited-English-proficient students.* Rockville, MD: Aspen Publishers.

Cheng, L. R. L. (1993). Asian-American cultures. In D. Battle (Ed.), *Communication disorders in multicultural populations* (pp. 38–77). Boston: Andover Medical Publishers.

Clement, C., & Wijnen, F. (1994). Acquisition of vowel contrasts in Dutch. *Journal of Speech and Hearing Research, 37,* 83–89.

Cole, P., & Taylor, O. (1990). Performance of working class African-American children on three tests of articulation. *Language, Speech, and Hearing Services in Schools, 21,* 171–176.

Creaghead, N. (1989). Development of phonology, articulation, and speech perception. In N. Creaghead, P. Newman, & W. Secord (Eds.), *Assessment and remediation of articulatory and phonological disorders* (pp. 35–63). Columbus, OH: Merrill.

Creaghead, N., & Newman, P. (1989). Articulatory phonetics and phonology. In N. Creaghead, P. Newman, & W. Secord (Eds.), *Assessment and remediation of articulatory and phonological disorders* (pp. 9–33). Columbus, OH: Merrill.

Eblen, R. (1982). A study of the acquisition of fricatives by three-year-old children learning Mexican Spanish. *Language and Speech, 25,* 201–220.

Fey, M. (1992). Phonological assessment and treatment articulation and phonology: Inextricable constructs in speech pathology. *Language, Speech, and Hearing Services in Schools, 23,* 225–232.

Gierut, J. (1989). Maximal opposition approach to phonological treatment. *Journal of Speech and Hearing Disorders, 54,* 9–19.

Goldstein, B. (1995). Spanish phonological development. In H. Kayser (Ed.), *Bilingual speech-language pathology: An Hispanic focus* (pp. 17–38). San Diego: Singular Publishing Group.

Goldstein, B., & Iglesias, A. (1996a) Phonological patterns in normally developing Spanish-speaking 3- and 4-year olds of Puerto Rican descent. *Language, Speech, and Hearing Services in Schools, 27*(1), 92–90.

Goldstein, B., & Iglesias, A. (1996b). Phonological patterns in Puerto Rican Spanish-speaking children with phonological disorders. *Journal of Communication Disorders, 29,* 367–387.

Goldstein, B., & Iglesias, A. (in preparation). *The effect of dialect on the analysis of phonological patterns in Spanish-speaking children.* Manuscript in preparation.

Grunwell, P. (1987). *Clinical phonology.* Baltimore: Williams & Wilkins.

Harris-Wright, K. (1987). The challenge of educational coalescence: Teaching nonmainstream English-speaking students. *Journal of Childhood Communication Disorders,* Fall–Winter, 209–215.

Haynes, W. O., & Moran, M. (1989). A cross-sectional developmental study of final consonant production in Southern Black Children from preschool to third grade. *Language, Speech, and Hearing Services in Schools, 21*(4), 400–406.

Hodson, B., (1986). *Assessment of phonological process—Spanish.* San Diego: Los Amigos Research Associates.

Howell, J., & Dean, E. (1991). *Treating phonological disorders in children: Metaphon—Theory to practice.* San Diego: Singular Publishing Group

Iglesias, A., & Anderson, N. (1993). Dialectal variations. In J. Bernthal & N. Bankson (Eds.), *Articulation and phonological disorders* (pp. 147–160). Upper Saddle River, NJ: Prentice Hall.

Iglesias, A., & Goldstein, B. (1998). Language and dialectal variation. In J. Bernthal & N. Bankson (Eds.), *Articulation and phonological disorders* (pp. 148–168). Boston: Allyn & Bacon.

Ingram, D. (1976). *Phonological disability in children.* New York: American Elsevier.

Jimenez, B. C. (1987). Acquisition of Spanish consonants in children aged 3–5 years, 7 months. *Language, Speech, and Hearing Services in Schools, 18*(4), 357–363.

Kupfer, M. L., & Kissel, J. (1990). *Bridging the dialect gap.* Austin, TX: Pro-Ed.

Ladefoged, P. (1993). *A course in phonetics* (3rd ed.). Fort Worth, TX: Harcourt Brace Jovanovich.

Linares, T. A. (1982). Articulation skills of Spanish-speaking children. In *Ethnoperspectives in Bilingual Education Series, Vol. III: Bilingual Education Technology* (pp. 363–387). Ypsilanti, MI.

Maez, L. (1981). *Spanish as a first language.* Unpublished doctoral dissertation. University of California, Santa Barbara.

Moran, M. (1993, July). Final consonant deletion in African American children speaking Black English: A closer Look. *Language, Speech, and Hearing Services in Schools, 24*(3), 156–166.

Myers-Jennings, C. (1994). *Onset of canonical babbling in environmentally at risk infants.* Unpublished doctoral dissertation, University of Florida, Gainesville, Florida.

O'Grady, W., Dobrovolsky, M., & Aranoff, M. (1993). *Contemporary linguistics: An introduction* (2nd ed.). New York: St. Martin's Press.

Oller, D. K. (1980). The emergence of the sounds of speech in infancy. In G. Yenikomshian, J. Kavanagh, & C. Ferguson (Eds.), *Child phonology, Vol. 1* (pp. 93–112). New York: Academic Press.

Oller, D. K. (1986). Metaphonology and infant vocalizations. In B. Lindblom & R. Zetterstrom (Eds.), *Precursors of early speech* (pp. 21–36). New York: Stockman Press.

Oller, D. K., & Eilers, R. E. (1982). Similarities of babbling of Spanish and English learning babies. *Journal of Child Language, 9,* 565–578.

Pandolfi, A. M., & Herrera, M. O. (1990). Produccio'n fonologica diastratica de ninos menores de tres anos (Phonological production in children less than three years old). *Revista Teorica y Aplicada, 28,* 101–122.

Pollock, K., & Keiser, N. (1990). An examination of vowel errors in phonologically disordered children. *Clinical Linguistics and Phonetics, 4,* 161–178.

Proctor, A. (1994). Phonology and cultural diversity. In R. Lowe, (Ed.), *Assessment and intervention applications in speech pathology* (pp. 216–228). Baltimore: Williams & Wilkins.

Secord, W. (1989). Articulation: Introduction. In N. Creaghead, P. Newman, & W. Secord (Eds.), *Assessment and remediation of articulatory and phonological disorders* (pp. 9–33). Columbus, OH: Merrill.

Seymour, H., & Ralabate, P. (1985). The acquisition of a phonological feature of Black English. *Journal of Communication Disorders, 18,* 139–148.

Seymour, H., & Seymour, C. (1981). Black English and Standard English contrasts in consonantal development of four- and five-year-old children. *Journal of Speech and Hearing Disorders, 46,* 274–280.

So, L., & Dodd, B. (1994). Phonologically disordered Cantonese-speaking children. *Clinical Linguistics and Phonetics, 8*(3), 235–255.

Steffersen, M. (1974). The acquisition in culturally diverse populations: The black child as a case study. In O. Taylor (Ed.), *Nature of communication disorders in culturally and linguistically diverse populations* (pp. 117–155). San Diego: College-Hill Press.

Stepanof, E. R. (1990). Procesos phonologicos de ninos Puertorriquehos de 3 y 4-snos evidenciado an ia prueba APP-Spanish (Phonological processes evidenced on the App-Spanish by 3- and 4-year-old Puerto Rican children). *Opphia, 8*(2), 15–20.

Stockman, I. (1991, November). *Constraints on final consonant deletion in Black English.* Paper presented to the meeting of the American Speech-Language-Hearing Association, Atlanta.

Stockman, I. (1995, November). *Early morphosyntactic patterns of African-American children.* Paper presented to the meeting of the American Speech-Language-Hearing Association. Orlando, FL.

Stockman, I., & Settle, M. S. (1991, November). *Initial consonants in young Black children's conversational speech.* Paper presented to the meeting of the American Speech-Language-Hearing Association, Atlanta.

Stoel-Gammon, C., & Dunn, C. (1985). *Normal and disordered phonology in children.* Austin, TX: Pro-Ed.

Taylor, O. L., Payne, K. T., & Anderson, N. B. (1987). Distinguishing between communication disorders and communication differences. *Seminars in Speech and Language, 8,* 415–427.

Vaughn-Cooke, F. (1986). Lexical diffusion: Evidence from a decreolizing variety of Black English. In M. Montgomery & G. Bailey (Eds.), *Language variety in the South* (pp. 111–130). Tuscaloosa: University of Alabama Press.

Wang, W. (1989). *Language and dialects of Chinese.* Palo Alto, CA: Stanford University Press.

Washington, J., & Craig, H. (1992). Articulation test performances of low-income African-American preschoolers with communication impairments. *Language, Speech, and Hearing Services in Schools, 23,* 201–207.

Weiner, F. (1981). Treatment of phonological disability using the method of meaningful minimal contrast: Two case studies. *Journal of Speech and Hearing Disorders, 46,* 97–103.

Welker, G., (1995). *The native web project.* World Wide Web: Syracuse University.

Wolfram, W. (in press). Language variations. In L. Cole & V. R. Deal (Eds.), *Communication disorders in multicultural populations.* Rockville, MD: ASHA.

Wolfram, W., & Fasold, R. W. (1974). *The study of social dialects in American English.* Englewood Cliffs, NJ: Prentice-Hall.

Yavas, M., & Goldstein, B. (1998). Phonological assessment and treatment of bilingual speakers. *American Journal of Speech-Language Pathology, 7*(2), 49–60.

# 10

# CLINICAL MANAGEMENT OF VOICE DISORDERS IN CULTURALLY DIVERSE CHILDREN: BACKGROUND AND DEFINITION

## RHODA L. AGIN

Interpersonal communication is the means by which the client-therapist relationship is discharged. As in all communication genres, interpersonal communication occurs in a sociocultural context. In voice therapy as in other behavior therapies, the success of the treatment session is dependent upon the existence of mutual *cultural norms;* those shared by the client and therapist. All the major elements of the client-therapist interaction including the case history, the assessment, interpretation of findings, and therapy planning and execution are subject to this mutuality of cultural norms. The norm or standard central to the therapeutic process is communication. For example, the Native American adult or child, whose custom it is not to speak upon meeting a new person and instead remain silent for a period of time, would obviously consider sharing personal information with a stranger inappropriate. Therefore, a more traditional Native American would find his or her communication norms, which include the use of silence for several different communication intentions, in direct conflict with the responsible speech pathologist seeking family and case history details for the benefit of his or her client. In this circumstance, communication would be strained at best.

Another example of a cultural norm at issue is Case Example 10.1 in the Study Questions and Activities. In Charlie's case, to speak of particular subjects and use a certain representative voice is a source of miscommunication. Several other pediatric cases from diverse linguistic and cultural backgrounds are also included in the study questions. In each case, reference will be made to a cultural norm influencing the voice client's behavior or the treatment method administered. A discussion of each Case Example follows the case.

It is the premise of this chapter that one's voice usage is an element of one's cultural communication norms and constitutes a feature of one's dialect. Vocal dynamics exhibit dialectal variations similar to phonology, syntax, prosody, proxemics, suprasegmentals, and other language features. It should be noted that suprasegmentals (intonation and stress) are not the only vocal dynamics to exhibit dialectal variation. Volume, pitch, quality, and perhaps vocal onset and vowel duration are also culturally influenced. It is because these vocal dialectal differences can be confused with vocal disorders that literature and case studies pertinent to both topics will be considered in this chapter. However, irrespective of whether a given vocal behavior is a minimal difference or a severe pathology, it may have a negative impression on a listener. Common perceptions of an aberrant voice ranges from temporary illness (hoarseness) to physical anomalies (unusual pitch, breathing, etc.). Lass, Ruscello, Stout, and Hoffman (1991) stated, "voice disorders appear to adversely affect peers' perceptions of certain personality and physical appearance traits of children." Consequently, management considerations for both populations will be considered.

Does cultural diversity imply linguistic diversity or vice versa? The answer is usually yes. Cultural diversity in the broad sense is ubiquitous in the United States even within the dominant Anglo-European Christian culture. For example, societal institutions such as the university have discrete cultures and associated linguistic "standards" and characteristics. Also, in the United States, the dominant culture and "standard" English vary according to geographic region.

In this chapter, whether a client's predominant communication mode is (1) a non-English language (children acquiring English as a second language), (2) a social or cultural dialect/variation of English, or (3) monolingual English from a family background practicing a culture different from the currently dominant Anglo-European Christian culture, he or she may use vocal features that are different from those characteristic of the dominant "standard" versions of English. These may be simply vocal differences or vocal disorders.

If we are to effectively assess and treat vocal disorders in this multicultural society, it seems necessary to determine the degree to which norms established on European peoples and cultures of the nineteenth century may remain the guideposts for service or must be adjusted to reflect the present and growing population diversity in the United States.

## CULTURAL AND LINGUISTIC DIVERSITY AND THE PEDIATRIC VOICE

The search for incidence data in the literature regarding laryngeal dysphonias in subjects from culturally diverse populations raises numerous questions. For example, how does the use or nature of the voice differ from one culture to another? Second, to what do we attribute these differences? Does vocal variability reflect physical diversity based on race? Third, are some vocal differences misinterpreted as vocal disorders? Do diverse cultural and racial groups vary in the type and incidence of vocal pathology? Lastly, how can treatment methods respect the cultural sensibilities of a diverse client population? Although the mandate of this chapter is to suggest treatment appropriate to children of diverse cultural groups, answers to most of those questions posed will be answered.

Unfortunately, studies of human vocal parameters, anatomy and physiology, and treatment techniques do not ordinarily delineate the racial or cultural identities of their subjects (e.g., Casper, Brewer, & Colton, 1987; Hollein & Jackson, 1973; Jacobson, Johnson, Gywalski, Silbergleit, Jacobson, Beninger, & Newman, 1997). Much of what we know about vocal diversity and pathology across cultures is based upon clinical observations, anecdotal evidence, and doctoral dissertations. Therefore, our current responses to even the most basic queries in this area of communication disorders are limited. In addition, all vocal dynamics and related disorders have not been the subject of clinical and/or research attention in this narrow literature—pitch and its objective correlate, fundamental frequency, appear to have garnered most of the focus.

## *Organic and Functional Dysphonias*

In the literature of laryngeal dysphonias, the traditional dichotomy of descriptors is organic versus functional. A review of approximately fifty years of literature in organic and functional dysphonias to date reveals scant research in voice disorders that includes subjects derived from culturally diverse populations. It is not unlikely that persons of non-white and non-European ethnic groups participated in surveys and large scale studies of voice disorders. However, it appears that the pertinence of cultural identity was not typically noted and/or reported. This situation is not surprising. Only in the last twenty years have journal papers and letters regarding cultural or ethnic influence on pathogenesis appeared infrequently in the medical literature (Blot, Fraumeni, & Morris, 1978; Diehl, 1988; Shaunak, Lakhani, Abraham, & Maxwell, 1986; Sorfman, 1986; Tashima, 1987). Almost all of these authors point out that racial, cultural, or religious data are rarely included in medical evaluations and reports. Consequently, the effect of these data on nutrition, attitude toward medicine and illness, and other pertinent health history is overlooked. Perhaps, the influence of the medical model of information gathering in the development of speech pathology specialties explains the neglect of sociocultural data in our discipline.

## Abuse, Overuse, and Misuse

Irrespective of age, the majority of dysphonias are attributed to one or more of the abnormal patterns of phonation known as abuse, overuse, and misuse. Abuse is typified by shouting (screaming), throat-clearing, and chronic coughing. Overuse is excessive periods of voice usage with insufficient periods of vocal rest. Misuse is the use of a breath control pattern, register, volume, or quality inappropriate for one's laryngeal mechanism. These vocal behaviors may cause a variety of vocal cord pathologies including vocal nodules, vocal polyps, hemangiomas, polypoid degeneration, chronic edema, and vocal fatigue. Additional studies are needed to identify epidemiologic factors including prevalence and establish efficacy of treatment. This knowledge should aid the development of preventive measures.

## Psychogenic Disorders of the Larynx and Upper Aerodigestive Tract

Psychogenic disorders of the larynx and upper aerodigestive tract occur frequently but are not well understood. They may be a primary disorder or secondary to a loss of communication skills. Disorders of a psychogenic nature include aberrant breath control, pitch, loudness, and quality, as well as spastic muscle behaviors, feigned vocal cord paralysis, and paradoxical vocal cord adduction. It is often difficult to distinguish voice symptoms caused by a psychogenic problem from those evidenced by an idiopathic organic disorder. Research is needed to permit clinical identification of the psychogenic components in the development and manifestations of a vocal disorder, and to determine how psychologic factors influence treatment outcome.

As yet, we do not have standards for counseling skills among voice therapists and referral guidelines. Although there is no literature suggesting differences in regard to psychogenic disorders in diverse cultures across the spectrum of clients receiving voice therapy, it is likely that counseling skills would harbor the greatest challenge for the voice therapist. It is known that stress, personality, anxiety, suppression, and so on are not culturally specific.

## Influencing Variables in Voice and Voice Therapy

There are several influencing variables in voice usage, including diet, gender, age, lifestyle, and the use of pharmaceuticals particularly for allergies in adolescents (Andrews, 1995). For example, normal maturation—specifically the onset of puberty and the subsequent drop in vocal pitch range—can be affected by diet. The laryngeal growth spurt followed by a vocal pitch decline (of as much as an octave) occurs at about two or more years after the pubescent transition, after physical and hormonal changes have occurred. Therefore, the occasional voice breaks in males that some youngsters exhibit occur at about 13.5 years of age, toward the end of puberty. The adult vocal pitch stabilizes at about 15 years of age (Agin, 1990). According to Stein (personal communication, 1987), where poor economic conditions exist and poor nutrition is rampant, puberty in adolescents is delayed. In J. S. Bach's Liepzig Boys' Choir the maturation rate of the voices of choir members reflected the abject economic conditions of war-torn Liepzig. In general, the boys left the choir at age 14. However, after the War of Accession (1740–1748), a period of severe economic conditions, the populace of Liepzig experienced poor nutrition. Meager food supplies meant that the boys did not have sufficient food or satisfactory quality of nutrition to mature into adolescence at the normal rate and experience the typical drop in vocal pitch range. Therefore, their voices remained high-pitched. The teenage boys participating in the choir remained in the group by as much as two years beyond age 14.

In developing nations where nutrition was good, the onset of puberty had been declining until about thirty years ago, when this progression stopped. The relationship between the onset of puberty and nutrition applies equally to girls (menstruation) in that the voice also drops, although only a few tones.

Another instance of an influencing variable that presents significant intercultural conflict is gender. For example, the "humming" technique is used for improving resonance and locating an optimal speaking pitch range. Teaching the technique requires placing fingers on the mask of the face and or the bridge of the nose to feel for vibrations. Depending upon the client's culture—for example, Afgani—a male teacher touching a female pupil on the face or a female therapist touching a female client would be taboo, both from the point of view of gender and bans on touching.

Of all the points of possible cultural conflict, the diet is most apparent. Today, it is generally known by voice therapists that drinking iced liquids and caffeinated drinks, as well as the use of decongestants, may cause drying of the mucous membrane of the inferior pharyngeal airway. Consumption of dairy products may cause excessive mucus and possibly subsequent throat clearing, causing abuse of the delicate mucosal covering of the vocal cords. Other dietary cautions include alcohol, spicy foods, and sugar (Agin, 1990). Each of the aforementioned food items is variably consumed across cultures, for example, the Asian American diet is generally devoid of dairy products.

## CULTURAL DIVERSITY IN VOCAL DISORDERS: SCHOOL-AGE CHILDREN

To date there is no evidence claiming that children from diverse cultural or racial backgrounds manifest vocal pathologies other than those currently in the established voice disorders literature. However, some research suggests that the incidence and severity of certain conditions might differ across cultures/racial groups.

New York City's Harlem Hospital Speech and Hearing Center is located in one of the largest black communities in the nation. Haller and Thompson (1975) screened 979 Harlem children ages 3 to 17 years for speech disorders. Voice problems accounted for 22 percent of the screening failures. The predominant dysphonia presenting was hoarseness. The relationship of articulation disorders to voice disorders was about 3:1 as compared to about 8:1 cited in the literature (on white or predominantly white populations). The authors do not explain this notable finding except to say that it may be a result of a higher prevalence of conditions causing laryngeal problems in children in Harlem than most other communities or the fact that speech therapists may be more sensitive to vocal quality deviations than most therapists because of a close working relationship with the otolaryngology discipline.

Barker (1984) screened 2153 13- and 18-year-olds for hoarseness and harshness in six schools in the Sweetwater Union High School District of San Diego County near the Mexican border. Of the total students screened, 950 were Mexican American (M-A) and 760 were Anglo-American (A-A). The result of the screening showed that 128 adolescents exhibited hoarseness and 47 had harshness. Forty-five of these symptomatic subjects had laryngeal examinations in which 26 Mexican Americans and 11 Anglo-Americans had "positive laryngeal examinations"; one subject had no findings. Barker concluded that Mexican American adolescents have a greater frequency of hoarseness and harshness than Anglo-American adolescents.

## CULTURAL DIVERSITY IN BASIC
## VOCAL FEATURES: PITCH, LOUDNESS, AND
## QUALITY ACROSS CULTURES

In the linguistics and speech pathology literature there is a focus on the intonation of discourse and the tonality of language. These features, as well as fundamental frequency, fall within the vocal parameter of pitch. Intonation and tonality are different modes of employing pitch change. Intonation is the pattern of pitch variability over time. We usually refer to the intonation of a phrase or sentence. However, it may also be used in regard to a word. Intonation is the earliest linguistic structure acquired by a child, regardless of what language may be spoken in his or her environment. In fact, intonation seems to be acquired by about the age of twelve months (Parker, 1986, p.159).

### *Pitch*

The primary function of intonation is the indication of attitude (Crystal, 1969, pp. 286–292). In English, when we alter the intonation of a phrase we may change the meaning or intent of the phrase without changing the words. For example, by varying the intonation pattern of "Joan is driving the car," the voice could indicate surprise, annoyance, uncertainty, or anger. Yet no matter how we vary the intonation and thereby invoke a different attitude, the specific word referents remain unchanged. Joan remains herself; a car remains a car as we know it, and so on. Chreist (1964) commented on the importance of native intonation in language learning:

> In his own native language he has absorbed the changing intonation patterns of his parents and associates as automatic reactions. When he seeks to speak the language of his new culture, these deeply ingrained habits of pitch change intrude. His native melody "shows through" . . . (p. 44)

Intonation, then, enters early in one's language development. In addition, English maintains a critical function in the expression of attitudes and is subject to misinterpretation. Although English speech intonation provides a variety of pitches, all speech pitches are included in one tonal level or range. In English, the word *tone* is generally used for a pitch, for example, a high tone or low tone.

All languages have intonation and tone (Taylor, 1993). However, English is not a tonal language. A tonal or tone language refers to those languages that make lexical use of tone (Cheng, 1991; Taylor, 1993). This means that a word meaning may be distinguished by the use of a tone. In a tonal language at least two tones (levels or mini ranges) are used, and its monosyllabic words change meaning when said in a higher or lower tone level. In addition, the tone applied may have a distinctive pitch pattern, for example, "mid tone rising," "high tone falling." For example, in the tonal system of Mandarin Chinese, which has four tones and a neutral tone, each syllable takes a particular tone plus a pattern of pitch movement in each tone. In this way, the word *ma* has 10 different meanings depending upon the tone pattern applied to the word (Cheng, 1991).

Cheng (1991) reports that there are six tones in Vietnamese and six tones in Laotian (pp. 43, 47), and there is some controversy as to whether Cantonese Chinese has seven or nine tones. Nevertheless, the effect on the referent meaning of a word when a tone is varied is apparent. For example, the syllable *si* in Cantonese, depending upon the tone applied to the word may be used as *poem, to think, history,* or *city* (pp. 28–29). Tshiluba, a dialect of Bantu from southern Africa, has fourteen tone levels; Oslo Norwegians use two tone levels and the Mandarin Chinese speakers use four (Chreist, 1964, pp. 54-55). By contrast, only one tone is used in Italian and Amharic, an Ethiopian language. Approximately 80 percent of the world's languages are tonal.

The influence of tones in the speech of many adults and children from diverse linguistic backgrounds or cultural dialect backgrounds may be a distinct disadvantage in a variety of standard English communication situations. First, the degree to which the presence of tonality or a non-English intonation pattern is considered a benefit or a detriment in a speaker's performance should be primarily dependent upon the speech standards of the audience of listeners. A second consideration is the presence of additional features of communication diversity such as the use of nonstandard syntax.

Few, but nevertheless interesting, reports have appeared in the speech pathology literature for over two decades that specific vocal standards and features reflecting group differences are culturally, regionally, and environmentally based (Fischer, 1975). Hollein and Malcik (1962) found that nineteen African Americans from the south ages 10, 14, and 18 had lower mean fundamental frequency in a 55-word reading task than comparable white subjects from the north studied in a similar earlier study. In a subsequent study, Hollein, Malcik, and Hollein (1965) corrected the oversight of comparing subjects from two different dialectal regions and found no differences between the subjects on fundamental frequency. However, in subsequent investigations comparing speaking fundamental frequency (Fo) of African American and white subjects, Fo was found to be lower in African Americans than in white subjects (Fitch & Holbrook, 1970; Hudson & Holbrook, 1981). Luchsinger and Arnold

(1965) offered anecdotal evidence that Puerto Rican teenage girls in New York City tend to speak in a rather high pitch (p. 100).

In 1972, Tarone compared the intonation of black vernacular English of the so-called "street culture," white English, and formal black English. The subjects were 16- to 24-year-old male and female blacks and whites studied during informal discussions, and an adult black male who was able to code switch between vernacular black English and formal black English. The results were:

1. The Black English data was characterized by a wider pitch range, extending into higher pitch levels than either the white English or the formal black English (p. 105).
2. There was a very high occurrence of the falsetto register in Black English, more often than in either white English or formal black English (p. 107). Both males and females used falsetto. It was used when a strong conversational point was being made and when passersby were greeted.
3. More rising and level final contours were used in black English, while white English and formal black English used more falling final contours (p. 108).

One of Tarone's conclusions was that intonation must be studied within the social situation. She found that the majority of the intonational characteristics in the black English data can be traced directly to systematic differences between black "street culture" and white "mainstream" culture. Speech events that occur in black street culture seem to call for specialized use of intonation patterns. These are a result of different "social rules" for speech within that culture (p. 118). Tarone also stated that "[i]f intonation indicates attitude and Black English differs from the standard dialects of American English, then there would likely be a misinterpretation of attitude and intonation in communication between speakers of different dialects" (p. 4).

## Loudness

There is further evidence that other differences exist in the speaking voice across diverse cultural populations. Loudness also plays a part in the use of vocal stress or emphasis. In Grant Fairbanks' (1960) classic text, he described intensity as one of three properties of stress:

Intensity is one of the elements of stress, along with duration and pitch. Large variation of intensity, between the stressed syllables and words on the one hand and the unstressed syllables and words on the other, is a mark of good speech. It has been shown experimentally that intensity, when good speakers are in question, is closely related to the grammatical functions of words. Words that carry the main burden of meaning, such as nouns and verbs, adjectives and adverbs, tend to have high intensity. Conjunctions, articles, prepositions, and pronouns are usually spoken with very low intensity in comparison. (p. 143)

It is interesting to note that a departure from the characteristic Standard English stress pattern has been documented in Puerto Rican English (Wolfram, 1988) and in black street speech (Baugh, 1983, pp. 1–4). Wolfram stated that "Puerto Rican English speakers will sometimes follow the Black English pattern of stressing the first rather than the second syllable." The examples he provides are *"police, hotel* and *July."* Baugh reported that black street speakers tended to put primary stress on bisyllabic words such as *"define"* and *"revise"* in informal settings. The implication of these findings is that syllable stress may give a listener the impression of loudness as a characteristic of speech in the English dialect of specific cultures.

In 1975, Fischer stated:

It is impossible to define good speech in all particulars, universal, cultural, regional and occupational differences work against a unitary definition. Japanese exchange students in America, for example, have resisted attempts to make them talk louder, because the level of loudness we consider good is in poor taste in Japanese society. (p. 9)

It is curious that Japanese culture permits vocal abuse in a competitive form. There is a "Year-End Shouting Contest in Tokyo, where participants yell out their joys and woes in throes of unbridled vocal expression." In 1994, the Associated Press reported that the winner's voice was recorded at 114.7 decibels (Associated Press, 1994).

In mainstream Anglo culture, a loud voice is usually associated with anger or hostility. A low volume or soft voice suggests shyness or embarrassment. These vocal dynamics can be relative to one's culture. Peñalosa (1981) included "loud-talking" as one of several "black verbal arts known in different geographical areas by various names such as signifying, rapping, . . . playing the dozens" (p. 148). Kochman (1981) indicated that a range of strong vocal intensity is utilized by African Americans, depending upon the degree of assertiveness/aggressiveness necessary. Wolfram and Christian (1989) said that some vocal features might be "molded by community norms. For example, a stylized use of raspiness among black males has been observed by some researchers. . . . Several studies have suggested that the range between high and low pitch used in black communities is greater than that found in comparable white communities."

Fairgray-Krofcheck (personal communication, 1993) described the strong cultural identity, language, and cultural customs maintained by the Maori (indigenous people of New Zealand) and Polynesian immigrants from the South Pacific Islands of Tonga, Samoa, Nuie, and the Cook Islands who live predominately in the city of Auckland. She estimates that "at least 50% of Maori and Polynesian boys aged between 5 and 10 years have dysphonia." She added that complete aphonia has also been observed and that immediate cause for both pathologies is typically vocal nodules. ". . . the incidence of childhood dysphonia is so high, most Maori and Polynesian parents do not perceive a problem. It is usually only when complete aphonia occurs that parents are concerned."

Maori and Polynesians have histories of singing/musical activities and highly vocal audience participation in sporting events such as rugby. Among the Maori

> the oral traditions were (and still are) a prominent feature of the culture. The gift of oratory is still esteemed and valued. Many young boys aspire to this skill and abuse their voices in attempts to address large audiences. . . . the "Haka" or ritual warrior challenge is frequently performed . . . by boys and involves a great deal of loud shouting at a very low pitch . . . to elicit intimidation. (p. 3)

Other "Haka" vocal features include

> excessively loud volume, hard glottal attacks at the beginning of most words . . . accompanied by body movements such as stamping the ground or throwing a symbolic implement, prolonged use of the voice in this manner for 10–15 minutes. (p. 3)

Kayser (personal communication, 1988) stated that a community of Mexican Americans in southern Arizona are known to use a loud and high-pitched voice called the "Sonoran Screech." Kayser explained that the use of this kind of voice is typical in the northern part of the Mexican state of Sonora. Consequently, Mexican residents from that state who have crossed the United States border and taken up residence in Texas, Arizona, and New Mexico continue to use this vocal style and pass it on to their children. According to Kayser, most Mexican Americans in the southwestern United States do not use the "Sonoran Screech," therefore, in her clinical experience "screeching" youngsters were provided with voice therapy to eliminate the aberrant vocal habits. In independent conversations, Jacobs (personal communication, 1988) and Murray (personal communication, 1988) reported their observations of an "inner city voice" exhibited by black youngsters in the Washington, DC and Baltimore inner city neighborhoods. Jacobs stated, "Kids in crowded Baltimore have a breathy hoarseness."

In a 1991 survey of greeting and addressing customs, conducted by Agin, Sakai, Fong, and Basu at California State University-Hayward, Asian Pacific students reported that a "low voice" (p. 24) (meaning low in volume and not pitch) or "a soft and gentle voice" (p. 27) is always used to speak with an elder or authority figures as a sign of respect. Ferrier (1991), in a study of foreign-born teaching assistants in universities, reported "some cross-cultural differences such as quieter speaking levels in Asians, particularly women." With some concern for the abandonment of their cultural attitudes and behaviors, the students pointed out that "in a classroom situation they may need to switch to louder speech or be considered lacking in confidence by mainstream native speakers. In investigations where fundamental frequency of black and white speakers (children as well as adults) are compared, speaking fundamental frequency of black speakers was consistently found to be lower than the white subjects (Fitch & Holbrook, 1970; Hudson & Holbrook, 1981; Wheat & Hudson, 1988).

## *Quality*

In the Southeast Asian language of Hmong, one of the seven tone levels is breathy. According to Huffman (1987), this means that normal and breathy phonation is used contrastively in Hmong. She found that laryngeal (source) differences, not vocal tract differences, are responsible for the breathy normal distinction in Hmong speech. The import of intercultural sensitivity is highlighted by Huffman's study. The Hmong speaker learning English is likely to apply his Hmong vocal skills to his new language. His or her use of breathiness as an element of meaning could easily be misinterpreted as a vocal disorder by an American speech therapist who has no knowledge of this particular tonal language.

## THE ROLE THAT VOICE PLAYS IN LANGUAGE VARIATION

Appreciation of vocal disorders in culturally diverse populations would not be complete without consideration of the role that voice plays in language variation. According to Parker (1986), a dialect is a systematic variety of a language specific to a region or a social class (e.g., American English, British English, Southern American English, Black English Vernacular) (p. 114). In general, dialects of a language are mutually intelligible, "absolutely rule-governed" behavior, and dialects are equally complex (p. 122). Parker stated that "regional dialects, at least in North America, differ primarily in terms of vocabulary and pronunciation (i.e., lexically and phonologically) . . . social dialects differ primarily in terms of pronunciation, word formation and sentence structure (i.e., phonologically, morphologically, and syntactically)" (p. 120). Taylor, Payne, and Anderson (1987) agreed:

> The most common rules that characterize a speech community are those that pertain to such surface structure features of language as phonology and grammar. These rules are part of the community's dialect. In addition to structural rules, every speech community has a set of rules that govern discourse and conversations. These rules govern, for example, the arrangement of sentences to achieve specific social functions and meanings . . . and appropriate conversational devices and their use (such as silence, interruptions, turn-taking, and nonverbal behaviors). (p. 416)

Neither Parker nor Taylor made mention of the role played by the voice in a dialect. However, Parker stated that linguists found it impossible to deal with language variation without acknowledging the fact that listeners judge a speaker according to the characteristics of the speaker's dialect (1986, p. 121). Although Parker's text does not consider vocal dynamics, other authors would probably apply Parker's comment to the vocal aspects in a speaker's dialect. For example, Chreist (1964) explained the influence of pitch patterns from a first language interfering in second language acquisition as an instance of a speaker's dialect distracting listener judgment from the message. Labov, Cohen, Robbins, and Lewis (1968, cited in Tarone, 1972), in a study of black and Puerto Rican speakers, stated that "voice qualifiers and intonational patterns are just as characteristic of Black English as grammatical and lexical features" (p. 12).

Vernacular and foreign language speaking adults and children learning standard English typically combine elements of English with those of their first communication system. Lately, on college campuses, this transitional or combination linguistic stage is colloquially referred to as "Spanglish" or "Chinglish," for example. Even though this expanding version of English may be become predominantly English, and may be generally understood by English speakers, the version of English heard (a dialect) could continue to reflect intonation patterns of the first language. Alleyne (1980) commented on intonation in black vernacular and offered tentative observations about the phatic and creative function that this dialect tends to emphasize.

> [It] serves to express the sentiments of brotherhood, community, and culture, which are said to be very strong among Blacks; the effect of this function on language form is well known. It is probably responsible for the preservation of tonal features in Black languages in Africa and in the New World. (p. 46)

Taylor (1988) stated that most sociolinguists think that Black English Vernacular reflects African influences that have been reinforced by such factors as social isolation, segregation, and group identity. Could these influences be vocal as well as semantic, syntactic and phonological? Alleyne clearly stressed the vocal characteristics of black communication when he said,

> It is customary to identify the dialect by means of a few high-recognition forms such as be as an auxiliary verb, double negative . . . ; but it may be that suprasegmental features, especially intonation and stress, are equally, if not more, typical. Certainly, the latter features remain even when Blacks adopt the Standard dialect at the syntactical and phonological (sequential) levels (p. 31).

In addition, for those speakers whose first language is tonal, the pitch pattern remnants in English would very likely be more difficult to eliminate than a nonstandard intonation pattern to which Alleyne refers. If we add Fairbanks' description of loudness as an element in word stress that varies with certain dialects, the answer to the question posed earlier is yes; the listener is influenced by vocal dialect features. Further support is affirmed by the substantial literature on prosody and discourse, a discussion of which follows later in this chapter.

As stated at the outset of the chapter, every society has its communication cultural norms. A breathy voice in a white American Anglo-Saxon Protestant culture is typically understood as implying sensuality or sexiness. A loud voice is usually associated with anger or hostility. A low volume or soft voice suggests shyness or embarrassment. These vocal dynamics can be relative to one's culture. Therefore, health service providers or clinicians need to be trained to recognize the diversity of cultural norms and acquire the ability to adjust their clinical skills as cultural imperatives change from one client to another.

## ETHNIC AND RACIAL CONSIDERATIONS

In addition to economic variables, gender and nutritional variables may contribute to vocal disorders. An ethnic rather than a cultural analysis might provide valuable insight into the manifestation of vocal abuse, misuse, and overuse in culturally diverse white and non-white populations in the United States. Ethnicity is the array of outward expressions of a culture such as clothing, customs, and so on. Ethnic diversity within a cultural group can also be reflected in diet, class values, education, religion, and health priorities (Shaunak et al., 1986).

An example of cultural heterogeneity within racial groups is the numerous cultural divisions included in the black race. African Americans of Haitian descent are ethnically diverse from rural African Americans in Louisiana, cosmopolitan African Americans in Atlanta or Washington, DC, and Hispanic blacks in Puerto Rico. These are a few of the divergent heritages within the black race. The same point can be applied to Hispanics, Asians, and other ethnic groups. Although similarities may exist among peoples of one racial group, it would be fallacious to assume cultural homogeneity for all blacks, all Asians, all Native Americans, or any other racial group. Based upon the introductory discussion of cultural norms, the therapist is alerted to expect linguistic diversity including vocal diversity and cultural diversity within the various branches of a large racial group.

## WORKING PHILOSOPHIES FOR THE THERAPIST

Speech clinicians/therapists possess a position of responsibility and authority in the realms of health services and education. We are entrusted by our clients and their families to direct significant behavior changes—changes so elemental to one's interface with the world that they affect the essence of the personality. Changing vocal behaviors has traditionally evoked trepidation among therapists for this reason. The concern for facilitating an inappropriate habitual pitch or quality, for example, has even caused therapists to avoid treating this population. Perhaps a holistic grounding in the precursors to successful voice therapy would assist therapists encountering individuals presenting voice disorders and voice differences.

In seeking culturally appropriate intervention strategies for voice therapy, the clinician's first hurdle might be the overriding philosophical bent that he or she uses in therapy. Understanding oneself as a conduit of change is a helpful starting point for the clinician. Whether or not we are aware of our fundamental outlook of the "true" or best way to do things, we have all assimilated such principles in the course of growing up. We may or may not be satisfied with the philosophy of our youth, but it behooves us to recognize it, and if necessary adjust it, in order to develop ethically sound and versatile therapy methods for an multicultural environment.

One's philosophy can sometimes evidence a vocal counterpart in clinician-client communication. Consider which of the following philosophical approaches and associated voice usage is yours.

1. *Authoritarian.* The authoritarian approach is an unquestioning obedience to certain practices and conduct. This pedagogical style can have ramifications for voice usage. For example, the intonational pattern in standard American English requires a drop in pitch at the end of a statement and a question (with the exception of questions requiring a yes/no answer). The therapist employing an authoritarian approach in therapy will likely use the downward intonational pattern suggesting that what he or she says or requests is unquestionable and expected behavior. Aside from vocal tendencies and because gender interactions are culturally specific, some male pupils will not respond well or not at all to a female authority figure, for example. This philosophical perspective provides insight into the seat of parental power in the family of our client. Is the family matriarchal or patriarchical? Assessing the organization of family power and responsibility is helpful information to gather during the case history.

2. *Interactive.* The interactive learning environment is less teacher-oriented and more collaborative and reciprocal. The therapist questions, seeks verbal responses, and, consequently, utilizes upward inflectional and intonational patterns with greater frequency. If this description reflects your philosophy, consider the interaction expectations for students and teachers in your client's culture.

Cultures vary in their style preferences regarding authoritarian versus interactive ways of learning. It is because learning, socialization, and the use of language are initiated in the home by the family that the clinician is urged to review his or her philosophical orientation. It may be ingrained and unconscious and not apparent to the therapist. However, of paramount concern is whether the clinician's philosophy is vastly different from the child-client's.

Your philosophy of therapeutic intervention segues into consideration of the style of therapy to be used: *formal versus informal.* Are there benefits to organizing a firm, rigorous, patterned clinical hour versus a casual, relaxed, non-routinized format? As a high school student, this writer recalls being told by a teacher that the class will not be taught while sitting under the tree outside on a particularly sunny spring day. The reason given was that we would focus better and therefore increase the efficacy of learning while at our desks. The multitude of distractions present while sitting outside on the grass decreases productivity. As a university instructor, the value of this maxim is reinforced each spring, when students understandably yearn to be outdoors. In the business sector of society, it is well-accepted that productivity at a meeting is improved when participants sit around a large table, have a reliable surface on which to write, and are able to view all speakers present.

The therapist might consider combining these philosophical approaches in an attempt to complement the child's home culture and create a bridge to a mutually acceptable mode of learning. A cautionary note regarding firmness and organization is pertinent at this point. Experienced therapists know that starting therapy using an informal approach will not easily permit change to a more structured style. Doing the reverse is likely to be more successful.

A striking departure from the authoritarian approach mentioned earlier is the *eclectic Sherlock Holmes approach* (Agin, 1990). If an educator or a medical professional does not know the etiology of a problem/disorder, it does not mean that one does not exist. Instead, the cause has not been determined, as yet. Therefore, viewing a differential diagnosis or diagnostic therapy as a puzzle to be resolved encourages the clinician's inventiveness and perseverance. This perspective is especially helpful when serving clients from multicultural backgrounds, given the frequency of communication difficulties in the gathering of case history information.

Determining the cause of certain problems is essential before appropriate therapy can ensue. For example, in the case of prosody difficulties and monotonous voice in a youngster using a social dialect or limited English proficiency, it is easy to assume that a confusion in the use of vocal dynamics in this youngster is generated by linguistic interference, much as we would observe in language interferences. However, an assessment of this child's hearing is a critical element of the management protocol, because it is a possible etiology for the youngster's vocal behaviors.

Another seemingly common case example warranting an eclectic investigatory stance is that of allergies masking vocal abuse. An airborne or food allergy, as well as allergies to certain medications, can cause vocal cord edema and/or inflammation of the mucosal lining of the vocal cords. Allergies often go undetected because the cause is not always present. The food trigger, for example, is not eaten consistently or daily. Consequently, the therapist might pursue vocal abuse as the likely etiology of the problem, overlooking the true cause of the edema. This was the case with a 12-year-old boy whose voice was fine in the morning but hoarse when he returned from jogging in the afternoon. It took three weeks for us to methodically review and experiment with the elimination of particular foods and plants in his environment. Eventually, we pinpointed the section of blooming trees that he passed on his afternoon jog near the local park. Once he changed his route, the vocal cord edema disappeared.

Last, recall an application of the eclectic Sherlock Holmes approach that went awry when I tried to be culturally insightful. A 6-year-old Samoan boy named Bob presented with severe hoarseness in all spheres of his life when he played with other children. He tended to yell when excited. Parental and teacher concern and monitoring failed to reduce the voice problem. After assessing the child, I was certain that traditional loud verbal celebrations at home were the source of vocal abuse, which in turn caused inflamed vocal cord mucosa and the subsequent hoarseness.

After two weeks of therapy, it became clear that the child was not sufficiently involved in his family's traditional celebrations and did not have vocal abusive behaviors. Instead, the child's throat-clearing for excessive mucus after drinking milk caused me to inquire about his hearing. In my experience, earaches and itchy external auditory canals are correlated with an intolerance to cow's milk. Although Bob passed a school screening four months earlier and only occasionally tugged at his ear, I thought another more thorough audiometric examination might be informative. Indeed, it was learned that Bob had mild bilateral otitis media. Two days after myringotomy tubes were inserted into Bob's eardrums, he stopped yelling during play and the hoarseness dissipated.

If we appreciate the value in the eclectic Sherlock Holmes approach, we are then encouraged to consider the merits of *alternative or complementary medical and therapeutic approaches*. Increasingly in my private practice, referrals of unusual or enigmatic cases are sent for evaluation and recommendations. Sometimes these individuals have suffered with their voice disorder for years and attempts to understand and treat their disorder have failed. When I or other professionals trained in current biomedical science can offer no better alternatives, I ask whether a nonallopathic or non-Western approach might be considered. In general, parents are understandably cautious about exploring unfamiliar health treatment for their children. However, frustration with the status quo and lack of treatment options sometimes allow them to try an alternative therapy.

It is not the purview of this chapter to review the array of alternative therapies available. The guides and research literature abound. However, there is a fundamental thread that permeates most alternative approaches: "Disease is dictated by personality and lifestyle" (Inglis & West,

1983, p. 9). Although many health professionals find this assertion lacking as a sound explanation for the cause of disease, those of us who work with the voice find this dictum useful, especially in cases of vocal abuse, misuse, overuse, and psychogenic voice disorders.

A corollary of this issue is if we do not know the cause, we cannot assume that therapy cannot be helpful. Sometimes treating the symptom(s) and showing the youngster that he or she can exert control over the breathing or vocal mechanism provides encouragement and/or a challenge that serves to motivate.

In sum, although the principles introduced here may apply to a variety of speech problems, they are nevertheless pertinent to effective voice therapy. In addition, diverse cultures may view these structural principles differently or not include them in their world view.

## THE VOICE TEAM: A HOLISTIC APPROACH TO THERAPY

When treatment is viewed as an integrated whole, it has the potential to be more effective than its individual elements functioning separately. Therefore, the intention of a team effort is to combine the skills of a several disciplines to optimize the assessment, planning, and treatment for a multifaceted problem. Application of the team approach to the treatment of voice problems provides the most efficient service for the client.

Moreover, the rehabilitation team is typically viewed as a medical construct. In other words, all team personnel are typically drawn from the medical or health professions with the occasional augmentation of a community social worker. Most textbook discussions of the now well-established framework for the habilitation of velopharyngeal and craniofacial anomalies known as the cleft palate team describe only health professionals as team members. However, another perspective, which provides opportunity for cultural input and disclosure, is to include the family and classroom teacher in the team (Agin, 1993).

A voice disorder is a family affair. Providing practical ways for parents or guardians and siblings to assist you in helping to improve your client's voice recognizes the ability and authority of the family in the child's welfare (Manolson, 1992, 1995; van Keulen, Weddington, & DeBose, 1998, pp. 264–275). A practical family-oriented intervention, taking advantage of parents/guardians and siblings as prime facilitators of the new voice, is advantageous to all concerned in the rehabilitation process. Family members spend large portions of the day together and therefore provide communication time with the client.

Furthermore, children are influenced by parental attitudes and comportment. A child's initial observations of parents and therapist interacting sets the stage for therapist-client rapport. The participation of family members on the voice team offers additional benefits, such as sharing valuable insights regarding the child and serving as a cultural resource. Recognizing the value of the family's contribution to the therapeutic effort and redirecting any guilt or defensiveness they may hold regarding their child's voice problem can be done constructively using the team configuration.

Last, it is clear that cultural and linguistic disparity between family and the therapy environment may be such that team membership by the family presents communication difficulties. In this instance, a translator, trained by the therapist in the goals and functioning of the team, is warranted.

The second essential member of the team is the voice client's classroom teacher. Teachers as allies is possibly the ideal perspective to facilitate compliance with therapy. Teachers in their roles as models of a "good" voice may be enlisted as helpful additions to the rehabilitation effort (Deal, McClain, & Suddeth, 1976; Filter & Poynor, 1982; Nilson & Schneiderman, 1983). Research has shown that children demonstrated positive changes in vocal abuse and in self-monitoring skills when teachers were trained as facilitators in a vocal hygiene program (Nilson & Schneiderman, 1983).

For the school-age child, the classroom teacher is not only the primary referral source but also a partner agent for change in behavior (van Keulen et al., 1998, pp. 250–264). A teacher, by virtue of the many hours he or she spends with your client, is a voice model, a motivator, a reinforcer of the desired behavior, and monitor of the carryover of new vocal behaviors. The teacher usually knows the voice client better than any other non-family member. Consequently, the teacher may recognize when a voice therapy technique is in conflict with a child's culture. The client's cultural preferences and biases are likely to be known to the experienced and conscientious classroom teacher. Additionally, teachers are at high risk for vocal problems and need to be models of good vocal behavior.

Intervention issues for the voice team include assumptions about the why and how of voice therapy, which may not be present in the world view of all cultures. For example:

1. Therapy as a way of changing behavior is not a pan-cultural concept.
2. The use of specific vocabulary to focus fundamental elements of therapy for the client is essential. Vocabulary function and usage often vary from culture to culture, increasing the likelihood of miscommunications.

Organizational matters for the team to consider invariably include:

1. The frequency with which the team meets
2. Selection of a day and time when all team members can meet regularly
3. A protocol for case presentations, examinations and discussion
4. Selection of a member to coordinate the teams activities, including the follow-up of decisions and recommendations

Small teams can easily determine these matters and avoid professional conflicts while maximizing efficacy. Other recommended members of the team are the family physician or nurse practitioner, pediatrician, and otolaryngologist, in the case of the presence of a laryngeal pathology. Last, if the client served by the team comes from a linguistic or culturally diverse background, then all team members would benefit from cultural informants and resources.

## A Model of Intervention Interaction

In 1985, under the mentorship of Dr. Orlando Taylor, this author drew a model of the interacting arenas of voice therapy. Basically, the model suggested that to succeed in changing vocal behavior in a youngster, the methods chosen would require penetration of three spheres of a child's life: home/family, school/teachers, and play/friends. In that model, the institution of church was subsumed in the home/family category. In retrospect, I was not culturally sensitive to the significance of the church in African American culture. The following revised model includes not only religious institutions, but takes into consideration the television and video media as well as, compact disc (computer) technology, and societal pressures in our youth-oriented culture.

Each sphere in the model may hold factors that variably affect the therapeutic process, and all areas will exhibit the vocal disorder as well as the improved voice. Consequently, therapy methods are best designed to penetrate each sphere of a child's life, the exception being psychogenic voice disorders, which may appear in one area and not another because of problems in interpersonal or situational psychodynamics.

Voice disorders cannot be managed in isolation. A therapist's success at facilitating effective cross-cultural voice therapy is the extent to which he or she seeks out alliances to encourage behavior change and motivate practice and reinforcement beyond the confines of the therapy room. A case in point is Carla, a 17-year-old high school student with chronic edema and bilateral true vocal cord nodules. It was apparent that Carla's choir participation had not been sufficiently reviewed by her school

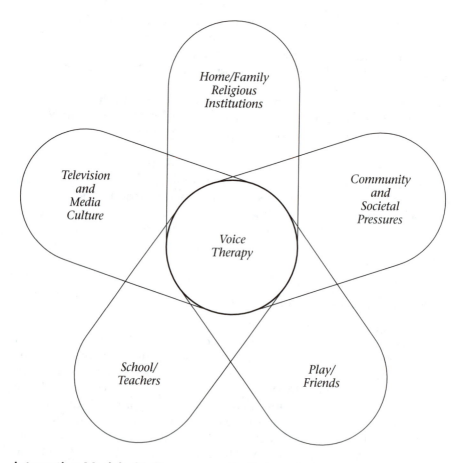

**Interaction Model of Influences on the Voice of Children**

speech therapist to ascertain the influence of choral singing on this teenager's chronic hoarseness and periodic aphonia.

In the presence of Carla and her mother, the school therapist reported that Carla had experienced five relapses in three years of voice therapy focused on vocal abuse. The ongoing goals for Carla's treatment included learning diaphragmatic breathing, avoidance of vocally abusive behaviors—such as hard glottal attacks and drinking five soft drinks daily—and reducing involvement in her church choir by one weekend per month. During the consultation session, open-ended questions posed to Carla and her mother revealed that Carla played a prominent role in the leadership of the youth in the choir. Also, she had a fine voice that

garnered admiration from her peers and frequent solo singing opportunities. When Carla described and exhibited how she sings and how
she responded to the choir leader's conducting cues, it became clear
that the choir conductor would need to be involved in Carla's therapy
for there to be a permanent or at least long-term elimination of the
voice disorder.

During rehearsals, when cued by the conductor for loudness, a sustained tone or sharp/"crisp" vocal onsets, Carla would give a performance
caliber effort instead of a rehearsal caliber effort. Taking her leadership role
very seriously, she was giving 110 percent in practice sessions, instead of
saving energy and effort for important rehearsals and performances. After
a telephone discussion of the situation and our findings with the choir
conductor, he became a member of our ad hoc voice rehabilitation team.
He monitored Carla's singing for "pushing" and "hard attacks" and ended
the drinking of cold sodas at all rehearsals. Creating treatment alliances to
facilitate carryover of newly learned behavior while at the same time respecting cultural allegiances was crucial in the achievement of treatment
goals for Carla. In sum, parent-teacher-therapist cooperation is the recommended alliance to facilitate therapy compliance.

## CONCLUSION

In a general communication context, Taylor (1988) stated, "Unfamiliar-
ity with cultural communication differences can lead to misinterpretation, misunderstanding, and even unintentional insult" (p. 10). If this
perspective of clinician responsibility is applied to voice disorders and
their management, vocal diversity across cultures should at least receive
the research and pedagogical efforts that language diversity currently enjoys. Until then, cautioning ourselves about misinterpreting vocal diversity as a disorder is warranted. It already seems likely that some clinical
methods and procedures traditionally employed in the treatment of dysphonic persons of most white cultures do not serve persons from other
cultures equally well. When we better understand normal vocal variability across cultures, vocal assessments and therapeutics are likely to increase in accuracy and success.

At present, the acquisition of knowledge regarding the influence of
cultural and racial diversity on vocal disorders is growing, but all too
slowly. The range of research issues has yet to be determined. All the pertinent research questions have not been raised. Specific cross-cultural
and cross-racial investigations of acoustic parameters, discourse variables,
anatomical and physiological bases for diversity, incidence and variability of disorders, and assessment and intervention methods are rarities in

the literature. The knowledge necessary to revise our protocols and thereby tailor our clinical services to the wider pluralistic society is at present a daily need in the speech clinics, hospitals, and schools across the country (Agin, 1992, 1995). Although the results of forthcoming research on this topic are eagerly awaited, it would be in the best interests of those we serve that we view the literature thoughtfully and critically, and in terms of its timeliness and applicability to culturally and linguistically diverse children.

## STUDY QUESTIONS AND ACTIVITIES

The case examples that follow are meant to raise points about cultural characteristics that may be preventing the successful execution of voice therapy for children of diverse cultural backgrounds. The aim of the study questions is to offer clinical insight and knowledge into the effect of normative cultural behaviors on voice therapy.

### Case Example 10.1

Charlie was an active, friendly 8-year-old boy who came from a Native American family living in a suburb of a small California city. He had two older siblings 11 and 13 years of age. Charlie was an average student in the third grade of the local elementary school. His voice was fine when he returned to school in September. Vocal quality began to deteriorate in October. By the time he was referred to the school speech clinician, he had mild hoarseness characterized by breathiness and a strained quality accompanied by low pitch for three months. An examination by an otolaryngologist found bilateral nodules at the anterior edge of the middle one-third of the true vocal cords. In previous sessions, Charlie learned how his vocal mechanism functions, what vocal abuse is, and the difference between various pitches. In his third week of voice therapy, Charlie's speech clinician taught him to differentiate between the qualitative differences in the voice to and combine his understanding of quality with pitch (e.g., a low rough voice, a medium pleasant voice, and a high squeaky voice). The therapist associated each of the voices with a photograph—a large brown bear with the first voice, a cow with the second, and a raccoon with the third. The session was going well until the bear voice was introduced. At that point, Charlie withdrew and stopped participating. The therapist was puzzled and after several unsuccessful attempts went on to the other animals and voices. Slowly, Charlie became responsive once again. What misunderstanding or lack of knowledge interrupted the session?

**Discussion:** Charlie's experienced but multiculturally unsophisticated speech therapist might have thought this youngster had realized that the example of the low-pitched growling type voice symbolized by the brown bear was indeed a representation of his own hoarse voice. Further, it would be reasonable to assume that the bear's voice had a negative connotation because the medium-pitched voice was described as pleasant. Therefore, the clinician might have thought that embarrassment caused Charlie to stop responding.

This was not the reason for his silence. In the religion of the Native American tribe from which Charlie's family is descended, animals have spiritual significance by virtue of special powers and are accorded respect. As an expression of that respect, the bear, known for its cleverness, physical strength, and persistence, is not spoken of during the winter months when it is in hibernation. Certainly, it would not be a negative attribute to have the voice of a bear—a highly regarded traditional symbol. In sum, it is helpful when choosing therapy materials to be mindful of the belief of indigenous peoples that all natural things, including trees, the sky, water, stones, and creatures, are alive and possess personalities and powers.

**Case Example 10.2**

When Terry was 14, he was in an accident in which he fractured the right thyroid cartilage with the handle bars of his mountain bike. Terry, who comes from an African American family, had a history of hoarseness that was never completely resolved. Terry's teachers reported that he was a good student and enjoyed talking and holding the attention of his friends. Also, he was thought to be a show-off and had a good sense of humor. As much as he tried, he was not able to totally rid himself of his mild to moderate hoarseness. The speech therapist reported that all the methods attempted could not permanently interrupt his pattern of vocal abuse. It should be noted that Terry was not concerned about his voice quality and his parents stated that they were used to it but preferred that his voice was clear. Before the accident Terry's voice was mildly hoarse. After the accident, a brief hospital stay and a few days of recuperation at home, Terry had a rough quality to his speaking and singing voice. A nasendoscopic examination by his otolaryngologist revealed a normal mucosal wave in both true vocal cords during isolated sound production. The cords were a slightly edematous. Terry was told by the physician to "take it easy and don't talk too much . . . the fracture will heal and your voice should be back to normal in a few weeks." Terry returned to school to find his former speech therapist waiting for him after his last class. At this point the speech therapist was concerned that Terry's voice would not return to "normal." A different treatment perspective was needed to prevent a chronically poor voice and the possible development of vocal nodules. What elements in Terry's speaking/vocal style were overlooked by the speech therapist? Why doesn't the hoarse quality bother him? What misunderstanding or lack of knowledge is revealed during this case?

**Discussion:** Terry's therapeutic experience is a good example of a clinician not having all the information necessary for the youngster to achieve the goals the therapist had set out for him. Two cultural imperatives were missed in this case. In African American culture, verbal skills and communication performance are highly valued (Taylor, 1986; van Keulen et al., 1998).

According to van Keulen and colleagues, one of the four basic values in African American culture is "uniqueness or individual style" (p. 78). The hoarse voice was not bothersome to Terry because he valued the novel voice. It set him apart from his peers. Second, loud-talking and shouting are considered acceptable assertiveness in communication (Kochman, 1981; Peñalosa, 1981). Observing Terry on the playground interacting with his friends, and discussing the value of the hoarseness to him could have alerted the clinician to esteemed cultural attitudes.

**Case Example 10.3**

Mai Li Chin was 2 years old when her family arrived from Mainland China in 1991. At the age of 5 she had her first surgery for the wart-like lesion called papilloma of the left true vocal cord precipitated by mild respiratory distress. Subsequently, she underwent four more surgeries—all accomplished by scalpel—for the same condition. The last surgery took place a month before Mai Li's mother contacted a speech therapist specializing in voice problems. Upon the recommendation of their otolaryngologist, the mother wanted to check on the possibility that a therapeutic approach to prevent the development of the lesions was not overlooked. Mai Li had completed prophylactic voice therapy in school and the family was aware of vocal abuse as only a contributory element in the condition. As the telephone conversation ensued, Mai Li's mother mentioned that her daughter would be visiting family in China for two months. She was concerned that a papilloma might begin while the child was out of the country. Given the singular treatment option offered by current American/western medical practice, and the limitations of the current supposition of viral etiology for the wart-like papillomatosis, the mother was asked if the family had ever considered a complementary medical approach such as Chinese medicine along with western treatment. Mrs. Chin reported that although the family was familiar with the medicinal use of herbs and acupuncture, they hadn't considered oriental medicine realistic nor appropriate any longer. She then elaborated about taking Mai Li to China for a four-month visit when she was 7 years of age. There, the child was treated by a practitioner of oriental medicine but ultimately, a papilloma developed again when she returned to California. Why did the therapist venture into a consideration of an atypical treatment approach that can claim only anecdotal evidence to support its efficacy in the realm of speech? What was the specific outcome of Mai Li's treatment in China?

**Discussion:** We know that Mai Li's papillomatosis is a life-threatening condition with a tendency to recur after surgical removal. Monitoring and maintaining the glottal airway by her otolayngologist is apparently the treatment of choice. However, the stress of surgery and the difficulty in preventing the growth of scar tissue on the surgerized cords encourages the health professional to leave no stone unturned in an attempt to reduce the frequencies of surgical interventions. The lack of definitive knowledge of the nature of wart-like lesions also encourages consideration of alternative therapeutics for this frustrating condition. A 1959 *Lancet* journal report described a study of ten subjects with warts on both sides of the face. In hypnotherapy, all subjects were told that warts on one side of the face would disappear; and they did (Inglis & West, 1983, p. 318)!

Chinese medicine is perhaps best known for its aid in pain reduction. Stimulating certain points on the body supposedly activates the release of the body's natural analgesics, endorphins, and enkephalins. According to Chinese medicine, the healing that occurs from stimulating these various points is a result of unblocking the movement of the chi, the life-force within each of us. Although the use of acupuncture and medicinal teas has a history of five thousand years and continues to be widely used in many Asian cultures, the influence of living in a new country and the natural tendency of the young to acquire the mores and customs of their adopted society can be potent. Mrs. Chin hesitated to share the family's attempt at employing Chinese medicine for Mai Li. When she did, it was learned that Mai Li had no growths of the now familiar lesions while in China and receiving regular acupuncture. It was when she returned home that the lesion began to grow again. The possibility of retarding the growth of the papilloma was emphasized as a positive effect of the acupuncture and should be pursued.

## REFERENCES

Agin, R. L. (1989). *Voice therapy for elementary, junior high, and high school pupils.* New Haven Unified School District Inservice Workshop, New Haven, CA.

Agin, R. L. (1990). *Voice disorders in culturally diverse populations.* Paper presented at ASHA Summer Institute on Multicultural Professional Education, Teaching Cultural Diversity Within the Professional Curriculum, Los Angeles.

Agin, R. L. (1992). *Voice disorders in culturally diverse populations.* National Institute on Deafness and Other Communicative Disorders (NIDCD) at National Institutes of Health (NIH), Testimony on Research and Training Needs of Minority Persons and Minority Health Issues, Bethesda, MD.

Agin, R. L. (1993). *Pediatric and teen voice problems and therapeutic methods: The Agin approach.* Workshop, San Mateo County Special Education Local Plan Area (SELPA). San Mateo, CA.

Agin, R. L. (1995). *Voice and voice disorders.* National Institute on Deafness and Other Communicative Disorders (NIDCD) at National Institutes of Health, National Strategic Research Plan. Chantilly, VA.

Agin, R. L., Sakai, S., Fong, C., & Basu, A. (1993). *Guide to the pronunciation of Asian Pacific names.* Hayward: California State University, Hayward.

Alleyne, M. C. (1980). Linguistic issues in black communication. In B. E. Williams & O. L. Taylor (Eds.), *International conference on black communication* (p. 46). Bellagio, Italy: Rockefeller Foundation.

Andrews, M. (1995). *Manual of voice treatment: Pediatrics through geriatrics.* San Diego: Singular Publishing.

Associated Press. (1994, April 26). Postscripts. *Jerusalem Post,* Israel.

Barker, M. (1984). *Voice disorders in Mexican-American and Anglo-American adolescents: A comparative study*. Doctoral dissertation, United States International University.

Baugh, J. (1983). *Black street speech: Its history, structure, and survival*. Austin, TX: University of Texas Press.

Blot, W., Fraumeni, S., & Morris, L. (1978). Patterns of laryngeal cancer in the United States. *The Lancet, 8091*, 674–675.

Casper, J. K., Brewer, D. W., & Colton, R. H. (1987). Variations in normal laryngeal anatomy and physiology as viewed fiberoptically. *Journal of Voice, 1*, 180–185.

Cheng, L. R. (1991). *Assessing Asian language performance*. Oceanside CA: Academic Communication Associates.

Chreist, F. M. (1964). *Foreign accent*. Englewood Cliffs, NJ: Prentice Hall.

Crystal, D. (1969). *Prosodic systems and intonation in English*. Cambridge University Press: London.

Deal, R. E., McClain, B., & Suddeth, J. F. (1976). Identification, evaluation, therapy, and follow-up for children with vocal nodules in a public school setting. *Journal of Speech and Hearing Disorders, 41*, 390–397.

Diehl, A. K. (1988). The melting pot: Examine before stirring. *Journal of General Internal Medicine, 3*, 90–91.

Fairbanks, G. (1960). *Voice and articulation drillbook* (2nd ed.). New York: Harper and Row.

Ferrier, L. (1991, April). Pronunciation training for foreign teaching assistants. *Asha*, 65–70.

Filter, M. D., & Poynor, R. E. (1982). A descriptive study of children with chronic hoarseness. *Journal of Communicative Disorders, 15*, 461–467.

Fischer, H. B. (1975). *Improving voice and articulation* (2nd ed.). Boston: Houghton Mifflin.

Fitch, J. L., & Holbrook, A. (1970). Modal vocal fundamental frequency of young adults. *Archives of Otolaryngology, 92*, 379–382.

Haller, R. M., & Thompson, E. A. (1975). Prevalence of speech, language and hearing disorders among Harlem children. *Journal of the National Medical Association, 67*, 298.

Hollein, H., & Jackson, B. (1973). Normative data on the speaking fundamental frequency characteristics of young adult males. *Journal of Phonetics, 1*, 117–120.

Hollein, H., & Malcik, E. (1962). Adolescent voice change in southern negro males. *Speech Monographs, 29*, 53–58.

Hollein, H., Malcik, E., & Hollein, B. (1965). Adolescent voice change in southern white males. *Speech Monographs, 32*, 87–90.

Hudson, A. I., & Holbrook, A. (1981). Fundamental frequency of characteristics of young black adults: Spontaneous speaking and oral reading. *Journal of Speech and Hearing Research, 25*, 25–28.

Huffman, M. K. (1987). Measures of phonation type in Hmong. *Journal of the Acoustical Society of America, 81*, 495–504.

Inglis, B., & West, R. (1983). *The alternative health guide*. New York: Alfred Knopf.

Jacobson, B. H., Johnson, A., Gywalski, C., Silbergleit, A., Jacobson, G., Beninger, M. S., & Newman, C. W. (1997). The voice handicap index (VHI): Development and validation. *American Journal of Speech-Language Pathology, 6*, 66–69.

Kochman, T. (1981). *Black and white styles in conflict.* Chicago: University of Chicago Press.

Lass, N. J., Ruscello, D. M., Stout, L. L., & Hoffman, F. M. (1991). Peer perceptions of normal and voice-disordered children. *Folia Phoniatrica, 43,* 29–35.

Luchsinger, R., & Arnold, G. E. (1965). *Voice-speech-language. Clinical communicology: Its physiology and pathology.* Belmont, CA: Wadsworth.

Manolson, A. (1992). *It takes two to talk: A parent's guide to helping your child learn.* Toronto: The Hanen Center.

Manolson, A. (1995). *You make the difference in helping your child learn.* Toronto: The Hanen Center.

Nilson, H., & Schneiderman, C. R. (1983). Classroom program for the prevention of vocal abuse and hoarseness in elementary school children. *Language, Speech, and Hearing Services in the Schools, 14,* 121–127.

Parker, F. (1986). *Linguistics for non-linguists.* Boston: College-Hill Press.

Peñalosa, F. (1981). *Introduction to the sociology of language.* Rowley, MA: Newbury House.

Shaunak, S., Lakhani, S., Abraham, R., & Maxwell, J. (1986). Differences among Asian patients. *British Medical Journal* [Clinical Research], *1,* 293(6555), 1169.

Sorfman, B. (1986). Research in cultural diversity: Unidimensional measures of ethnicity. *Western Journal of Nursing Research, 8,* 467–468.

Tarone, E. (1972). *Aspects of Black English intonation.* Doctoral dissertation, University of Washington, Pulham.

Tashima, C. (1987). Americans whose forbears were Japanese. *New England Journal of Medicine, 317,* 1209.

Taylor, D. S. (1993). Intonation and accent in English: What teachers need to know. *International Review of English in Language Teaching, 31,* 1–21.

Taylor, O. L., (1986). Historical perspectives and conceptual framework. In O. L. Taylor (Ed.), *Nature of communication disorders in culturally and linguistically diverse populations.* Boston: Butterworth-Heinemann.

Taylor, O. L. (1988). *Cross cultural communication: An essential dimension of effective communication.* Washington, DC: The Mid-Atlantic Center for Race Equity, The American University.

Taylor, O. L., Payne, K. T., & Anderson, N. B. (1987). Distinguishing between communication disorders and communication differences. *Seminars in Speech and Language, 8,* 415–427.

van Keulen, J. E., Weddington, G. T., & DeBose, C. E. (1998). *Speech, language, learning and the African American child.* Boston: Allyn & Bacon.

Wheat, M. C., & Hudson, A. I. (1988). Spontaneous speaking fundamental frequency of 6-year-old black children. *Journal of Speech and Hearing Research, 31,* 1–3.

Wolfram, W. (1988). Puerto Rican speech. In L. Cole & V. R. Deal, (Eds.), *Communication disorders in multicultural populations.* Rockville, MD: American Speech-Language-Hearing Association.

Wolfram, W., & Christian, D. (1989). *Dialects and education.* Englewood Cliffs, NJ: Prentice Hall.

# 11

# CLINICAL MANAGEMENT OF VOICE DISORDERS IN CULTURALLY DIVERSE CHILDREN: THERAPY AND INTERVENTION

### RHODA L. AGIN

Therapeutic approaches are numerous and varied. The selection and application of a given method is reflective of the therapist's education, experience, and skill. The following suggestions for therapeutic techniques to eliminate or reduce voice disorders may be used with a diverse population of children from toddlers to 18-year-olds. A description of each technique is followed by considerations of cultural sensibilities that might be at risk for offense or conflict. Until such time as we have data on the efficacy of various therapeutic techniques for specific diverse populations, treatment plans based upon known and tried methods are recommended.

The array of helpful professional texts offering a rich variety of voice therapy suggestions has grown significantly in recent years (Andrews, 1995; Dworkin & Meleca, 1997; Fawcus, 1992). The therapy ideas offered can be useful in the multicultural environment with the caveat of the need for alertness to cultural sensitivity. The successful completion of vocal behavior change may not be a reaction to the method chosen but rather the degree to which there was compliance (Verdolini-Marston, Burke, Lessac, Glaze, & Caldwell, 1995). As always, the likelihood of achieving compliance is influenced by the motivation of the client.

## CREATING AN ARCHITECTURE FOR
## MAXIMIZING THERAPY OUTCOME

Every therapist develops with experience. Many of the techniques we use as speech therapists are extensions or revised applications of what "worked" with another client. Therefore, the reader may find some of the following fundamental points relevant to treatment for other speech disorders, and as experienced therapists you may have developed your own structure for optimizing children's therapy experiences. The following holistic perspective is an element of this author's teaching style and tendency toward comprehensiveness. It is recommended that the following elements be discussed with the voice team in all cases, irrespective of cultural orientation. However, it is incumbent on the therapist to appreciate the unfamiliar or strange nature of some of these points and the total acceptability of others given a particular cultural milieu. Informed judgment is the therapist's ally when serving a culturally diverse population.

*Treatment enablers* are those elements of the therapeutic process that serve to facilitate productivity. Optimizing the learning experience for each client is the therapist's paramount consideration. Inexperienced clinicians seek to follow a progression of steps in a series of techniques to rehabilitate a particular client. Seasoned therapists learn to appreciate the overall shape or structure of the therapy hour and experience. Several enablers follow with commentary about the cultural imperatives that may influence them. Incongruence in the therapist's selection of the following treatment enablers with the client's culture may render therapy ineffective as a result of frustration and misunderstandings. As always, heterogeneity in personality, range of individual abilities, and personal preference will play a part in the adaptation of any method to the client.

## ORGANIZING THE TEMPORAL LEARNING
## ENVIRONMENT

How to engage in the best professional practice for pediatric voice disorders in cross-cultural environments such as schools, hospitals, and community clinics is also not evident in the professional literature. Adoption of a strategy of viewing the voice difficulty and the need for treatment from the child-client perspective will aid compliance. With increasing frequency, we as clinicians are encouraged to examine our own cultural experiences and through analysis gain appreciation of how tradition, religion, folk-beliefs, and other cultural cornerstones characterize our communication (Cheng, 1996). We all have a natural tendency to prefer our own culturally infused linguistic style.

Although a worthy ideal, bias-free communication is not natural. Each of us experiences the world filtered through our own culture. Both learning styles and cognitive styles are culture-bound. In addition, we see individual variation in learning styles, for example, reflexive versus impulsive. What we are able and expected to do is create a respectful and productive learning environment through a wider knowledge of the features of the diverse cultures present in our work settings today.

## Time of Day

Selecting the *time of day for therapy* requires some consideration of vocal quality during the course of a day. In the average adult, the normal voice tends to alter during the course of the day. It tends to be weak, low-pitched, and poor in quality during the hour or so after awakening. Within a few hours it is strong and clear, and remains so until the late afternoon or early evening when pitch may drop slightly and general vocal energy may wane. Although we have no research to support this thinking, children may experience the same cycle to a lesser degree. Young children may nap in the afternoon and the voice may be fatigued before the nap and restored shortly thereafter.

It has been a practice in my therapy method to routinize the schedule of the therapy hour until the last few appointments for treatment. At that time, the therapy hour is varied to test the reliability of the new behaviors at other times of the day. At the outset of therapy, it is best to see and hear the voice at its worst. In this way, the clinician learns how poorly the voice sounds and how difficult it is for the client to modify the voice problem.

Since all human cultures vary in their communication attributes and define them differently, be prepared to experience cultural conflicts in the form of tardiness, forgetting to come to therapy, absences for family obligations and work, and choosing not to attend speech therapy because of concern for missing out on classroom activities, especially language learning.

## Length of Therapy

The *length of the therapy session* is variable with one exception: It must be long enough to assure time for sufficient correct productions of the behaviors to be changed. If the client does not experience sufficient trials or opportunities to "do it right," the correct behavior will be extinguished.

This topic has generated vigorous controversy, especially with regard to children under eight years of age. The anecdotal evidence suggests that young children have difficulty concentrating.

## Structure of Therapy Time

*Structuring the therapy session* (Agin, 1989) is an often-neglected enabler providing several advantages for the learning process. By structuring each therapy session to include a beginning, middle, and end, expectations are kept in check and accomplishments become apparent. The following progression of tasks is recommended:

1. *Spontaneous speech.* Casual conversation to note carryover of previously learned behaviors.
2. *Review of homework.* Monitor, reinforce, and reward practice.
3. *New material.* Introduce one to three new behaviors in varied activities.
4. *Assign new homework.* Fifteen to twenty minutes of daily practice is essential for progress; therefore, homework is specifically written or taped into the child's speech notebook. Instructions and objectives of each exercise in the assignment are simply and precisely written to the client. If the child is unable to read the assignment, a sibling or parent is enlisted for this role.
5. *Ending the session.* Complimenting the child in front of a parent or other member of the voice team at the session's end gives the child a feeling of success. A small reward for good participation assures motivation to practice and return again.

Goals, tasks, conditions, and results are each pertinent elements of the session, too. However, the organization of the time spent with the child-client can optimize the productivity and smooth functioning of the hour.

## Consistency

Allied with a structured design for the therapy session is *consistency*. Therapy is not ordinarily a familiar learning process to children or their families. The small group or one-to-one relationship plus seemingly unusual exercises may be particularly suspect to parents from diverse cultures. It can make any child anxious. Therefore, building consistency or a routine progression from one part of the session to the next is comforting to the client. This orderliness would also apply to the regular appearance of certain activities, for example, blowing bubbles to improve breath control and breath focus. Young children, especially, look forward to an enjoyable task or game during each session.

## Criteria for Success

*Criteria for success* are often a point of contention among university supervisors. Student clinicians frequently note the disparity between supervisors when deciding about both the accuracy level and when to the upgrade therapy tasks. Working at high level of accuracy generates the following controversy: Is the skill level good enough for most communication needs? or Should the youngster achieve the highest possible skill level to increase the likelihood of average usage on "off days"?

All individuals occasionally experience an off day. These times usually occur when we are distracted, ill, moody, or fatigued. If one works to maximum potential in polishing a new vocal or breathing skill, then on the off days, the skill is utilized at an average level. If one's best performance is only at an average skill level, then an off day will leave the client with a less than average or unsatisfactory vocal habit.

## Client Notebook/Taking Notes and Drawing Pictures

The child's speech book serves multiple roles. It is the record of the progress made in treatment, the depository of all the materials and rewards earned during the course of the child's therapeutic experience, and a means of keeping the parents informed of the substance of therapy. To assure the arrival of homework at the home and the preservation of materials given to the child, a hard-covered notebook with lined pages is recommended. All games, drill sheets, drawings, pictures, stamps, and so on are securely taped or glued or stapled onto the pages therein.

## Practice aka Homework, Homework, Homework

The experience of *practicing* a newly learned vocal behavior is the primary facilitator of applying the new voice in daily communication or what is typically referred to as "carryover." The importance and effect of doing this routinized experience cannot be overemphasized. Not only does practice provide speed and smooth adjustments of apparent technical skill, it can induce inner changes as well. Acton (1984), stated

> Not only does personality and emotional state show in pronunciation . . . , but the converse is also true: Speakers can control their nerves and inner states by speaking properly. This is a basic tenet of successful programs in voice training and public speaking

(Lessac, 1967). By focusing on posture breathing and general body tension, or by using biofeedback techniques for controlling heart rate and blood pressure, the speakers' perception of their internal, emotional, or affective states are changed, and these changes, in turn, serve to influence those same internal states even further. (p. 75)

Thus, the ramifications of practice are at least twofold and beneficial, if not critical, for carryover. However important the benefits might be, effectuating practice in a child's daily life is often difficult. Practice often competes with a variety of sports and social activities or household responsibilities. In addition, practice tends to be informal with regard to when it is to occur, how long or how often to do it, where one should practice, and who is responsible for remembering to practice. When practice is structured into a homework assignment, it has the best chance of being put into effect.

It is a basic proposition of this author's voice therapy method that the degree to which a youngster does his or her homework corresponds to the pace at which he or she completes therapy. Therefore, if homework becomes the client's accepted responsibility, it puts the client in control of concluding voice training and returning to "normal." Homework is best accomplished when specifically and simply assigned in writing to be approximately 15 minutes in length and done twice each day, once before leaving the home in the morning and again before dinner each evening. In some households, homework is not a customary learning method.

## *Awareness*

Often a youngster has a little or no awareness of the various respiratory and vocal dynamics that are not serving him or her well. For example, breath control and breath support may be uncoordinated or insufficient for the child's speech needs. We see this problem when a child continues to talk on one breath without resupplying the airstream by pausing and taking a breath at appropriate points in an utterance. Instead, the child goes on until he or she is breathless (a bit red in the face), and pitch as well as volume and quality has degenerated. To reverse this lack of awareness, *heighten sensitivities* to the changes that you seek. "Feel, See, Listen, and Move" are the bywords this author typically uses with young children to increase awareness of respiratory and vocal dynamics. "Feeling the voice" might include the movement of the stomach outward for inhalation or the placement of the thumb and forefinger over the right and left lamina of the thyroid cartilage to feel vocal cord vibration.

Just as voice therapy techniques are often thought to be universally appropriate, so too are *learning modalities*. Elsewhere in this text, the reader will find an overview of diversity and learning styles. Suffice it to say here that a child may prefer one learning modality versus another and some cultures have a tendency toward the use of one learning modality versus another. For example, most people are familiar with the importance of visual skills among Native American cultures and the importance of reading and book learning among Jewish people. In the absence of information about a preferred modality for a given youngster, a multimodality approach should be considered. In addition, a multimodality approach is helpful when attempting to teach behaviors generated from a source which is difficult to see and understand, such as the larynx.

The use of multiple modalities activities such as same/different, identification, auditory contrast, visual contrast, kinesthetics, and tactile contrast could all be utilized when teaching the meaning and appearance of relaxation. A significant number of youngsters with voice problems caused by vocal abuse are often tense when speaking, exhibiting taut laryngeal strap muscles. One helpful exercise that may teach a child how relaxed muscles feel is the following: After confirming that touching and holding the child's hand by the clinician is an acceptable behavior in his or her culture, the therapist would ask the child to raise his or her arm straight out in front and make a tight fist. Then the therapist, holding up the wrist of the outstretched arm with an open hand, asks the child to release the fist and drop the arm. The weight of the arm falls into the therapist's hand and the child feels the tension dissipate immediately. With several repetitions and modeling by the therapist, the feeling of relaxation can be learned and subsequently applied to the muscles of the neck. The matter of touching is considered later in this chapter.

Learning modalities may also be affected by socioeconomics and health; thus, we should be cautious about using them without checking the condition of the modality. We customarily use the audio-perceptual mode to train a new pitch or vocal quality. However, hearing acuity may vary significantly among different racial groups. Therefore, all children cannot be relied upon to respond exactly the same way when the therapist models a particular pitch, volume, or quality to be imitated by a given child. For example, we know that the Native American population has more otitis media than Asian Americans, Caucasians, and African Americans. They have increased otorhea, perforated eardrums, and complications to ear infections. Among African Americans, hypertension and sickle cell anemia are related to ear disease (Agin, 1992). This information alerts us to the possibility that certain racially/culturally diverse youngsters will not have the same preferences in learning modality. In both examples, relying upon auditory skills to teach new vocal behaviors to children from two cultural groups could undermine a youngster's success in learning. Additionally, these youngsters may not typically complain about the poor health of their ears or vision because they are accustomed to its poor functioning.

## Self-Monitoring

In the context of therapy, once a new behavior is taught, the client needs to continue to use it correctly. The process referred to as self-monitoring is the way the client compares his or her incorrect pattern to the desired one. More specifically, *self-monitoring* is the ability to consciously use a new behavior and reflect on it, judging the extent to which the new behavior was incorporated into a given utterance. Successful training of self-monitoring should start in the first therapy session. By so doing, the client learns that, ultimately, he or she is the therapist outside the therapy room. This means that the client is responsible for the application of new behaviors and the arbiter of correctness in all environments.

Most of the literature about the training of self-monitoring is found in the articulation literature pronunciation training literature (Acton, 1984). When training the youngster to use a new pitch or diaphragmatic breathing, for example, often the subtlety of the behavior makes for difficulty in monitoring. Therefore, it is reasonable to seek assistance to enable the child to succeed in this practice. So, in addition to auditory self-monitoring, it is recommended to use visual, tactile, or kinesthetic (Acton, 1984) self-monitoring.

An example of tactile self-monitoring highlights the need for varied ways of regulating oneself. A youngster with a weak voice caused by low vocal energy characterized by mild breathiness learned that by placing the pads of two fingers on the neck slightly above the thyroid notch, she will feel the vibration of the true vocal cords. Once she learns to increase and decrease the vibration at will, monitoring the strength of the vibration is made easy via the tactile feedback of her fingers. To rely on an auditory assessment for every youngster would not respect the different ways we prefer to learn. Acton (1984, p. 78) summarizes, "as long as they can 'remember' the physical sensations, they can be led to practice the 'feel' of the distinction until they themselves begin to hear it."

## TREATMENT METHODS FOR VOICE DISORDERS

For the purposes of this chapter, it is assumed that prior to selecting a treatment approach, the clinician has (1) taken a case history of the disorder; (2) recorded a self-description of the voice; (3) inquired about medical or pharmacological intervention to the head, neck, or chest (e.g., breathing can be disturbed by allergies); (4) evaluated all vocal dynamics by perceptual measure, acoustic analysis, and aerodynamic measures; (5) noted vocal hygiene, including participation in speaking and/or singing activities/clubs; (6) tape recorded samples of speech in reading, conversation, and singing; (7) inquired about previous therapy/singing lessons; (8) checked stimulability for changing vocal behavior; (9) determined appropriate treatment goals; and (10) determined a prognosis for behavior change.

The realities of otolaryngological opinion should not be overlooked (Haller & Thompson, 1975; Haynes & Pindzola, 1998). A pre-therapy laryngological examination, either indirect (mirror) or direct (endoscopic), provides a baseline to serve as a comparison for the changing condition of the vocal mechanism as therapy progresses. A routine report of a laryngeal examination should include the appearance and function of the true and false vocal cords at rest and in phonation, as well as the condition of supraglottic contours and mucosa. A laryngostroboscopic visualization will provide details about the nature of vibration, including the condition of the glottic wave. Although skills and choice of viewing instrumentation vary among physicians, an ear, nose, and throat consultation may be the key to a successful voice evaluation and subsequent treatment (Glaze, 1996).

The successful voice diagnostician and therapist should understand the cause, nature, and extent of the vocal symptoms that interfere with communication and/or pose a danger to one's health. At this point in this chapter, it is clear that culture can influence the perception of symptoms. Gandour and colleagues' (Gandour, Weinberg, Petty, & Dardaranda, 1988) work on the "normal" breathiness in Thai and Loveday's (1981) study of pitch in Japanese speakers are examples of the relative subjective nature of these perceptions. It follows then that there is also diversity in problem-solving systems. In other words, our present assumptions underlying current clinical practices with respect to voice therapeutics may not always be appropriate. If we are to effectively assess and treat vocal pathologies in this multicultural society, we need to determine the degree to which the norms established on European peoples and cultures of the nineteenth century may remain the guideposts for service or must be altered to reflect the present and growing population diversity in the United States (Agin, 1990).

Will all parents/guardians follow through on a recommendation to secure an otolarngologic examination? The answer to this question is dependent upon the family's orientation to western medical intervention, the other options they have available to them, the cultural worldview - vis-à-vis the handling of illness, and the impression of the authority figure making the referral.

## THERAPEUTIC TECHNIQUES

Almost all voice therapies begin with two therapeutic objectives, depending upon whether hoarseness is present. The first objective is to *establish the healthiest vocal mechanism* possible before vocal exercises and other activities begin. If the cause of the voice disorder is vocal abuse or misuse, it might be possible to improve the health of the vocal cords without formally resting the voice or not speaking. If a misuse is the predominantly presenting vocal behavior or the condition of the cords is poor, then *vocal rest* is recommended (Agin, 1993). This author uses the analogy of the injured baseball player to explain the concept of vocal rest to children. Once the athlete has hurt his arm, he must rest it before it can be exercised back into playing condition. He should not exercise a painful or weak arm. Resting the arm will permit it to heal. Children usually understand and appreciate this analogy.

Although controversial, the interruption of speech has two benefits to the client with a voice disorder. First, vocal rest offers significant healing of abused true vocal cord mucous membrane. Appropriate application of vocal rest depends upon the severity of the pathological condition of the cords and the age of the child. A game-like format for vocal rest can be used, such as rewarding the child for each 30 minutes of rest. Should the child slip into speech inadvertently, a brief reminder by the listener would easily return the youngster to rest.

The second objective is *awareness of the aberrant symptom and how it differs from the norm:* how we make a youngster aware of his or her unpleasant voice or a potentially dangerous vocal behavior, and how we talk about it. Andrews (1975) suggested the avoidance of negative descriptors such as "wrong" or "bad," because the voice is so closely associated with a child's identity. Instead, the word "different" or a similarly neutral word be used. However, a Japanese or Chinese child might not find the term "different" dispassionate. Being separated from one's peers is not valued and may be a source of concern. Contrastingly, an African American child may even value being exceptional. Here again, the therapist's word choice may be the initiator of a supportive or a biased attitude in the therapeutic session from the outset.

As we seek to accomplish therapy objectives and subsequent goals, it is helpful to be reminded of influential variables considered in Chapter 10 including sensitivity to cultural diversity in matters of gender, age appropriate behavior, and comfort level in the therapy process. To be specific consider the following issues.

Some techniques may seem universal, for example, clapping the hands for two to three minutes or more to give the client a sense of the fatigue caused by ongoing vocal hyperfunction (Greene, 1998, p. 23). At first glance, this behavior appears suitable and quite benign to the mainstream Anglo therapist's orientation. However, it may seem odd to the Cambodian child who comes to the United States after three years in a refugee camp in Thailand. The Cambodian child may associate clapping the hands with praise; however, not having had the American kindergarten and first-grade experience, which is known for lots of clapping to rhythms and music to facilitate learning, the Cambodian child may need to learn about other kinds of clapping.

Let us proceed through a brief survey of voice therapy techniques often used for the pediatric population and note areas of cultural conflict that may interfere with therapy.

## Breathing Exercises

Breathing exercises carried out in various positions often comprise the foundation task to improve the voice for many youngsters with voice disorders. As the reader will recall, there are three types of breathing: clavicular, thoracic, and diaphragmatic. Although diaphragmatic breathing is our natural breathing method, breathing method is dependent upon the activity in which the body is engaged. In aerobic activities, clavicular and thoracic breathing provide a fast and increased volume of air. Diaphragmatic breathing is generally accepted as best for speech and singing. It provides the most efficient and beneficial use of the breath. However, we usually do not take full advantage of the method and breathe shallowly. Further, individuals use the other breathing methods for speech in addition to diaphragmatic breathing. If a child is asked to take a breath, he or she will probably raise the shoulders and expand the chest in an exaggerated fashion. Often, if asked to breath and say a phrase, the child will breathe and then exhale the air before speaking. There is little awareness that air is the medium for speech (voice followed by articulation). If it is exhaled before speech begins, then voice cannot be made. Therefore, most intervention plans target breathing before attempting changes in pitch volume or quality.

When we teach diaphragmatic breathing, we show the technique, pointing out the absence of clavicular and thoracic activity, and model the anterior movement of the stomach and abdomen by putting one hand on the stomach and the other on the abdomen. Then the therapist asks the child-client to place his or her hands on the stomach and abdomen as modeled by the therapist, and the therapist applies gentle hand pressure on the child's hands, reinforcing the in and out desired movement.

One way to challenge the newly learned breathing skills is to breathe for various lengths of time and in various positions, adding arm and trunk movements—for example, the "rag doll," or what this author calls the "bending" exercise. The slow roll-down of the head and shoulders to a position of hanging from the waist in this kind of exercise requires less-than-dignified body movements that may be perceived as odd for adolescents who may feel to old for that kind of physical activity. Certainly, the name of the activity could be at odds with cultural sensibilities. These exercises serve as a foundation for subsequent vocal exercises. Note anxiety-based or "trying too hard" efforts to accomplish a particular task, for example, holding the breath while thinking.

## Mouth-opening Exercises

Mouth-opening exercises can be used in various ways: with or without sound, for syllables or words, and in association with other activities. Most voice therapists use the "yawn-sigh" technique to resolve tension problems in the facial musculature, improve oral resonance, and reduce the extra tension that trying hard sometimes causes. Exaggerated mouth opening is the key to the yawn. Most Asian and Southeast Asian women would tend to be uncomfortable with these exercises. In Japan and Vietnam, for example, women tend not to be as verbal and outspoken as American and European women. Lip movement is minimal and laughing among women typically initiates the hand being brought up to cover the lips. Indeed, yawning in front of a venerated authority figure such as the voice therapist may be quite impolite and embarrassing for an Asian American child.

An activity that requires watching a particular part of the face for specific movements, such as in mouth opening, can be problematic for those children who are taught not to look directly at an adult of the opposite sex. Looking at the models provided by the therapist is essential to learn accurate positions; looking away from the therapist's models could cause the client to miss a helpful cue. Problems can arise in the African American community, where it is a sign of respect to look down when spoken to by an adult. In addition, in Native American cultures, an adult female teacher inadvertently looking at the eyes of a male child to shape specific vowels can imply sexual overtones.

## Sighing, Gliding Vowels, and Exercises to Widen Pitch Range

Sighing, gliding vowels, and other exercises used to widen a narrow pitch range typically require exaggerated high-pitch activity. Using a high pitch for any purpose might be uncomfortable for a male youngster who originates from a traditional male-dominated society such as in the Hispanic and Japanese cultures. In these cultures women have traditionally developed a relatively high and soft voice. The following example of a gliding exercise employs a series of phonically written English vowels. Please note that in the instance where one is working with a child whose first language is not English, it may be easier to use fewer and/or more familiar vowels in the child's first language. The point of the activity is to begin the widening of the vocal range by utilizing a natural voice behavior such as sighing.

1. Begin by asking the child for a light sigh as if he or she has been carrying something heavy and just put it down. Accompany the request with your model.
2. Gradually shape your mouth into the vowels—ah, eh, oo, oh, ay, ih, uh, aeh, ee—and ask for three imitations of each.
3. Convert the light breathy sigh to a phonated glide and apply to each vowel.
4. For increasing the upper pitch range, start at the top of the client's present range and glide downward in small increments, one of two tones at a time. This is always difficult for those of us who do not have an ear for the musical scale and have limited ability to carry a tune. However, pitch direction (when to go up and when to go down) is the significant point here and not the accuracy of the pitch.

## Voice Projection Exercises

Voice projection activities such as the "calling" technique require exaggerated mouth opening during the learning process and usually some permanent increase in mouth opening. The calling technique gives the speaker the impression of loudness and increased oral resonance. The preparation for succeeding at a projection exercise includes activities to

1. Increase breath support.
2. Raise pitch.
3. Increase duration of vowels.
4. Exaggerate lip movement.
5. Raise volume as a last resort, if the previous changes in behavior have not succeeded in obtaining the desired improvement in projection.

An example of a calling exercise follows:

1. Try to apply each of the elements in the voice projection activities above, one at a time, to the following words/phrases and note the effect on projection. Each word receives three attempts:

| | | |
|---|---|---|
| GO | SAIL | AWAY |
| HELLO | TOMORROW | BEHIND ME |
| WHERE ARE YOU | LEAVE IT ALONE | OPEN UP THE BOX |

2. Repeat step 1, but this time project the voice to three different marked distances in the room.
3. Last, repeat the exercise incorporating three, then four, then five of the elements above, always starting with increased mouth opening.
4. Apply the newly learned behavior to different and longer stimuli.

A caution: Culturally sensitive directives could be attached to each of the tasks in the previous projection technique. For example, a teenage Hispanic male from Mexico might find high-pitched exercises as unseemly for a male. Children of the Thai culture, who tend to be quieter in demeanor than mainstream Anglo-American youngsters, would probably be uncomfortable doing a projection exercise. Last, a Native American youngster might be unfamiliar with the repetitive nature of the voice training process—learning and refining several progressive tasks to achieve the final goal of a well-projected voice.

## Units of Practice

### Rote Drills
Counting and alphabet recitation provide rote, easy words to practice the accuracy of the new voice or breathing pattern. Words, phrases, and sentences, known and then unknown, provide a progression of difficulty with which to apply the new behaviors. Here again, cultural sensitivity is a requisite for effective voice therapy. Just as every child does not play chess or monopoly, so too drills and word lists may not be customary learning approaches in a given culture. Careful preparatory explanation and gradual shaping of the technique, particularly increased mouth opening, would be essential.

### Dialogue, Reading Aloud, Storytelling, and Psychodrama
Creative drama and language learning experiences provide effective clinical techniques to promote speech and language learning for many disorders including voice (Bush, 1978). Practicing dialogue, reading aloud, speaking on the telephone, storytelling, psychodrama, and communicating in public are all activities designed to facilitate carryover. Reading aloud trains the auditory and kinesthetic modalities. Psychodrama helps therapists to be guided by the clients' concerns and interests. Roles may

be reversed by suggesting to the child, "you be the teacher and I'll be the pupil." Active and naturalistic methods promote the learning and reinforcement of contemporary patterns. According to Weiss (1992), the use of acting for vocal exercises can help an individual sound more like a native speaker in the second language. Physically or psychologically taking the child out of the therapy room for carryover activities provides a reality check for the new vocal and/or breathing skills.

## Cueing

In therapy, cueing provides a suggestion or a hint of the behavior sought. Clinicians use a variety of cues to facilitate or retrieve the correct response. We might move our lips, raise a finger, utter a sound or initial syllable, tap part of a pattern on the table, touch the arm or hand, and so on. Obviously, a particular movement that is quite acceptable in one culture may be taboo in another. For example, while sitting in therapy or at a parent conference with one leg crossed, it is likely that the sole of your shoe would face upward in view of others present and thus be considered rude by a traditional Arab family. Also, certain hand waving and finger movements used for animals in Southeast Asian cultures could be misconstrued if used with children and considered vulgar. According to van Keulen, Weddington, and DeBose (1998), among African Americans touching is reserved for family and very close friends (p. 217). According to Adler and King (1994), "in some Asian cultural groups, a smile is reserved only for very close friends or a spouse, and individuals do not smile casually at one another" (p. 84). Therefore, it appears that the assistance cueing provides is best moderated by cultural guidelines and verified in consultation with knowledgeable individuals.

Voice therapy also benefits from the aid of the cueing technique, and similar culturally specific cautions are applicable. For example, a spirited vocal style using a loud voice for emphasis might be acceptable usage in an African American interaction but seem boisterous and inappropriate with Chinese youngsters.

## Discourse Strategies

In communication the voice adds a peculiar complexity beyond the status of the laryngeal tone. Each language system includes changes in vocal and temporal dynamics, such as pitch, volume, rate, rhythm, and stress, which serve to inform persons in conversation about discourse strategies. These dynamics are typically applied in combination quite automatically. The vocal cues that signal when to start talking and when to stop are examples of language-specific discourse patterns. Catherine John Lewis (1986) considered these and other elements of discourse and the prosodic features that function as cues in the management of spoken interaction. In Lewis's review of the literature and papers included her text, she reported on studies indicating that low vocal key signals finality, and pitch height and loudness are two features that are used to effectively take over the speaking turn in English.

Understanding that there are approximately 32 million inhabitants of the United States who speak a non-English language at home (U.S. Bureau of the Census, 1995), more than 760,000 speakers of an estimated Native American languages (Leap, 1981), and unknown numbers of citizens who speak social dialects, it is likely that the pediatric population requiring therapy services for vocal disorders included in these statistics will also present diverse prosodic patterns. If we use our current knowledge of the concept of "interference" in language and language-specific schemas that are present in one language and not another and apply these to prosody, we soon realize the complexity of voice therapy in the multicultural context.

Most speakers have little formal knowledge about the discourse patterns of their own language and the prosodic features used to effect those patterns. We learn the basis of communication as toddlers and young children and they become automatic. The literature in prosody management does not alert speech therapists to the complexity of training a child with an other than English first language or social dialect.

## Silence in Communication

One notably different means of interaction is the use of silence as a communication device. Most non-Anglo-American cultures and non-English linguistic systems assign significant value to no exchange of greeting utterances and silent pauses. In many Native American cultures, it is customary to sit together for a part of an hour and work in parallel activities before engaging in conversation. A warm and vociferous greeting of the Native American parents of your client could give a negative impression.

Some children work slowly and carefully to perfect a task and others compete for speed of completion. Either practice may be a reflection of a youngster's personality or cultural norms.

As reported earlier in this chapter, voice therapy literature does not prepare clinicians to manage vocal pathology in linguistically diverse populations. We can see that fundamental activities employed in most therapeutic plans for vocal change afford the potential for a panoply of cultural hurdles to be overcome. However, we lack any incidence data to provide definitive solutions.

## CULTURALLY SPECIFIC PROGRAMS
## AND MATERIALS

Certainly, we are guided by our general knowledge of the young learner in the primary schools. He or she has robust curiosity, short memory, limited attention span, responsiveness to approval, a tendency to learn by doing, creativity, and linguistic skills appropriate to his or her age within his or her cultural milieu (Ohana, 1991). However, the experienced reader recognizes that knowing age-appropriate fundamentals and augmenting them with the best of intentions does not assure successful therapy. We are often stymied and disappointed when our clinical information does not seem to suffice and therapy fails. With culturally and linguistically diverse youngsters, the reason for this may be neglecting to apply cultural diversity to what we know.

In general, the literature includes recommendations to help minimize cultural conflicts for children with Limited English Proficiency (LEP). Cheng (1986) suggested that when working with children with LEP, therapy should utilize naturalistic interactions, incorporate the child's classroom subject matter, and infuse cross-cultural perspectives into therapy themes. Adler (1993) and Kayser (1995) reminded the reader of the importance of creating culturally sensitive, functional, motivating, and linguistically accessible material for youngsters with social dialects. Although specific references to vocal skills or voice therapy are not offered by these authors, these recommendations are applicable to the dysphonic pediatric client. And we can also extrapolate from children with LEP to those with social dialects.

Speech therapists typically use reading passages, poems, stories and the like as modes for practicing a new vocal behavior. Is the passage culturally relevant? How helpful is it for Haitian youngsters newly arrived in America to be reading about Paul Revere's ride in colonial American history as a practice text? Culturally specific programs and materials for children with language and phonology disorders have increased in availability. Catalogues such as Bilingual Speech Source (1997) and portions of the Academic Communication Associates (1998, pp. 89–100) are examples of these resources. The most notable increase has been in assessment materials rather than in intervention programs. Lists of these have been compiled and periodically updated by the American Speech-Language-Hearing Association and advertised in the assortment of catalogues of published materials serving the profession. However, multicultural voice improvement offerings continue to be minimal or nonexistent.

Choosing therapy materials for a culturally diverse caseload requires exploration of ethnic bookstores, neighborhood museums, and community centers. The educational materials sold in such places provide

reinforcement of the values, symbols, and history of the immediate surrounding community. Look for ethnic storybooks (for example, the Multicultural Infusion Series, edited by L. Cheng), games, toys, and charts
under the guidance of a knowledgeable salesperson. Choose pictures or
objects about holidays, known household practices, and representations
of traditional arts, crafts, and music. For example, when working with
Mexican American children and looking for culturally relevant clinical
materials, the author happened upon a toy shop in a Hispanic neighborhood. One wall of the store was filled with dolls, statuary, key chains,
puppet-like hangings, and storybooks of skeletons! The scene would very
likely seem quite odd to the average non-Mexican speech therapist. However, once the significance of the Mexican religious holiday called Day of
the Dead was explained, that wall of merchandise became meaningful
and useful.

The increased utilization of visual feedback (Fawcus, 1992, Volin,
1998), and specifically computer technology, in all therapies is also evident from the professional materials catalogues of recent years. We know
that children enjoy interaction with a computer. As yet, the greater portion of computer-generated speech therapy programs are for phonology
and language problems, not voice disorders. Minimal multicultural orientation is seen in the software technology developed for applied clinical
assessment and intervention in adult accent modification, such as Speech
Works by Blackmer and Ferrier (n.d.). A computer offers the advantages
of computer voice modeling, auditory and sensory feedback, and an interactive system to promote accelerated learning. According to Schwartz,
Brogan, Emond, and Oleksiak (1993), "By both seeing and hearing comparisons of their approximations to model utterances, speakers develop a
better understanding of what is meant by the terms such as stress, intonation, timing, or voicing. Speakers can, therefore, assume much greater
control over the modification of their own speech patterns" (p. 44).

Indications of improvement and success are essential elements of a
good learning environment. Praise, reinforcement, and student progress
charts are well known to the experienced clinician. They provide feedback to facilitate accuracy of the new behavior and motivation to continue to participate in the behavior change process. Do these indications
need to be culturally appropriate or are they universals—implying that a
pat on the shoulder or a gift of a toy or similar actions are recognized similarly by all cultures? Here again, clients from particular cultural traditions may find that strong or frequent praise of a youngster's efforts
clashes with the family's communication style. In some Asian societies,
desired behavior is expected and not especially rewarded or recognized,
and punishment is the recourse when the child exhibits unacceptable
behavior.

Last, discipline methods and standards, as well as consequences, vary notably today, even within one culture or community. In this author's twenty-five years of supervisory experience in a busy university-community clinic, approximately 60 percent of normal-hearing Anglo-American children under 6 years of age in therapy, when asked to "please sit down" by an experienced student therapist, do not do so after the first or second request. This suggests that the youngster has no expectations of negative consequences for ignoring the request from an authority figure.

## VOCAL HYGIENE

The promotion and maintenance of health and the prevention of disease is referred to as hygiene. Avoiding poor vocal hygiene is a challenge for an adult, let alone a child. Misuse, abuse, and overuse, as described at the outset of chapter 10, would be examples of poor vocal hygiene. It is easy to drift into these negative behaviors and habitualize them. The primary responsibility for changing poor vocal hygiene often rests on the engaging nature of the treatment and a highly desirable reward system. However, family involvement can provide the monitoring and encouragement necessary to guide the child when using the voice inappropriately. For example, using the voice when the larynx and pharynx are symptomatic, can cause a temporary illness to become chronic. When the voice is involved in the illness, obviously *resting the vocal mechanism* is paramount.

Overuse of a normal voice can be abusive to the vocal cords. Unfortunately, overuse is difficult to quantify because of its relativity. Making specific recommendations to guide the therapist, in the context of this chapter, is therefore impractical. It is quite possible that overuse of the voice is personality bound.

Teenagers are notorious for poor vocal hygiene. Their consumption of two to six cold soft drinks daily is ubiquitous. The drinking of warm fluids can increase circulation to the throat and facilitate healing in that area. Cold and/or carbonated drinks will decrease circulation and cool the neck and body. This state can cause dryness of the throat and retard the healing of the delicate membrane covering the vocal cords as in vocal cord nodules.

Another matter in vocal hygiene is the *use of negative behaviors* such as whispering or breathiness as part of a training method. Not all cultures recognize the progressive nature of therapy or the western logic that structures the way American therapists go about rehabilitation. For example, to eliminate the hard glottal attack, which is often the vocal abuse causing true vocal cord nodules, some therapists may encourage the use of a mild whisper, also known as a stage whisper. It could be difficult for someone from a non-mainstream Anglo culture to appreciate the benefit of doing something wrong as an initial behavior to reduce or eliminate another less desirable behavior.

In sum, the therapist is encouraged to extend his or her management skills to embrace the cultural norms of a wider diversity of clients. In all likelihood a portion of the conceptual and practical therapeutic recommendations presented here is familiar to the reader. Several of the activities described are not disorder specific but, rather, pertinent to behavior training in general. Many applications of therapeutic concepts await the scientific scrutiny of experimental verification. Nevertheless, the suggestions provided offer the experienced clinician a practical framework and specific therapy ideas for the resolution of voice problems among culturally and linguistically diverse children—an area yet to be formally addressed in the profession.

## CONCLUSION

The model for clinical encounter as presented in this chapter is client-centered. It is an eclectic and dynamic process in which the therapist responds to the child-client's need or desire to improve the voice. By virtue of this flexible stance, we are afforded the opportunity to learn from our clients. The cultural insights that we gain reinforce our ability to effectively respond to our clients' needs. Indeed, the clinical experience is also shared. Through education, experience, and intuition we as therapists plan long-term goals and short-term objectives, select therapy methods, and upgrade to more challenging tasks. The eclectic clinical process is in consonance with the multicultural environment and diverse clientele.

## STUDY QUESTIONS AND ACTIVITIES

The following case example is meant to raise points about cultural characteristics that may be preventing the successful execution of voice therapy for children of diverse cultural backgrounds. The aim of the discussion is to offer clinical insight and knowledge into the effect of normative cultural behaviors on voice therapy.

Case Example 11.1

Luis's family comes from a small city outside Manila. He was born in California to a traditional Phillipino family. A few months earlier, Luis's larynx was hit on the left side by a baseball while he was playing in the schoolyard.

Although an otolaryngologist repositioned the traumatized larynx and a minute left thyroid lamina fracture had healed, his left vocal cord appeared to be paretic. After a month of compensation therapy to reduce breathiness, 7-year-old Luis entered the speech therapist's room with his mother for a parent-therapist conference. No significant improvement in his voice had been made. Luis seemed reluctant to participate in therapy activities, although Mrs. Billman, his classroom teacher, reported that he was more responsive in her class. The rules of communication use appeared to be in conflict in the therapy room. He routinely arrived for his session at the wrong time, he would not speak the therapist's name, and there seemed to be a lack of concern by the family for the hoarseness. The therapist reviewed her methods and found them to be routine and appropriate. Out of frustration with the lack of progress, she telephoned the family's physician, Dr. Gomes, who is also of Phillipino descent. After a lengthy conversation reviewing the therapy stalemate, the therapist learned that at least three cultural norms were in conflict. What cultural issues were overlooked and how might they be discussed with the child's mother? What changes would be necessary to facilitate progress?

**Discussion:** The Philippines is said to be ethnically the most diverse country in Asia. Urban residents are often said to be very sophisticated, well-educated, and multilingual. In the region of the capital city of Manila, the use of English and Spanish are commonplace as well as Tagalog/Pilipino. However, 80 percent of the populace lives in rural areas. Luis's family came from such a town in a farming community. They came to take advantage of America's educational opportunities.

Dr. Gomes explained that the three apparent cultural norms in conflict with the therapy setting were the concept of punctuality, God's role and responsibility in life, and the informality in the student-teacher relationship. Arriving at the therapy room on time was routinely left to each pupil. In Luis's case, punctuality was not a value at home, which is characteristic of the Philippines. In general, he knew that he needed to be in therapy in the midmorning, so he always appeared, but he viewed the specific time as not important. Second, Luis's mother, although concerned, viewed the accident and subsequent voice problem in terms of destiny. In Filipino culture, God's mercy is sought to solve problems. Her seemingly inattention to her child's therapy experience was in actuality Filipino division of power of sorts. The therapist encouraged the informal use of her first name in the sessions. Status and title as well as age are valued in Filipino culture. Luis was confused as to how to regard the therapist, an authority figure and elder. Not wanting to be rude, he chose to be silent.

Once the therapist shared her understanding of these cultural norms with the parent, it was easy to make the necessary adjustments to reduce the conflicts. The clinician told Luis her last name and asked to be addressed that way. She assigned another student to pick up Luis at therapy time and invited family members to therapy to train them to reinforce new behaviors and monitor homework.

# REFERENCES

Acton, W. (1984). Changing fossilized pronunciation. *Tesol Quarterly, 18,* 71–84.

Adler, S. (1993). *Multicultural communication skills in the classroom.* Boston: Allyn & Bacon.

Adler, S., & King, D. A. (Eds.). (1994). *Oral communication problems in children and adolescents* (2nd ed.). Boston: Allyn & Bacon.

Agin, R. L. (1989). *Voice therapy for elementary, junior high, and high school pupils.* New Haven Unified School District Inservice Workshop, New Haven, CA.

Agin, R. L. (1990). *Voice disorders in culturally diverse populations.* Paper presented at ASHA Summer Institute on Multicultural Professional Education, Teaching cultural diversity within the professional curriculum, Los Angeles.

Agin, R. L. (1992). Voice disorders in diverse cultural populations. In *Testimony on research and training needs of minority persons and minority health issues.* Bethesda, MD: National Institute on Deafness and Other Communication Disorders (NIDCD) at National Institutes of Health (NIH).

Agin, R. L. (1993). *Pediatric and teen voice problems and therapeutic methods: The Agin approach.* Workshop, San Mateo County Special Education Local Plan Area (SELPA). San Mateo, CA.

Andrews, M. (1975). Some common problems encountered in voice therapy with children. *Language, Speech, and Hearing Services in the Schools, 6,* 183–187.

Andrews, M. (1995). *Manual of voice treatment: Pediatrics through geriatrics.* San Diego: Singular Publishing.

Blackmer, E. R., & Ferrier, L. (n.d.). *Speech Works: The accent reduction tool.* Campton, NH: Trinity Software.

Bush, S. (1978). Creative drama and language experiences: Effective clinical techniques. *Journal of Language, Hearing, and Speech Services in the Schools, 9*(4), 254–258.

Cheng, L. R. (1986). Intervention strategies: A multicultural approach. *Topics in Language Disorders, 9,* 84–93.

Cheng, L. R. (1996). A quest for cross-cultural communicative competence. *Topics in Language Disorders, 16,* 4.

Dworkin, J. P., & Meleca, R. J. (1997). *Vocal pathologies: Diagnosis, treatment, and case studies.* San Diego: Singular.

Fawcus, M. (Ed.). (1992). *Voice disorders and their management* (2nd ed.). San Diego: Singular.

Gandour, J., Weinberg, B., Petty, S. H., & Dardaranda, R. (1988). Tone in Thai laryngeal speech. *Journal of Speech and Hearing Disorders, 53,* 23–29.

Glaze, L. E. (1996). Treatment of voice hyperfunction in the pre-adolescent. *Language, Speech and Hearing Services in the Schools, 27,* 244–250.

Greene, J. (1998). *Once upon a just right voice.* Advanced Vocal Rehabilitation Project, California State University, Hayward.

Haller, R. M., & Thompson, E. A. (1975). Prevalence of speech, language and hearing disorders among Harlem children. *Journal of the National Medical Association, 67,* 298.

Haynes, W. O., & Pindzola, R. H. (1998). Laryngeal voice disorders. In W. O. Haynes & R. H. Pindzola (Eds.), *Diagnosis and evaluation in speech pathology.* Boston: Allyn & Bacon.

Kayser, H. (Ed.). (1995). *Bilingual speech-language pathology: A Hispanic focus.* San Diego, CA: Singular.

Leap, W. (1981). American Indian language. In C. Ferguson & S. Heath (Eds.), *Language in the USA* (pp. 116–144). New York: Cambridge University Press.

Lessac, A. (1967). *The use and training of the human voice: A practical approach to speech and voice dynamics* (2nd ed.). New York: DBS Publications.

Lewis, C. J. (1986). *Intonation in discourse.* San Diego: College Hill Press.

Loveday, L. (1981). Pitch, politeness and sexual role: An exploratory investigation into pitch correlates of English and Japanese politeness formulae. *Language and Speech, 24,* Part I, 71–89.

Ohana, J. (1991). For the new teacher in primary school. *English Teachers' Journal (Israel), 42,* 68–70.

Schwartz, A. H., Brogan, V. M., Emond, G. A., & Oleksiak, J. F. (1993, September). Technology-enhanced accent reduction. *Asha, 44–46,* 51.

U.S. Bureau of the Census. (1995). *Statistical abstract of the United States* (110th ed.). Washington, DC: U.S. Department of Commerce.

van Keulen, J. E., Weddington, G. T., & DeBose, C. E. (1998). *Speech, language, learning, and the African American child.* Boston: Allyn & Bacon.

Verdolini-Marston, K., Burke, M. K., Lessac, A., Glaze, L., & Caldwell, E. (1995). Preliminary study of two methods of treatment for laryngeal nodules. *Journal of Voice, 9,* 74–85.

Volin, R. A. (1998). The relationship between stimulability and the efficacy of visual biofeedback. *American Journal of Speech-Language Pathology, 7,* 81–90.

Weiss, W. (1992). Perception and production in accent training. *Revue-de-Phonetique-Applique, 102,* 69–82.

# 12

# MULTICULTURAL ISSUES AND SPEECH FLUENCY

## TOMMIE ROBINSON, JR. and THOMAS CROWE

The possible influence of cultural factors on speech fluency has been investigated in numerous studies. Cultural groups that have been studied include: Native Americans (Clifford, Twitchell, & Hull, 1965; Johnson, 1944a, 1944b; Lemert, 1953; Snidecor, 1947; Steward, 1960; Zimmerman, Liljeblad, Frank, & Cleeland, 1983), African Americans (Anderson, 1981; Brutten & Miller, 1988; Conrad, 1985, 1987; Ford, 1986; Goldman, 1967; Leith & Mims, 1975; Nathanson, 1969; Robinson, 1992; Robinson & Crowe, 1998), Asians (Lemert, 1962; Toyoda, 1959; Wakaba, 1983), Hispanics (Bernstein-Ratner & Benitez, 1985; Dale, 1977; Jayaram, 1983; Nwokah, 1988; Travis, Johnson, & Shover, 1981), and other speaker groups (Aron, 1962; Bullen, 1945; Ralston, 1981). Results of these studies generally suggest that cultural differences influence speech fluency and that there are differences in perceptions, beliefs, values, and norms about speech fluency and fluency disorders among various cultural groups. One possible significance of these suggestions is that cultural factors might appreciably affect the outcomes of clinical intervention with fluency disorders.

Each day clinicians are faced with providing speech and language services to culturally and linguistically diverse populations. Clinicians and researchers have attempted to address this issue by providing models for service delivery in various clinical settings and with various cultures (Seymour, 1986; Seymour & Seymour, 1977; Taylor, 1986, 1987; Taylor &

Payne, 1983; Taylor & Samara, 1985; Vaughn-Cooke, 1983, 1986). These models, for the most part, have been discussed relative to non-biased assessment of speech articulation and language development and disorders with little reference to the treatment process. More recently, attention has been given to the influence of cultural factors on the evaluation and treatment of stuttering (Cooper & Cooper, 1993; Watson & Kayser, 1994).

The purpose of this chapter is to provide clinicians with tips and techniques that have been and can be used to address the differences that are seen among various cultural groups when providing assessment and treatment for stuttering. While the examples presented in this chapter are specific to African American children, the intervention model described is appropriate for use with clients of any culture.

## ISSUES IN SERVICE DELIVERY

Although a limited number of models have been developed for service delivery to multicultural populations, there have been several that are noteworthy. The focus of these models is summarized in Table 12-1.

Taylor and Samara (1985) offered a model for service delivery that addresses underserved persons of color in developing nations. They cite cultural, political, health, educational, and professional domains as barriers to service delivery. They indicate that within some societies, it is believed that little or nothing should be done about communication disorders, except to keep them hidden from the public. Although this model does not include suggestions for clinical application, it serves to increase clinicians' awareness of critical issues in service delivery to multicultural populations.

Taylor (1986) stated that there are four processes that operate within the constraints of culture to influence clinical outcomes. They are (1) developmental issues, (2) precursors of communication pathology, (3) assessment/diagnosis, and (4) treatment. The first two processes concern the nature of communication disorders within a cultural group, while the other two address issues of clinical intervention. Taylor indicated that within any cultural group, developmental processes provide the foundation for understanding the nature and most effective treatment of communication disorders. Two levels of development were presented: (1) development within the indigenous culture and (2) optional development of external cultural, cognitive, language, and communication behavior. Taylor then described the two major precursors to the emergence of communication pathology as "culturally defined pathological behaviors" (p. 12) and abnormal or unsatisfactory biological, social, psychological,

**TABLE 12-1** Various Models of Multicultural Service Delivery

| Author(s) | Evaluation | Treatment | Counseling | Transfer | Application to Stuttering |
|---|---|---|---|---|---|
| Taylor & Payne (1983) | √ | | | | Suggests a thorough examination and understanding of the culture prior to the speech fluency evaluation process. |
| Taylor & Samara (1985) | √ | | √ | | Expands clinicians' knowledge of critical issues in service delivery to multicultural populations, especially barriers that may impact on stuttering, such as political, cultural, health, educational, and professional. |
| Taylor (1986) | √ | | √ | | Suggests understanding the nature of stuttering within the cultural groups and involves the community in determining acceptable and nonacceptable stuttering patterns. |
| Taylor (1987) | √ | √ | | | Clinicians must be aware of cultural differences—both verbal and nonverbal—that are brought to the clinical encounter by the clinician and the client. |
| Vaughn-Cooke (1983, 1986) | √ | | | | Develops alternative ways to assure that a representative sample of the child's stuttering is presented and suggests ways to eliminate penalties. |
| Cooper & Cooper (1993) | | √ | √ | | Evaluates attitudes and values relative to the client's culture in order to provide effective treatment. |
| Watson & Kayser (1994) | √ | | | | Suggests techniques for the evaluation of bilingual/bicultural children and adults who stutter. |

nutritional, and genetic factors that are known to contribute to the development of communication pathology. The issue of assessment is addressed by Taylor, calling for culturally and linguistically valid testing to determine the communication pathology in specific cultures or language groups. He recommended that treatment be approached within the context of the client's culture with respect to culture-based values, beliefs, learning style, and attitudes.

Later, Taylor (1987) expanded the components of the model described above to include intercultural dimensions of service delivery to multicultural populations. This frequently cited model asserts that clinicians must maintain a cross-cultural perspective in order to provide accountable services. Taylor suggested that in every clinical encounter there exists the potential of underlying cultural influences that is represented equally by the client and the clinician and is reflected in their interaction. Three major aspects of this potential cultural influence were addressed: (1) cultural assumptions—for example, values, beliefs, attitudes, perceptions, and communicative norms; (2) [a] verbal behaviors—for example, language or dialect, prosodic features, speech acts, and so forth; [b] nonverbal behaviors—for example, eye behaviors, body movements, spatial relationships, and so forth; and (3) rules of interaction that include turn-taking, interruption, silence, conversation, and so forth.

# SERVICE DELIVERY MODELS

## Assessment

Vaughn-Cooke (1983, 1986) provided a model for assessing language in minority children. She points out a number of issues to consider in the evaluation of nonmainstream English speakers, such as including a small percentage of minorities in the standardization sample when developing a test, using a language sample when assessing the language of non-mainstream speakers, and using criterion-referenced measures when assessing the language of nonmainstream speakers. Vaughn-Cooke's suggestions for resolving these issues can easily be applied to the assessment of stuttering. However, this model was designed to address evaluation only and does not include suggestions for the treatment process.

Taylor and Payne (1983) presented a model that represents a proactive approach to evaluation of communication disorders. This suggests that culturally valid or nonbiased assessment can be achieved by preventing situational bias in testing, bias in presenting test directions or test format bias, culture/social value bias, and linguistic bias. The authors provide clinical examples of how to address these issues in the evaluation process; however, limited attention is given in this model to treatment of communication disorders.

Watson and Kayser (1994) presented a comprehensive differential assessment model for dealing with bilingual and bicultural children and adults who stutter. The premise of their approach is to assess the client and his or her environment relative to: (1) identifying a potential problem that would persist without intervention; (2) understanding the nature of the problem in a variety of communicative contexts in light of the influence of physiological, sociocultural, and linguistic variables; and (3) developing a course of action for intervention. The authors stressed that throughout the course of intervention, clinicians must address (1) the client's environment and cultural information; (2) the client's communication skills, including fluency; and (3) the attitudes of the client and significant others.

## Intervention

One of the earliest models for addressing a culturally diverse population was developed by Seymour and Seymour (1977). They designed a therapeutic model for interacting with children who speak African American English and who have communication disorders. This model is based on a framework in which normal communicative behavior encompasses linguistic features that characterize African American English. Children's utterances are classified as variant or invariant with Standard English or African American English and are determined to be developmental or pathological based on normative referents.

Seymour (1986) expanded on the earlier model and proposed clinical principles upon which clinical intervention strategies may be established for children who are language disordered and who are also of nonstandard English environments. The six principles assert that intervention strategies represent language models that are (1) multidimensional, (2) interactive, (3) generative, (4) child-centered, (5) bidialectal, and (6) diagnostic.

Cooper and Cooper (1993) presented a model that can be applied to the stuttering treatment process. Their culturally sensitive stuttering therapy process involves four stages that are applied during use of the *Personalized Fluency Control Therapy-Revised* (Cooper & Cooper, 1985) program. The four stages are as follows: (1) Structuring Stage—the clinician assists the client in enhancing fluency-facilitating feelings, attitudes, and behavior; (2) Targeting Stage—the clinician asks the client to modify the behaviors identified in the first stage; (3) Adjusting Stage—the clinician reinforces appropriate feelings and attitudes as well as fluency; and

(4) Regulating Stage—the clinician guides the client into using treatment techniques during life situations. The focus on client attitudes in these stages of treatment conforms with Taylor's (1986) suggestion that attitudes and values identified with specific cultures are important to consider in treatment design.

## A DECISION MODEL FOR ADDRESSING MULTICULTURAL VARIABLES IN STUTTERING INTERVENTION PROGRAMMING

This chapter presents a model for evaluating and treating stuttering in African American children. Although this chapter focuses on African American children, the model can be used with multicultural populations in general. Figure 12-1 provides an overview of this model in which decisions about multicultural programming are represented in six levels of counseling and therapy (Robinson & Crowe, 1994). In the schematic in Figure 12-1, the solid arrows represent the possible directions through the intervention process. The broken arrows indicate that a client's progress through the levels is not necessarily linear, in that previous levels may often need to be revisited to address additional cultural factors. At each level decisions are made about which cultural factors should be addressed at that level.

Clinicians should be cautious in interpreting and applying the information presented in this model so as not to stereotype clients and their families. Clinicians should remember that individual differences within cultures do exist (Taylor, 1986; van Kleeck, 1994) and realize that this chapter's content is not intended to recommend a cookbook approach to intervention with all African American clients and their families.

Consideration of cultural variables should begin when clients or their families first contact clinical centers to schedule evaluations or merely to obtain information. Clinical intervention for treatment of stuttering should be structured within the context of each client's cultural system and cultural environment in order for therapy to be maximally effective and also for therapy to be efficient in regard to time spent setting and achieving goals. Clinicians' attention to these cultural dimensions of the therapy relationship also will increase the probability that counseling for prevention of stuttering will be effective (Crowe, 1995).

*Cultural system* pertains to all that comprises the belief systems of clients. This includes values, attitudes, perceptions, myths, and so on, and to a large extent these culture-based factors determine the perceived reality in which clients operate. The client's perceptions of reality may or may not match the clinician's; if their perceptions do not match, there is

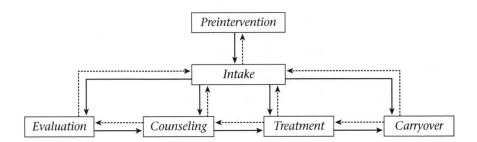

DECISION LEVEL I
Preintervention

---

• Cultural identification
• Age and gender
• Communication norms

DECISION LEVEL II
Intake

---

• General disorder typing
• Specific cultural variables relative to stuttering
  • Myths
  • Attitudes
  • Terminology
  • Beliefs

DECISION LEVEL III
Evaluation

---

• Cultural adjustment modification
  1. Nonverbal behaviors
  2. Verbal language/interaction
  3. Visual stimuli
• Cognitive learning styles
• Parental-child interaction styles
• Client clinical interaction styles

DECISION LEVEL IV
Parent/Client Counseling

---

• Rules for interaction
• The family unit
  1. Relative to cultural identity
  2. Relative to residential history
  3. Relative to generational factors
• Importance of language spoken in the home

DECISION LEVEL V
Treatment

---

• Build cultural-based factors into therapy goals/techniques

DECISION LEVEL VI
Carryover/Generalization

---

• Utilize the home unit
• Utilize peers
• Utilize the client

**FIGURE 12-1  A Decision Model for Inclusion of Multicultural Variables in Stuttering Intervention Programming**

a high likelihood that therapy, and especially counseling, will not be maximally effective. Of course, cultural variables account for only one of the reasons that a client's and clinician's phenomenal field may not match, but different cultural systems present a frequent reason why they do not. Phenomenal field in this context refers to the comprehensive experiences and belief systems of individuals.

*Cultural environment* is also important to take into consideration when structuring a plan for fluency counseling or therapy intervention. This includes all aspects of the client's environment: his or her phenomenal field, access to experience, semantic environment, relationships with significant others, and language environment. In the case of child clients, it is important for clinicians to remember that parents are the chief architects of their child's environment and should be counseled to be active in designing an environmental gestalt for their child that is conducive to speech fluency and normal personality development (Crowe, 1994). The environment of the disfluent child should be conducive to his or her developing coping use of ego functions, which might in turn help prevent the stuttering syndrome from developing, rather than developing defensive reactions to speech disfluency.

## *Decision Level I—Preintervention*

This is the first decision level for clinicians: Do cultural differences come into the evaluation/therapy picture, and, if so, how might they influence subsequent client-clinician interaction? First, in order to answer these questions, during client intake the *cultural identity* of the client must be explored. This is at times obvious but at other times must be queried. Clinicians must be mindful that cultural identity goes beyond the race of individuals and that just because a culture has been assigned to a client does not mean that the client identifies with that particular culture. Second, after the cultural identity of the client has been determined, his or her age and gender must also be considered prior to evaluation or therapy, because in some cultures these variables influence the communicative norms that are expected by clients or parents of clients. At this point, clinicians will have enough information to make generalizations about the culture-based beliefs and values about communication that the clients and their significant others bring to the clinical setting (Watson & Kayser, 1994). A factor that should be considered when gathering culture background information about a client is his or her degree of *cultural assimilation*. This is the idea that although a client may identify with a given culture, they may not be fully assimilated into the culture. The degree of assimilation in a particular culture may vary from client to client.

*Example:* African Americans typically place a high premium on oral performance. In order to achieve the desired effect in oral performance, they often use speech disfluency for emphasis. (Labov, 1972; Smitherman, 1977)

## Decision Level II—Intake

Counseling begins at the second level of intervention, which is intake/case history. Counseling continues throughout the intervention process as needed, although it is indicated in the model as a distinct level between evaluation and treatment. At this level, the nature of the disorder is discussed as well as specific cultural variables relative to stuttering. This discussion should help clinicians identify myths and attitudes clients may associate with stuttering. Clients can then be counseled about attitudes, myths, beliefs, and values that might prevent optimal success from being achieved in the next intervention level. It is also important at this level to establish conformity of meaning in terminology used by clinicians and clients in reference to stuttering.

*Clinical Implication 1:* Relative to general cultural variables about stuttering, clinicians should be mindful of attributes such as silence, interruptions, topic maintenance, and verbal expectations. These are important to consider in dealing with both children and their parents. Oftentimes children and parents are penalized for interaction styles that clinicians judge to be inappropriate. What clients evidence may in fact be a culturally specific interaction style that may have no deleterious effect on speech.

*Clinical Implication 2:* It is important for clinicians to be familiar with the myths of the culture group relative to etiological factors and approaches to intervention for stuttering. A number of such myths have been gathered by the first author from African American families. Clinicians must take these myths very seriously because they represent the parents' honest understanding of stuttering. A sample list of myths African Americans hold about stuttering is presented in Appendix 12A.

*Clinical Implication 3:* It is important to have the parents or clients describe what they perceive is the problem. With African American families, the problem may not be stuttering. Because of the cultural emphasis on verbal expectations, when parents note some disruption in speech, they attribute it to abnormalities with the flow of speech. In many cases, the child will demonstrate a language or articulation problem rather than a fluency problem.

*Clinical Implication 4:* Standardized assessment and many treatment programs often do not consider cultural information, so clinicians should add this information component to the clinical protocol.

## Decision Level III—Evaluation

Evaluation is conducted at the third level, but here again not before considering possible necessary cultural adjustments and modifications that should be made to the intervention process. For example, modification of test items or testing procedures might be made to make visual stimuli more culturally specific, to incorporate recording of meaningful nonverbal behaviors of clients, and to account for cultural differences in the cognitive learning styles of clients. Terrell and Hale (1992) state: "African American children are more physically active, and thus profit from the incorporation of more physical activity, movement, and variation in the learning environment." (p. 6).

Clinicians should also be sensitive to cultural differences in parent-child interaction styles and client-clinician interaction styles. African Americans have been described as highly affective and people-oriented; this leads to more interpersonal characteristics, which foster a less independent learning style (Hale-Benson, 1987; Terrell & Hale, 1992).

*Clinical Implication 1:* Clinicians, during their interactions with children, should be mindful of nonverbal behaviors such as silence, eye contact, and physical activity level (e.g., excessive gross motor behavior, constant body movement, and out-of-seat behavior). These are often misconstrued as secondary mannerisms or avoidance behaviors when they are in fact cultural differences in nonverbal behaviors. Cultural influences on verbal behavior and interaction also should be noted as clinicians elicit speech samples in a variety of speaking contexts, with emphasis placed on narrative discourse. This will allow clinicians to address issues often raised by parents relative to their children's stuttering behavior being more prominent "when they are trying to tell events of a story."

*Clinical Implication 2:* Children's cognitive learning styles should be considered during the evaluation process. With African American children, physical activity levels, language use, and whole-to-part/, relational learning should be given close attention. Hilliard (1976) and Hale-Benson (1987) described relational learning styles in opposition to analytic learning styles. They indicated that characteristics of analytical cognitive styles may include: stimulus-centered behavior, parts-specific learning, long attention span, standard English language style, formal and stable rules for language organization, and long concentration span. Aspects of relational cognitive style may include: self-centeredness; global orientation; fine descriptive characteristics; fluent spoken language; short attention span; short concentration span; gestalt learning; and language dependent upon unique context, interactional characteristics of the communicants, time and place, inflection, muscular movements, and other nonverbal cues. African American children tend to use relational learning styles.

*Clinical Implication 3:* During observation of parent-child interaction, clinicians should take note of differences based on cultural background. Particular attention should be given to issues such as directive behaviors, child rearing practices, and verbal expectations that often influence parent-child interaction (Conrad, 1985, 1987).

*Clinical Implication 4:* Commercial programs, such as *The Fluency Development System for Young Children* (Meyers & Woodford, 1992), *Stuttering Prevention: A Clinical Method* (Starkweather, Gottwald, & Halfond, 1990), and *Stuttering Therapy for Children* (Gregory & Hill, 1980), call for the observation of parent-child interaction. Clinicians should be mindful that modifications can easily be made so that cultural expectations can be observed, noted, and not subjected to penalty (Conrad, 1985, 1987; van Kleeck, 1994). This can be done by adjusting for these expectations in light of the client's cultural background.

## Decision Level IV—Parent/Client Counseling

After the fluency evaluation is completed, counseling should begin. This is an especially important level in clinical intervention with multicultural clients, because it is here that the stage is set for therapy, ideally with the complete comprehension and support of clients and their supporting others. Rules for interaction are identified and agreed to here that will define the nature of the client-clinician relationship and remove potential sources of miscommunication between clients and clinicians. It is important to involve the entire family unit, including grandparents, at this stage and to explore with them the possible significance of cultural identity, residential history, and generational factors.

Clinicians should be mindful of the three aspects of counseling that occur at this level. The first aspect is that counseling should begin, when possible, as soon as stuttering develops and definitely before stuttering becomes severe. The second aspect of counseling concerns the interpretation of test results to clients, definition of the disorder and its treatment, and explanation of prognosis. The third aspect of counseling addresses personal adjustments of the client and significant others as an ongoing part of the treatment process.

> *Clinical Implication 1:* It is important that clinicians understand rules for interacting with individuals from diverse backgrounds. Important attributes such as touching, establishing eye contact, and observing levels of emotion are crucial to the counseling session. Clinicians must be able to adjust to cultural differences in order to win the trust of clients and parents so that counseling with them will be maximally effective.
>
> *Clinical Implication 2:* Clinicians should keep in mind that residential history and generational factors are germane to the counseling process for individuals who stutter. This information provides a clear picture of the family with whom work is to be done. Generational factors may influence counseling and treatment expectations and general understanding of the treatment process, especially if family members other than the parents will accompany the child to treatment.

## Decision Level V—Treatment

Therapy for fluency disorders begins at intervention level five with culture-based factors built into therapy techniques and goals. These factors include variables previously discussed: values, beliefs, attitudes, interaction styles, cognitive learning style, environmental factors, and so forth.

A sample list of strategies used to build culture-based factors into therapy goals and techniques is presented in Appendix 12B. When using a commercial fluency treatment program that involves specific activities and materials, clinicians may have difficulty developing strategies to enhance the cultural sensitivity of the program. However, clinicians may find that the program's concepts can be preserved and used with other activities for cultural enrichment. For example, a component of *The Fluency Development System for Young Children* (Meyers & Woodford, 1992), can be adjusted to substitute characters familiar to the client rather than "The Tortoise and the Hare" story as a basis for establishing the cognitive-linguistic components of the therapy program. For programs that do not require adherence to specific activities and materials, modification for inclusion of culturally sensitive materials can easily be made. For example, when using the *Fluency Rules Therapy Program for Young Children* (Runyan

& Runyan, 1986) with an African American school-age child, clinicians can use sports activities to adjust for physical activity level and can easily incorporate narrative discourse activities.

## Decision Level VI—Carryover/Generalization

The sixth and last level of intervention is perhaps the most challenging to all clients and clinicians, especially when working with multicultural populations and with stuttering. It is at this stage that carryover and generalization of therapy results are effected or at least attempted, and clinicians will need to utilize all resources at hand to achieve maximal success. Clinicians should structure carryover and generalization strategies within the cultural context of clients by utilizing the home unit, peers, and the clients themselves.

> *Clinical Implication:* Clinicians may find that using individuals from the home as well as peers will aid in establishing and maintaining fluency. The use of peers and the home unit should be implemented as soon as the therapy process is initiated. Clinicians may have situations where direct contact with the parents or caregivers may be impossible. Video- or audiotaping therapy sessions and sending them home with a responsible individual will aid in the carryover process by keeping parents informed of procedures, techniques, and strategies used in the treatment process. Clinicians can use this mechanism as a means to communicate with working parents and caregivers.

## SUMMARY AND DISCUSSION

In this model, designed to address stuttering when dealing with multicultural populations, decisions are made at each intervention level as to the relevance of cultural variables in the intervention process. At each level the decision also is made whether to revisit previous levels or to expedite progress through a given level.

In order to maximize the positive outcome of intervention with stuttering, evaluation and treatment of clients should take place within the context of each client's cultural system and cultural environment. Beginning at the intake and preintervention levels, clinicians should consider cultural variables and continue to incorporate culture-based content and strategies into the intervention process until carryover and generalization of therapy results have been achieved. Culture considerations are of particular importance to the process of parent/client counseling;

cultural factors relative to the entire family unit should be integrated into this process. While this model was designed specifically for intervening with individuals who stutter and addresses use with African American children, it can be easily adapted by clinicians for clinical use in dealing with other communicative disorders and with other cultural groups.

## STUDY QUESTIONS AND ACTIVITIES

1. Watson and Kayser (1994) stressed that throughout the course of fluency intervention with bilingual and bicultural children and adults who stutter, clinicians must address three things. They are:

   a.

   b.

   c.

2. Explain why the *Personalized Fluency Control Therapy Program-Revised* (Cooper & Cooper, 1985) may be considered to be a culturally sensitive stuttering therapy process.

3. What is a cultural system and a cultural environment? Why is it important to understand these concepts in order to use culturally appropriate strategies in fluency control therapy?

4. Discuss the six levels of counseling and therapy presented by Robinson and Crowe (1994).

5. Why is carryover/generalization an especially challenging level of intervention when working with multicultural populations?

6. Read the following case example and answer the questions at the end.

   Mark Dell is an African American student at Riley College. He was referred to the fluency clinic at nearby Carey University during the first semester of his junior year in college. He was in the ROTC program and had been told that he would not qualify to enter the Army as an officer if he did not improve his communication skills. They would only allow him to continue in the program if he enrolled in speech therapy. On the first day of therapy he advised the staff that he believed it to be the will of God for him to stutter.

   Mark exhibited severe episodes of tense pauses and other nonverbal aspects of stuttering such as lip tremors, unusual eye movements, and movements of his hands and legs when he attempted to speak. Few audible nonfluencies were displayed.

   Each semester Mark was assigned to work with a different student clinician but with the same supervisor. The supervisor made the same assignment for the first day of therapy for each student clinician. The student was told to engage Mark in conversation about the ROTC program and about his previous stuttering therapy. Notes were to be made of the nature, type, and frequency of stuttering observed. Every clinician made a similar report after interacting with Mark for the first time. When they were asked how the session went, the common response was "Fine, but he is not a stutterer. I did not hear him stutter a single time." The next time the student was scheduled to meet with Mark, the supervisor would accompany the student clinician to the session. After some initial interactions, the supervisor would remind Mark that he must not use any of the devices to conceal stuttering. He was told to use the strategies to increase fluency. During the times the supervisor was in the room Mark showed some disfluent behaviors but was able to use the newly acquired strategies to modify, reduce, or eliminate the stuttering. There were far fewer verbal disfluencies during the supervisor's absence. The student clinicians reported that his other behaviors were "odd" when the supervisor was not present.

Mark's course of treatment was an eclectic approach designed to teach him methods to increase fluency, eliminate the various devices he used to conceal stuttering, and control or manage stuttering during difficult moments. The approach was quite successful within the clinic setting. However, there was very little transfer or generalization to other situations.

- Discuss some cultural variables that may have been factors in Mark's therapy experience.
- How might things have been different if the clinic staff had used the model of intervention presented in this chapter?

## APPENDIX 12A: AFRICAN AMERICAN MYTHS ABOUT STUTTERING

### *Etiology Myths*

Stuttering is caused by:
- The mother's eating improper foods when breast feeding the infant.
- Allowing an infant to look in the mirror.
- Tickling the child too much.
- Cutting the child's hair before he or she says his or her first words.
- The mother's seeing a snake during pregnancy.
- The mother's dropping the baby.
- Being scared as a baby.
- The child's being bitten by a dog.
- The work of the devil.

### *Remediation Myths*

- Stuttering is something that can be controlled by the child.
- Stuttering can be controlled by telling the child not to move his or her feet when talking.

- Stuttering can be cured by hitting the child in the mouth with a dish towel.
- Stuttering can be cured by having the child hold nutmeg under his or her tongue.

## APPENDIX 12B: EXAMPLES OF WAYS TO BUILD CULTURE-BASED FACTORS INTO THERAPY GOALS/TECHNIQUES

1. **Client-Child Interaction**
   - Use silence as a means for setting the stage for slow and easy talking.
   - Incorporate physical activities into the therapy session (for example, basketball, baseball, soccer, or video games).
   - Study client's secondary mannerisms to distinguish them from "normal" high energy/physical activity behaviors.
   - Have the client begin using some form of narrative discourse as soon as the treatment process begins.
   - Expand the treatment program by using peers and the family unit as a part of remediation.
2. **Clinician-Family Interaction**
   - Understand and correct myths.
   - Present counseling information orally in addition to in written form. More emphasis should be placed on the oral presentation than on the written.
   - Incorporate parents as active participants in the intervention process during the treatment sessions.
3. **Cognitive Learning Style**
   - Change activities frequently and use the entire room rather than the table. This will address the African American child's need for physical activity when trying to learn.
   - Change names and description of the characters in commercial treatment programs to reflect the cultural experiences of the child.

## REFERENCES

Anderson, B. (1981). *An analysis of the relationship of age and sex to type and frequency of disfluencies in lower socioeconomic preschool black children.* Unpublished doctoral dissertation, Northwestern University, Evanston, IL.

Aron, M. (1962). The nature and incidence of stuttering among a Bantu group of school going children. *Journal Speech and Hearing Disorders, 27,* 116–128.

Bernstein-Ratner, N., & Benitez, M. (1985). Linguistic analysis of a bilingual stutterer. *Journal of Fluency Disorder, 10,* 211–219.

Brutten, G., & Miller, R. (1988). The disfluencies of normally fluent Black first graders. *Journal of Fluency Disorders, 13,* 291–299.

Bullen, A. K. (1945). A cross cultural approach to the problem of stuttering. *Child Development, 16,* 1–88.

Clifford, S., Twitchell, M., & Hull, R. (1965). Stuttering in South Dakota Indians. *Central States Speech Journal, 16,* 59–60.

Conrad, C. (1985). *A conversational act analysis of black mother-child dyads including stuttering nonstuttering children.* Unpublished doctoral dissertation, Northwestern University, Evanston, IL.

Conrad, C. (1987). Fluency in multicultural populations. In L. Cole & V. Deal (Eds.), *Communication disorders in multicultural populations.* Rockville, MD: American Speech-Language-Hearing Association.

Cooper, E. B. & Cooper, C. S. (1985). *Cooper personalized fluency control therapy-revised.* Allen, TX: DLM.

Cooper, E. B., & Cooper, C. S. (1993). Fluency disorders. In D. Battle (Ed.), *Communication disorders in multicultural populations* (pp. 189–211). Boston: Andover Medical Publishers.

Crowe, T. A., (1994). Preventative counseling with parents at risk. In C. W. Starkweather & H. F. M. Peters (Eds.), *Proceedings of the First World Congress on Fluency Disorders* (pp. 232–235). Nijmegen, The Netherlands: University Press.

Crowe, T. A. (1995, December). *Counseling for fluency disorders: Rationale, strategy and technique.* Paper presented as part of short course (with W. H. Manning and G. W. Blood) at the American Speech-Language-Hearing Association Convention, Orlando, FL.

Dale, P. (1977). Factors related to dysfluent speech in bilingual Cuban-American Adolescents. *Journal of Fluency Disorders, 2,* 311–314.

Ford, S. (1986). *Pragmatic abilities in black disfluent preschoolers.* Unpublished master's thesis, Howard University, Washington, DC.

Goldman, R. (1967). Cultural influences on the sex ratio in the incidence of stuttering. *American Anthropology, 69,* 78–81.

Gregory, H., & Hill, D. (1980). Stuttering therapy for children. *Seminars in Speech, Language and Hearing, 1*(4), 351–363.

Hale-Benson, J. E. (1987). *Black children: Their roots, culture, and learning styles.* Baltimore: The Johns Hopkins University Press.

Hilliard, A. (1976). *Alternative to IQ testing: An approach to the identification of gifted minority children.* Final report to the California State Department of Education.

Jayaram, M. (1983). Phonetic influences on stuttering in monolingual and bilingual stutterers. *Journal of Communication Disorders, 16,* 287–297.

Johnson, W. (1944a). The Indians have no word for it: I. Stuttering in children. *Quarterly Journal of Speech, 30,* 330–337.

Johnson, W. (1944b). The Indians have no word for it: II. Stuttering in adults. *Quarterly Journal of Speech, 30,* 456–465.

Labov, W. (1972). *Language in the inner city: Studies in the Black English vernacular.* Philadelphia: University of Pennsylvania Press.

Leith, W. R., & Mims, H. A. (1975). Cultural influences in the development and treatment of stuttering: A preliminary report on the Black stutterer. *Journal of Speech and Hearing Disorders, 40,* 459–466.

Lemert, E. M. (1953). Some Indians who stutter. *Journal of Speech and Hearing Disorders, 18,* 168–174.

Lemert, E. M. (1962). Stuttering and social structure in two Pacific societies. *Journal of Speech and Hearing Disorders, 27,* 3–10.

Meyers, S. C., & Woodford, L. L. (1992). *The fluency development system for young children.* Buffalo, NY: United Educational Services.

Nathanson, S. (1969). *A study of the influence of race, socioeconomic status and sex on the speech fluency of 200 nonstuttering fifth graders.* Unpublished doctoral dissertation, Northwestern University, Evanston, IL.

Nwokah, E. (1988). The imbalance of stuttering behavior in bilingual speakers. *Journal of Fluency Disorders, 13,* 357–373.

Ralston, L. (1981). Stammering: A stress index in Caribbean classrooms. *Journal of Fluency Disorders, 6,* 119–133.

Robinson, T. L., Jr. (1992). *An investigation of speech fluency skills in African American preschool children during narrative discourse.* Unpublished dissertation, Howard University, Washington, DC.

Robinson, Jr., T. L., & Crowe, T. A. (1994, November). *A model for inclusion of multicultural variables in fluency intervention programming.* Paper presented at the American Speech-Language-Hearing Association Convention, New Orleans, LA.

Robinson, Jr., T. L., & Crowe, T. A. (1998). Culture-based considerations in programming for stuttering intervention with African American clients and their families. *Language Speech and Hearing Services in the Schools, 29,* 172–179.

Runyan, C. M. & Runyan, S. E. (1986). A fluency rules therapy program for young children in the public schools. *Language, Speech and Hearing Services in the Schools, 17,* 276–284.

Seymour, H. N. (1986). Clinical principles for language intervention. In O. L. Taylor (Ed.), *Nature of communication disorders in culturally and linguistically diverse populations* (pp. 115–133). Austin, TX: Pro-Ed.

Seymour, H. N., & Seymour, C. M. (1977). A therapeutic model for communicative disorders among children who speak Black English vernacular. *Journal of Speech and Hearing Disorders, 42,* 247–256.

Smitherman, G. (1977). *Talkin' and testifyin'.* Boston: Houghton Mifflin Company.

Snidecor, J. C. (1947). Why the Indian does not stutter. *Quarterly Journal of Speech, 33,* 493–495.

Starkweather, C. W., Gottwald, S. R., & Halfond, M. M. (1990). *Stuttering prevention: A clinical method.* Englewood Cliffs, NJ: Prentice Hall.

Stewart, J. L. (1960). The problem of stuttering in certain North American Indian societies. *Journal of Speech and Hearing Disorders (Monograph Supplement 6),* 87

Taylor, O. L. (1986). Historical perspectives and conceptual framework. In O. L. Taylor (Ed.), *Nature of communication disorders in culturally and linguistically diverse populations* (pp. 1–17). Austin, TX: Pro-Ed.

Taylor, O. L. (1987). Clinical practice as a social occasion. In L. Cole & V. R. Deal, *Communication disorders in multicultural populations.* Rockville, MD: American Speech-Language-Hearing Association.

Taylor, O. L., & Payne, K. T. (1983). Culturally valid testing: A proactive approach. *Topics in Language Disorders, 3,* 8–20.

Taylor, O. L., & Samara, R. (1985). *Communication disorders in underserved populations: Developing nations.* Paper presented at the National Colloquium on Underserved Populations, American Speech-Language-Hearing Association, Washington, DC.

Terrell, B. Y., & Hale, J. E. (1992). Serving a multicultural population: Different learning styles. *American Journal of Speech-Language Pathology: A Journal of Clinical Practice, 1,* 5–8.

Toyoda, B. (1959). A statistical report. *Clinical Paediatrica, 12,* 788.

Travis, L. E., Johnson, W., & Shover, J. (1981). The relationship of bilingualism to stuttering. *Journal of Speech Disorders, 2,* 185–189.

van Kleeck, A. (1994). Potential cultural bias in training parents as conversational partners with their children who have delays in language development. *American Journal of Speech-Language Pathology: A Journal of Clinical Practice, 3*(1), 67–78.

Vaughn-Cooke, F. B. (1983) Improving language assessment in minority children. *Asha, 25,* 29–34.

Vaughn-Cooke, F. B. (1986). The challenge of assessing the language of nonmainstream speakers. In O. L. Taylor (Ed.), *Treatment of communication disorders in culturally and linguistically diverse populations* (pp. 23–48). Austin, TX: Pro-Ed.

Wakaba, Y. (1983). Group therapy for Japanese children who stutter. *Journal of Fluency Disorders, 8,* 93–118.

Watson, J. B., & Kayser, H. (1994). Assessment of bilingual/bicultural children and adults who stutter. *Seminars in Speech and Language, 15,* 149–164.

Zimmerman, G., Liljeblad, S., Frank, A., & Cleeland, C. (1983). The Indians have many terms for it: Stuttering among the Bannock-Shoshoni. *Journal of Speech and Hearing Research, 26,* 315–318.

# 13

# MANAGING HEARING IMPAIRMENT IN CULTURALLY DIVERSE CHILDREN

## DIANE M. SCOTT

## INTRODUCTION

### Audiologist/Speech-Language Pathologist in a Culturally Diverse World

Being an audiologist or a speech-language pathologist in a culturally diverse world is not an easy task. Audiologists and speech-language pathologists and the children and families they serve may not share a common cultural system or even a common language. Lack of a common language and differing cultural systems can lead to difficulties in establishing rapport between the audiologist, or speech-language pathologist, and the child or family and in finding language-appropriate test materials. As Mary Lane (1984) stated,

> Great cultural diversity still exists on our planet, even as modern technology pushes for more uniformity and as McDonald's and Coca Cola spread everywhere. In ecological terms, we accept the principle of diversity for plants and animals. We protect endangered species—too late sometimes—in most of the civilized world. But if humankind is to maintain itself, the valuing of diversity must increase in our own lives also. (p. 76)

Recent data on the prevalence of hearing impairment in children show some significant changes in terms of racial and ethnic diversity. According to data from the Office of Special Education and Rehabilitative Services (OSERS) and the 1993–1994 Annual Survey of Deaf and Hard of Hearing Children and Youth (Schildroth & Hotto, 1995), the number of children identified with hearing impairment or deafness appears to be decreasing (Table 13-1). While the total number of children with hearing impairment or deafness may be decreasing, the representation of children from racial/ethnic minority populations is increasing. Examination of the data from the Annual Survey shows dramatic shifts due to race and ethnicity (Table 13-1) and matches the general population data obtained by the U.S. Bureau of the Census. If the numbers reported by the states to the federal Office of Special Education Programs (OSEP) are accurate, then the Annual Survey collects information on 60 to 65 percent of all deaf and hard-of-hearing children receiving special education services in the United States (Schildroth & Hotto, 1995).

Between 1974 and 1994, the number of Asian/Pacific Islander children reported to the Annual Survey increased by 500 percent. One-third of the Asian/Pacific Islander children in the 1993–1994 survey were reported from California with 10 percent from Minnesota. In five states, Asian/Pacific Islander children outnumbered both African American and Hispanic children. Fifty-seven percent of African American children in the 1993–1994 Annual Survey were reported from the South. Only 8 percent were from the West. The number of Hispanic children increased from under 3000 in 1973–1974 to almost 7400 in 1993–1994 Annual Survey. Hispanic children outnumbered African American children in eighteen states in the Annual Survey. California, Texas, and New York

**TABLE 13-1    Racial/Ethnic Background from 1973–1974, 1983–1984, and 1993–1994 Annual Surveys of Deaf and Hard of Hearing Children and Youth**

|  | 1973–1974 (N = 41,070) | 1983–1984 (N = 52,330) | 1993–1994 (N = 46,099) |
|---|---|---|---|
| Asian/Pacific Islander | <1% | 2% | 4% |
| African American | 16% | 18% | 17% |
| Hispanic | 7% | 11% | 16% |
| Other | <1% | 2% | 3% |
| White | 76% | 67% | 60% |
| Total | 100% | 100% | 100% |

*Source:* Schildroth & Hotto (1995).

reported two-thirds of all Hispanic children to the survey (Schildroth & Hotto, 1995).

## Cross-Cultural Competence

Cross-cultural effectiveness is an essential skill for professionals to possess. Developing cross-cultural competence requires commitment, desire, and time. It also requires: (1) lowering one's defenses, taking risks, and practicing behaviors that may feel unfamiliar and uncomfortable; (2) a flexible mind and willingness to accept alternative perspectives; (3) self-awareness; (4) cultural-specific awareness and understanding; and (5) communication competence (Lynch, 1992). Audiologists and other service providers must avoid stereotyping children and families based on group identity.

The rationales for becoming cross-culturally competent have been outlined by Brislin, Cushner, Cherrie, and Yong (1986). Becoming cross-culturally competent will assist service providers to (1) feel comfortable and effective in their interactions and relationships with families whose cultures differ from their own, (2) interact in ways that enable families from different cultures to feel positive about the interactions and the service providers, and (3) accomplish the goals that are established jointly between the family and service provider.

In order to build cross-cultural competence, service providers must (1) clarify their own values and assumptions, (2) collect and analyze ethnographic information related to the community in which families they serve reside, (3) determine the degree to which each family operates transculturally, and (4) examine each family's orientation to specific child-rearing practices (Hanson, Lynch, & Wayman, 1990). Cross-cultural competence is necessary in order for audiologists and other service providers to do their jobs appropriately, effectively, and ethically.

Self-awareness is the first step in building cross-cultural competence. Self-awareness begins with an exploration of one's own heritage. All people have a cultural, ethnic, and linguistic heritage that influences their current beliefs, values, and behaviors. Sources, such as Lynch (1992), provide questions service providers can ask themselves to learn more about their own heritage. This knowledge then helps service providers separate ways of thinking, believing, and behaving that may be universal from those that are based upon different cultural beliefs and biases. Service providers also need to gather culture-specific information. They can accomplish this task by studying and reading about the culture of interest, talking and working with individuals from the culture who can act as cultural guides, and venturing out into the community itself. Guidelines on determining family structure, child-rearing practices, and language and communication styles can be found in Wayman, Lynch, and Hanson (1990).

Effective communication is the foundation for the appropriate provision of services. Cultural differences make effective communication more challenging but even more important. Communication effectiveness is improved when the communicator respects individuals from other cultures, makes continued and sincere attempts to understand the world from others' points of view, is open to new learning, is flexible, has a sense of humor, tolerates ambiguity well, and approaches others with a desire to learn (Lynch, 1992).

## SERVICE PROVISION IN GENERAL

### Case History Information

The usual case history form may not ask all the questions that an audiologist may need to have answered in order to obtain culturally relevant information. For example, information may be needed about (1) both race and ethnicity (Hispanic is a designation of ethnicity and not of race; some etiologies for hearing losses occur more frequently in some racial groups); (2) place of birth as well as year of birth (assists in determining if a person is an immigrant and how long he or she has lived in the United States; see Case Example 13.1); (3) natural healing methods used as well as medications prescribed and taken (assists in determining if a person believes in alternative methods of healing, and if the person is actually taking prescribed medication); and (4) language(s) spoken in the

---

**Case Example 13.1**

JL was a 3-year-old boy suspecting of having a hearing loss. He was not developing speech and language appropriately. His family was Hmong and had immigrated to the United States to live in a Hmong community in Michigan. The case history form had only asked a question about date of birth. It had not asked about place of birth, which for JL was a refugee camp in Thailand where he had lived most of his life. JL had been exposed to a variety of diseases and had rarely, if ever, seen a toy. Behavioral assessment of his hearing status was difficult because he did not know how to interact with toys, and, in some instances, was frightened of them. JL made "clicking" sounds during the hearing assessment; however, these "clicking" sounds were not a normal means of communication among the Hmong.

home (assists in determining if the family is multilingual or if the language spoken in the home is other than English even though the family may speak English). For more in formation on modifying the case history form, see Orque, Block, and Monrroy (1983).

As audiologists or other service providers read over the case history information, they need to know if specific auditory disorders are more common in certain racially/ethnically diverse populations than in others. Otitis media, sickle cell disease, and the etiologies of hearing impairment in children are examples of auditory disorders that may differ in rate of occurrence by race/ethnicity.

Differences have been found in the incidence rates of otitis media among racial groups (Reis, 1986). Though the actual rates differ from study to study, American Indians/Alaskan Natives have the highest rates, while African Americans have the lowest. Hispanic and White incidence rates fall between the other two. Asian/Pacific Islander rates may match American Indian incidence rates due to a common gene pool. Ancestors of present day Asian/Pacific Islanders are believed to be American Indians who crossed the Bering Strait into Asia before the oceans separated the continents of Asia and North America.

Differences in rates of otitis media may be caused in part by differences in the structure and function of the Eustachian tube among racial groups (Beery, Doyle, Cantekin, Bluestone, & Wiet, 1980; Doyle, 1977). Intraracial differences also exist, such that not all American Indian tribes have the same incidence rates of otitis media. Individual variability, familial and genetic factors, climate, exposure to antibiotics, and (child's) inclusion in daycare all must be taken into account in examining rates of otitis media.

Sickle cell disease (SCD) is a blood disease that results from a hereditary abnormality of the hemoglobin molecule found in red blood cells. SCD is recognized as a world health problem predominantly affecting people of African descent in the United States, Africa, and the Caribbean, and to a lesser extent Hispanics and selected populations generally adjacent to the Mediterranean Sea and Indian Ocean, such as Greeks and Sicilians. One of the clinical manifestations of the disease is that sickle-shaped cells tend to occlude smaller veins and capillaries, possibly including those supplying blood to the cochlea. In addition, central nervous system (CNS) manifestations, which include the auditory pathways, are frequent in SCD. Children with SCD therefore may present with higher rates of peripheral and central auditory impairment compared to children developing normally.

The Annual Survey of Deaf and Hard of Hearing Children and Youth (Schildroth & Hotto, 1995) collects data on the etiology of hearing loss (see Table 13-2). As indicated by the authors, the "cause of hearing loss"

**TABLE 13-2    Racial/Ethnic Background and Etiology of Hearing Loss from 1993–1994 Annual Survey of Deaf and Hard of Hearing Children and Youth***

| | Maternal Rubella (N = 893) | Heredity (N = 6034) | Meningitis (N = 3626) | Prematurity (N = 2171) | CMV (N = 621) | Otitis Media (N = 1754) |
|---|---|---|---|---|---|---|
| Asian/Pacific Islander | 3% | 2% | 2% | 2% | 2% | 5% |
| African American | 18% | 10% | 26% | 25% | 15% | 10% |
| Hispanic | 28% | 14% | 11% | 14% | 9% | 12% |
| Other | 4% | 2% | 3% | 3% | 2% | 2% |
| White | 48% | 72% | 58% | 58% | 72% | 70% |
| Total | 100% | 100% | 100% | 100% | 100% | 100% |

*Because some children were reported with more than one cause of hearing loss, there is a very small amount of duplication within the percentages.

*Source:* Schildroth & Hotto (1995).

question in the Annual Survey is not answered by many of the respondents to the survey, which is usually the school. The question is often left blank or receives the response "data unavailable" or "cause unknown." This large amount of missing data is a limitation of the Annual Survey. Given that caution, the data do provide some information. Meningitis and heredity were the primary causes of hearing loss across all racial/ethnic groups reporting in the 1993–1994 survey. Among African Americans, Hispanics, and whites, prematurity was the third major cause of hearing loss, while among Asian/Pacific Islanders it was otitis media. Hispanic children were represented disproportionately in all causes of hearing impairment except cytomegalovirus (CMV), while African Americans were represented disproportionately in the categories of maternal rubella, meningitis, prematurity, and CMV.

## Assessment

Audiologists cannot rely solely on pure tone, immittance, and electrophysiologic testing to determine a child's hearing status. At some point audiological speech tests will need to be administered to a child.

There is a growing number of persons in the United States who do not speak English as a first language. School systems have seen an explosion in the number of languages spoken by their students. The U.S. Bureau of the Census estimates that 14 percent of school-age children (more than 6.3 million) speak a non-English language at home and that 4 percent of school-age children live in households that are "linguistically isolated," that is, in households in which no member age 14 or older speaks English at least "very well." Most of the children speak either Spanish or an Asian language. Being able to communicate with a child and the family in their first language helps establish rapport. Multilingual professionals or the use of interpreters, therefore, are needed to effectively communicate with these children.

With this growing number of children who do not speak English as a first language, the use of English-language speech test materials becomes a critical issue, and the use of these materials would be inappropriate. Spanish-language materials for children are available along with materials in a few other languages. Audiologists must look at the norming of any non-English tests used and at the country of origin of the speaker if using recorded speech materials to determine the cultural and linguistic backgrounds of the populations used for norming and of the speaker. Unless an audiologist is qualified to provide bilingual or multilingual services (see ASHA's definition of a bilingual speech-language pathologists or audiologist, 1989), the use of non-English language materials would be outside of the audiologist's scope of practice. Interpreters who speak the languages most commonly spoken in the surrounding community then can be hired and trained. Interpreters can be found within the community itself at community centers or places of worship, even at local colleges and universities.

When hiring an interpreter, audiologists and other service providers should seek an individual who meets a minimum level of qualifications. Family members, friends, or "the secretary from down the hall" should not be used as interpreters. Among the qualifications for an effective interpreter are: (1) a high degree of oral and written proficiency in both the first and second language; (2) the ability to convey meaning from one language to the other; (3) the ability to adjust to linguistic variations within different communities (dialects exist); (4) knowledge of the cultures of the people who speak the languages; (5) familiarity with the specific terminology used in audiology and speech-language pathology; and (6) understanding of the function and role of the interpreter on the team (Roseberry-McKibbin, 1995).

## Cultural Views of Chronic Illness and Disability

Culture frames how people view the world. It can assist professionals in anticipating and understanding how and why individuals and families make certain decisions regarding intervention. In order to provide culturally relevant and successful intervention services with culturally and linguistically diverse populations, some judgment or measurement of acculturation and biculturalism must be made. Acculturation (to traditional or mainstream culture) should not be viewed as a predictor of success. It should be viewed as a tool for determining what assessment techniques and interventions might be appropriate for the child and family.

Acculturation can initially be determined by reviewing the (modified) case history form, which should include questions on country of origin, time of residency in the United States, language(s) spoken in the home, and use of alternative healing methods as well as "modern medicine." Information needs to be obtained concerning family practices related to childrearing, health care, and socialization. Discussion is needed concerning the family's beliefs regarding the causes of hearing loss.

Nonetheless, three almost universal issues have been identified concerning the social implications of chronic illness and disability (Groce & Zola, 1993). The first is that the culturally perceived cause of a chronic illness or disability is significant in all cultures. The reason for the presence of a disability will play a significant role in attitudes toward the individual with the disability. The disability can be viewed as a form of punishment, a family curse, or an indication of an imbalance in the body. If a disability is viewed as unacceptable by a culture, the family may feel pressured not to seek services even though they know the need exists. In addition, for new immigrants to the United States, the concept of early intervention may not exist in their native countries.

The second issue is that expectations for survival (usually conceptualized as actual physical survival) for the individual with an illness or disability will affect both the immediate care the individual receives and the amount of effort expended in planning for future care and education. The final issue is that the social role(s) deemed appropriate for children with disability will determine the amount of resources a family and community invest in an individual. This includes education, training, and social life. As an example, a gender bias in favor of males is found in many cultures (Groce & Zola, 1993). Fewer resources and attention may be given to girls and young women with disability from traditional families (see Case Example 13.2).

> **Case Example 13.2**
>
> HK and BK were a young sister and brother whose family was from India. Both were diagnosed with bilateral sensorineural hearing impairment and fitted with hearing aids. At his regularly scheduled hearing aid reevaluation, BK was wearing one of his sister's hearing aids. BK's own hearing aid was in need of repair. When asked why BK was wearing his sister's hearing aid, the parents replied that BK was a boy, and it was more important that he hear well than his sister.

Audiologists may need to consult with individuals within the family's community to enlist their cooperation in the assessment and intervention process. Role models and support groups from the same racial/ethnic/cultural group as the family can be very helpful. Audiologists must acknowledge the family's beliefs and perspectives. In order to accomplish the goals of both the family and the audiologist, the assessment and intervention process (case history, counseling, etc.) may take more time than many audiologists are accustomed to.

## Intervention

As stated previously, audiologists and other service providers may need to change the way they carry out the intervention process when serving culturally diverse children and families. Some examples of behavior that may need to be changed follow. Remember that interpreters can play a role throughout the intervention process, and it would be advantageous to both the audiologist and the family to have trained interpreters available.

The definition of family needs to be broadened to include single parents, gay and lesbian parents, fictive kin, and large extended families.

Audiologists must be flexible and prepared for all kinds of families in scheduling sessions, accommodating observers of therapy sessions, and training primary care givers.

The color of hearing aids and earmolds is important; flesh tone comes in many different shades. For children, the use of colorful hearing aids (e.g., colors that match their favorite football teams' colors) can be helpful (see Case Example 13.3). Audiologists may need to help families tap into sources of funding for their child's hearing aids and assistive listening devices (ALDs) if they are unfamiliar with the health and education systems.

The use of cochlear implants on children who are deaf can raise some important issues. Parents who are deaf may have differing viewpoints from parents who have normal hearing. Cochlear implants are viewed with suspicion by many in the Deaf community. The Deaf community tends not to believe that a deaf child's hearing needs to be "fixed." It is their belief that the child does not need to hear; the child has a communication system, American Sign Language (ASL). The family will decide the method and means of intervention, though the audiologists and other service providers can provide the family with a variety of materials to assist them in making an informed decision.

The choice of language or communication system for (re)habilitation needs to be made by the family. Too often in the past, English has been the language of intervention with little or no consideration given to the home language or signing system, or to language dominance should the child be bi- or multilingual.

---

**Case Example 13.3**

SB was an 11-year-old African American girl with a history of sensorineural hearing impairment. She had worn bilateral hearing aids successfully for most of her life. SB was scheduled for a hearing aid reevaluation because she had "accidentally on purpose" lost both of her hearing aids. In order to increase her acceptance of the new hearing aids (through her teenage years), the colors of the hearing aids and earmolds were chosen to compliment the color of her skin and hair. (Her original hearing aids were a beige color.) The new hearing aids were smoke-colored, while the color of the earmolds matched the color of her hair. SB's mother was excellent in encouraging her daughter to wear the hearing aids and create this "fashion look." SB heard her new baby sister for the first time once she was fitted with the new aids, which helped immensely in her accepting the hearing aids. The new hearing aids also allowed SB to make use of assistive listening devices.

The fields of first- and second-language acquisition, bilingualism, and special education recommend that parents continue using their native language at home, even if it is different from the school language. There are several reasons for this recommendation, including the fact that children's brains have the capacity and facility to learn more than one language; children who have been diagnosed with language/learning problems by bilingual professionals have been observed to acquire and use more than one language; language acquisition theory suggests that human brains need consistent, complete language models that offer the opportunity to acquire linguistic rules and cognitive concepts (therefore, families need to communicate in the language they know best); and, most importantly, the native language of the family and child is the "language of love" and the language of socialization.

Audiologists should be able to refer families to support groups. All hearing parents of deaf children need early intervention and support in order to adjust to the deafness. Some programs may be inaccessible to non-English speaking families due to linguistic and cultural obstacles. If support groups for non-English speaking families do not exist, audiologists and others can assist in forming them. Families should be provided with information describing hearing impairment and auditory (re)habilitation in writing in their native language. Most parents do not remember much of what was said once someone tells them their child has a hearing impairment. They need written information. Audiologists can receive assistance in developing the written material by contacting bilingual audiologists and speech-language pathologists or professional associations such as the American Academy of Audiology or the American Speech-Language-Hearing Association. Videotapes (in the native language) could be provided instead. Some parents may be unable to read in their native language. For many parents a "one-stop shopping" center for intervention services can be very helpful and reduce the "no-show" rate. If various service providers, such as audiologists, speech-language pathologists, psychologists, physicians, and other professionals, are located at the same site, families would not need to leave the site and travel to other locations to see the professionals. Multiple appointments could be made for the same day.

## Collaboration with Other Professionals

Audiologists who are not multilingual should collaborate with other professionals who are multilingual and who have specific cultural knowledge. As an example, monolingual audiologists should collaborate with bilingual audiologists or speech-language pathologists who can provide information on tests in other languages and on developing local norms for tests. A directory of bilingual audiologists and speech-language pathologists is published by the American Speech-Language-Hearing Association.

Audiologists have knowledge about auditory function and hearing intervention services, while other professionals may have knowledge in other areas of possible interest to them. Audiologists could collaborate with teachers of the hearing impaired and English as a Second Language (ESL) professionals in developing appropriate intervention services for culturally and linguistically diverse children.

Audiologists also may need to find cultural guides, sometimes called cultural brokers. Cultural guides can provide information on feelings, beliefs, and practices that are unfamiliar to the audiologist. The guides can relate their experiences in living bi- or transculturally. Friends, colleagues, and acquaintances can be cultural guides. The audiologist and cultural guide must have trust and respect for one another and for each other's culture. Families also must trust and respect cultural guides.

## SERVICE PROVISION TO SELECTED PEDIATRIC POPULATIONS

### Sickle Cell Disease

Sickle cell disease (SCD) is a genetically inherited abnormality of the hemoglobin molecule, which is responsible for carrying oxygen in red blood cells (RBCs). Normal RBCs are always soft and flexible and have no problems squeezing through capillaries. Inside normal RBCs, hemoglobin is dissolved in a watery solution and remains dissolved under all conditions. Inside the RBC of a person with SCD, hemoglobin stays dissolved under some conditions and not under others. Instead of remaining liquid, hemoglobin forms crystals that twist the RBC out of shape. The RBC is no longer soft and flexible. Hemoglobin crystals also damage the membrane of RBCs. Crystallized hemoglobin and damaged RBC membranes have the following consequences:

1. RBCs clog blood vessels and blood flow backs up. Oxygen does not get delivered to organs that need it.
2. When an organ has its oxygen supply cut off, it is damaged and it produces pain. Damage can be serious and pain can be severe (referred to as painful episodes or crises).
3. When RBCs are damaged, the body destroys them. So many RBCs are damaged and destroyed in people with SCD that they suffer from chronic anemia.

**4.** People with SCD are not hardy. They are in danger of getting infections; they are frequently incapacitated; they do not grow and develop as well as their peers; and they are not likely to live as long. (Bloom, 1995)

Over 50,000 African Americans in the United States have SCD. One in 375 who are of African ancestry is born with SCD (HbSS) (see Table 13-3). One in twelve carries the sickle cell gene (HbAS). About one in 835 African Americans is born with an HbS and a HbC gene, referred to as sickle cell-hemoglobin C disease; it is milder than SCD. About one in 1667 African Americans is born with a HbS gene and a beta thalassemia gene. This disease is variable, ranging from being indistinguishable from ordinary SCD to being almost symptom-free, depending upon the nature of the thalassemia mutation (Bloom, 1995).

The largest proportion of SCD cases occurs among blacks, both in Africa and in countries with a slave-trading history. Individuals from these countries are among the many immigrants to the United States. Within the United States, there is a regional variability in SCD cases. There is a lower frequency of cases in the North than in the South, probably due to the greater numbers of blacks who have lived and still live in the South. SCD occurs among whites and other races from the Middle East, India, and the Mediterranean. The gene is common, for example, among Israeli Arabs, Saudis, Turks, Greeks, Sicilians, and Cypriots. The sickle hemoglobin gene has become less common among American blacks than it was among their African forebears, probably due to racial mixing and natural selection.

People with SCD now live longer, fuller, and more comfortable lives. In 1973, the average lifespan was 14 years. Now, it is 42 years for men and 48 years for women. For individuals with sickle cell-hemoglobin C disease, the lifespan is 60 years for men and 68 years for women (Bloom, 1995).

Sickle cell screening programs for newborn infants exist in forty states and in Puerto Rico and the Virgin Islands. As of 1994, universal screening was provided in 34 states. At birth 50 to 95 percent of hemo-

## TABLE 13-3   Types of Hemoglobin

| | |
|---|---|
| HbA | Normal hemoglobin gene |
| HbS | Sickle hemoglobin gene |
| HbC | Gene for another hemoglobin or hereditary blood disease; found primarily among people from West Africa |
| beta thalassemia | Amount, rather than kind, of hemoglobin is abnormal; found primarily among people from around the Mediterranean Sea; "thalassa" is the Greek word for sea |
| HbF | Fetal hemoglobin |

globin is fetal hemoglobin (HbF). After birth the percentage drops off at a rate of 3 to 4 percent each week, changing to HbA, HbS, or another hemoglobin. Thus, by 4 to 5 months of age, RBCs in children with SCD are capable of sickling.

Children with SCD routinely are given prophylactic (preventive) antibiotics (drugs that kill microorganisms) to prevent infections. They are especially susceptible to *Streptococcus pneumoniae* (which can cause septicemia or meningitis), *Hemophilus influenzae* (which can cause nose, throat, and ear infections), *Salmonella* (which can cause osteomyelitis—bone inflammation), and *Escherichia coli* (which can cause septicemia or osteomyelitis). Penicillin is generally begun at 2 months of age; erythromycin may be given if the child is allergic to penicillin. The dose is 125 mg twice a day every day until the child is 3 years old, then it is increased to 250 mg twice a day until the child's physician decides to discontinue the use of the drug.

It must first be understood that the sickle cell gene expression and the severity of the disease are variable due to the interactions of hereditary and environmental factors. Taking this awareness into account, the early life cycle of children with SCD may look something like this. After birth, HbF production is replaced by HbS production in babies with SCD. During early infancy, the babies are usually without symptoms. Infections start after two to three months, but many children remain symptom-free for a year or more. In the absence of prophylactic antibiotics, children die of infections between the ages of 1 and 3 years. Early deaths should decrease as screening of newborns becomes prevalent. In early childhood, hand-foot syndrome (blocked blood flow in the bones of the hands and feet causes local swelling accompanied by pain and fever) is often the first presenting problem. Infections, especially of the lungs and kidneys, begin at the same time, though their incidence can be modified by the administration of prophylactic antibiotics. Infections are often associated with painful episodes or crises. Painful episodes can produce organ damage. By mid to late childhood, strokes increase in frequency, and physical growth is retarded.

The effects of SCD on speech and language development have not been thoroughly investigated. Vaso-occlusive crises in the CNS can cause strokes in individuals of any age, and the strokes can adversely affect speech and language abilities. Early case studies by Cook (1930), Arena (1935), and Kampeier (1936) identified children admitted to hospitals during a crisis with aphasia and slurred speech. Baird, Weiss, Ferguson, French, and Scott (1964) studied eight children for neurological symptoms and found evidence of motor and sensory aphasia, as well as weakness of the mouth, tongue, and facial muscles.

Cummings (1976) studied 34 children with and without SCD. Those with SCD had no history of neurological disorders. No significant differences in speech and receptive and expressive language skills were found between the two groups. Those children with the greatest number of crises and hospitalizations generally did not perform as well as those with SCD and fewer complications. In a pilot study reported by Waengler and Bauman-Waengler (1992), the language skills of preschoolers with SCD were compared to those of preschoolers with and without language disorders. The children with SCD performed as a group similar to preschoolers with language disorders.

Studies examining the auditory function of children with SCD have found some evidence of auditory dysfunction. Friedman, Luban, Herer, and Williams (1980) examined 43 children with SCD ages 7 to 18 years plus 23 controls. Five of the children with SCD exhibited a mild unilateral or bilateral high frequency sensorineural hearing loss. Three of the five children had a history of cerebrovascular accidents of varying severity and possible CNS involvement. Forman-Franco, Karayalcin, Mandel, and Abramson (1982) examined 54 children with SCD and a control group of 30 children. Almost 4 percent of the children with SCD had sensorineural hearing impairment, while 7 percent had conductive hearing impairment. None of the control group had any hearing loss. Thirteen of 28 children with SCD tested showed evidence of mild central auditory dysfunction on the Staggered Spondaic Word (SSW) test, compared to only one of the control subjects (see Table 13-4).

The aim of a study conducted by Scott (Crawford, Burch-Sims, Scott, & Turner, 1994) was to longitudinally assess auditory function in a group of pediatric subjects (ages 5 months to 16 years) with SCD. Twenty-four subjects received comprehensive audiologic evaluations (pure-tone and speech audiometry and immittance measurements), while eight subjects received electrophysiologic testing (ABR). Six children exhibited a mild bilateral conductive hearing impairment, one exhibited a slight high frequency sensorineural hearing impairment, and one exhibited both a mild conductive impairment in the low frequencies and a slight sensorineural impairment in the high frequencies (see Table 13-4). Some of the children also exhibited abnormalities on acoustic reflexes and acoustic reflex decay and ABR waveforms and latencies.

From the various studies, it can be concluded that there is evidence of peripheral and central auditory dysfunction in children with SCD. Permanent peripheral dysfunction is most likely to manifest itself as a high-frequency sensorineural hearing impairment. The incidence of conductive hearing impairment may vary because children with SCD are susceptible to infections, but at the same time they are being administered prophylactic penicillin to prevent infections. Central auditory dysfunction is not uncommon, but shows no consistent pattern. Children

**TABLE 13-4    Selected Pediatric Studies on Hearing Impairment and Sickle Cell Disease**

| Investigator | Number of Subjects | Age in Years/Disease | Number (Percent) Sensorineural Loss | Number (Percent) Conductive Loss |
|---|---|---|---|---|
| Friedman, Luban, Herer, & Williams (1980) | 43 | 7–18    HbSS | 5 (12%) | 0 (0%) |
| Forman-Franco, Karayalcin, Mandel, & Abramson (1982) | 54 | Mean = 12 HbSS | 2 (3.7%) | 4 (7.4%) |
| Crawford, Burch-Sims, Scott, & Turner (1994) | 24 | 5 mo.–16  HbSS (17) | 2 (8%) | 7 (29%) |
| | | HbSC (4) HbSD (1) Hb-thalassemia (2) | | |

HbSS = sickle cell disease
HbSC = sickle cell-hemoglobin C disease
HbSD = sickle cell-hemoglobin D disease
Hb-thalassemia = sickle cell-beta thalassemia disease

should undergo periodic audiologic testing, including some form of central auditory testing. The use of otoacoustic emissions could provide useful information on site of lesion.

## HIV/AIDS

HIV is the human immunodeficiency virus that causes acquired immunodeficiency syndrome (AIDS). HIV is a retrovirus that infects white blood cells, the brain, the bowel, the skin, and other tissues (Simonds & Rogers, 1992).

Approximately six thousand infants are born to HIV-positive women each year, with 25 to 35 percent becoming HIV positive themselves (Ellerbrock, Bush, Chamberland, & Oxtoby, 1991). HIV affects children from all cultural groups, socioeconomic levels, family structures, and regions of the country. The majority of the children with HIV infection are born to mothers who are intravenous drug users (IVDUs) or mothers who were sexual partners of IVDUs. A disproportionate number of these women and their children are African American, Hispanic, and members of lower socioeconomic groups.

The number of American children contracting AIDS from their mothers at birth dropped 43 percent between 1992 and 1996 because women are getting tested earlier and beginning drug treatment. The Centers for Disease Control and Prevention (CDC) reported that 516 children were found to have AIDS in 1996, down 43 percent from 905 in 1992. The rate of infants found to have AIDS before age 1 has fallen 39 percent, from 8.4 per 100,000 births in 1992 to 5.1 in 1995 (CDC: Rate of babies, 1997).

Doctors believe most mothers who pass HIV to their babies do so during delivery, when the infant is exposed to the mother's blood and other fluids. Nationwide, the antiviral drug AZT has been given regularly during pregnancy since a successful 1994 experiment. As stated previously, without treatment, more than 25 percent of HIV-positive mothers will pass the virus to their newborns. With AZT, the rate drops to approximately 8 percent (CDC: Rate of babies, 1997).

In 1989, 55 percent of the children with reported perinatally acquired AIDS were African American, 33 percent Hispanic, and 12 percent white. Fifty percent were male, and 42 percent were diagnosed before 1 year of age (Simonds & Rogers, 1992). The percent of cumulative pediatric AIDS cases reported through June 1991 by ethnicity included 52.7 percent African Americans, 25.1 percent Hispanics, 21.3 percent whites, 0.5 percent Asian/Pacific Islanders, and 0.2 percent American Indians (Fleming, Gwinn, & Oxtoby, 1992). Most women (73%) and children (78%) with AIDS are African American and Hispanic. African American women are 13.8 times more likely to contract AIDS than white women. African American children are 12.8 times more likely to contract AIDS than white children (Jenkins, 1992). The greater incidence of AIDS among African American children is due to the higher rates of infection in African American women, which in turn is due to their higher rates of IV drug abuse and higher rates of infection among their drug-using sexual partners. AIDS is the eighth leading cause of death among African American women 15 to 44 years of age (Jenkins, 1992). African American children are far more likely to be orphaned at the death of both parents from AIDS (Rothenberg, Woefel, Stoneburner, Milberg, Parker, & Truman, 1987).

Hearing impairment associated with HIV/AIDS is generally viewed as a secondary disorder arising from at least three primary etiologies: (1) direct infection of the hearing mechanism by HIV itself; (2) other opportunistic infections that attack the hearing mechanism (e.g., an acquired viral illness, such as CMV); and (3) damage to the hearing mechanism due to toxic side effects of medications prescribed to treat the HIV or any associated opportunistic infections (Lalwani & Sooy, 1992; Madriz & Herrera, 1995). The hearing impairment can be manifested as a conductive, sensorineural, or central auditory disorder (Lalwani & Sooy, 1992).

Hearing impairments are prevalent when accompanied by the presence of developmental delays. At a university-affiliated program where a special multiprofessional team was established to serve children with HIV infection and their families, 50 percent of the children seen had conductive hearing loss and 5 percent had severe to profound sensorineural hearing impairment (Diamond & Cohen, 1992). Audiological evaluations, therefore, are crucial and should be conducted at least annually. Central auditory tests should be included in the test battery.

Children with HIV infections require the array of services needed by any children with chronic health conditions. Their individual needs should be assessed by an interdisciplinary team of professionals. The needs of the children with chronic infections change and therefore must be monitored regularly so that current needs can be addressed. Because some children with HIV infection who had been asymptomatic can later present with developmental changes, including loss of developmental milestones and limited expressive language, there is a need to test these children and monitor their growth and development closely. The children's caregivers can be provided with pamphlets describing developmental milestones and what behaviors they should be monitoring.

## The Deaf

A culturally and linguistically diverse child who also is deaf is dealing with at least three cultures—the culture of the ethnic or racial group, the culture of the Deaf community, and the mainstream culture. As mentioned previously, the numbers of culturally and linguistically diverse deaf students have increased significantly over the years. The most rapidly growing group of culturally and linguistically diverse deaf students is Hispanic. In the 1979–1980 Survey of Hearing-Impaired Children from Non-Native (English) Language Homes conducted by the Center for Assessment and Demographic Studies at Gallaudet University, it was estimated that 7 percent of deaf children came from linguistically diverse homes.* It was assumed, however, that schools have underreported the actual numbers of deaf children from linguistically diverse homes (Delgado, 1981, 1984). Many of the linguistically diverse children are from racial/ethnic minority populations that historically have been undercounted, and many schools probably did not know if their children came from linguistically diverse homes.

Diverse deaf children come from homes with languages such as Spanish, Vietnamese, Laotian, Hmong, and Navaho. Among school personnel Spanish is probably the non-English language most likely to be spoken. Yet, there are few teachers of the deaf who speak Spanish fluently, are familiar with the cultures of their Hispanic deaf students, or are trained in bilingual methodology, in addition to being fluent in ASL and familiar with Deaf culture (Gonzales, 1990). The same situation would exist for children whose home languages were other non-English languages.

The academic performance of Hispanic and African American deaf children is significantly worse when compared to their white deaf peers. African American deaf children achieve less than white deaf children, and Hispanic deaf children achieve at the lowest level of all (Cohen, Fischgrund, & Redding, 1990). An analysis of the issues that face culturally and linguistically diverse hearing children indicates that culturally and linguistically diverse deaf children may fail in school for many of the same reasons that their hearing culturally and linguistically diverse peers do (Gerner de Garcia, 1990; Simmons de Garcia, 1988).

Linguistic diversity within the Deaf community presents some challenges. It is accepted that deaf children with deaf parents will use ASL, but what about deaf children who are exposed to languages other than English and ASL? Deaf people from other countries do have their own sign languages. Examples are French, Russian, Puerto Rican, Dominican, Mexican, Colombian, Venezuelan, and Cuban Sign Languages (Gerner de Garcia, 1992).

What happens to children who are exposed to languages other than English or ASL? Spanish will be used in this chapter as the exemplar for all non-English languages. When a deaf child is from a Spanish-speaking home, questions of language dominance and language proficiency in Spanish, English, and a signed language must be considered. The dominant language should be used for assessing the child, although it is

*The language used in the deaf or hard of hearing child's home is collected on an occasional basis in the Annual Survey (Schildroth & Hotto, 1995).

important to know the child's proficiency in Spanish, English, and a signed language in order to plan a program and decide placement (Gerner de Garcia, 1993). If the child is Spanish dominant, then the evaluator should try to determine the child's expressive and receptive abilities in Spanish (Payan, 1989), as well as language proficiency or competence in English. Most deaf children of hearing parents begin school with no fluency in any language (Johnson, Liddell, & Erting, 1989). Hispanic deaf children from Spanish-speaking homes who begin school in the United States vary in their language preference. Deaf children who begin their education in a Spanish-speaking country may be Spanish dominant. However, programs for the deaf in Spanish-speaking countries vary in quality, and almost all of them are oral (Gerner de Garcia, 1993).

In order to perform an appropriate assessment of a culturally and linguistically diverse child, a team of professionals may be needed. This team should consist of multilingual professionals including, bilingual audiologists, bilingual speech-language pathologists, and psychologists who have knowledge of the deaf and/or who are bilingual, fluent ASL signers, and individuals who can provide information about other countries' deaf education programs.

Schools for the deaf can better meet the needs of the growing number of Hispanic deaf children by doing the following: promoting a positive attitude toward diversity at all levels of the school by embracing a multicultural curriculum, and working to involve and empower parents of Hispanic deaf children by providing ASL classes taught in Spanish and setting up parent groups for Spanish-speaking families (Gerner de Garcia, 1993). Inservices can be provided to school personnel on bilingual and trilingual education, English as a Second Language, multicultural literature and other resources, cross-cultural communication, and Spanish for educators.

Audiologists and speech-language pathologists can work as a member of a team and advocate for the deaf child. Audiologists and speech-language pathologists once again must be cognizant of the Deaf community's beliefs regarding the use of cochlear implants and its preference for the use of ASL. These beliefs can differ based on the racial/ethnic or linguistic background of the family. Therefore, audiologists and speech-language pathologists must take the cultural and linguistic background of the child into consideration during the assessment and intervention process and in making recommendations.

## SUMMARY AND RECOMMENDATIONS

Audiologists and other service providers must become cross-culturally competent. To do so is a lifelong process. No one can ever know everything there is to know about all cultures, but they can learn about the cultures of the community they serve. Cultural ignorance and an unwillingness to learn can actually harm culturally and linguistically diverse children and their families. For example, culturally and linguistically diverse children may not receive appropriate assessment and intervention services and the entire family's quality of life may suffer. Audiologists need to educate themselves about the relationship between race/ethnicity and auditory disorders and about cultural views of disability. They must be willing to change their case history forms, use of interpreters, interactions with the surrounding community, and, ultimately, themselves in order to serve culturally diverse children and their families.

Nevertheless, audiologists and other service providers must be aware that cultural identity is not the only critical influence on a person's life. Other factors also shape children and their families' lives and how they identify themselves. These factors include socioeconomic status, educational level, age, gender, language proficiency, length of residency and time of arrival in the United States, and proximity to their own cultural or ethnic group as well as proximity to other cultural or ethnic groups. Each child and family is different, and culture-specific information cannot be assumed to apply to every situation.

Audiologists, speech-language pathologists, and other service providers must bear in mind the "platinum rule." They must remember to treat the family not as they would want to be treated but as the family would want to be treated.

## STUDY QUESTIONS AND ACTIVITIES

1. You have taken a new job in a Spanish-speaking community in Washington, DC. What steps might you take to become more cross-culturally competent and serve the community better?

2. A 4-year-old child with SCD is being seen for the first time by you, the audiologist. What would be some of your concerns regarding the child's speech, language, and hearing skills?

3. A 2-year-old Chinese American child who is deaf has been referred to you for a hearing assessment. What kinds of questions do you need to have answered (on the case history form) before conducting the evaluation? What kinds of information do you need to obtain during the evaluation? Who should participate in the evaluation?

4. You have noticed a change in your client (patient) caseload recently. You now are testing large numbers of children who speak Russian. What can you do to better assess and communicate with them and their families?

# REFERENCES

American Speech-Language-Hearing Association. (1989). Bilingual speech-language pathologists and audiologists. *Asha, 31,* 93.

Arena, J. M. (1935). Vascular accident and hemiplegia in patients with sickle cell anemia. *American Journal of Diseases in Children, 47,* 722–723.

Baird, R. L., Weiss, D. L., Ferguson, A. D., French, J. H., & Scott, R. B. (1964). Studies in sickle cell anemia, XXI. Clinical pathological aspects of neurological manifestations. *Pediatrics, 34,* 92–100.

Beery, Q. C., Doyle, W. J., Cantekin, E. I., Bluestone, C. D., & Wiet, R. J. (1980). Eustachian tube function in an American Indian population. *Annals of Otology, Rhinology and Laryngology, 89*(Suppl. 68), 28–33.

Bloom, M. (1995). *Understanding sickle cell disease.* Jackson: University Press of Mississippi.

Brislin, R. W., Cushner, K., Cherrie, C., & Yong, M. (1986). *Intercultural interactions: A practical guide.* Beverly Hills: Sage Publications.

CDC: Rate of babies born with HIV down 43 percent in 4 years. (1997, November 21) *News & Record* (Greensboro, NC), p. A6.

Cohen, O., Fischgrund, J., & Redding, R. (1990). Deaf children from ethnic, linguistic, and racial minority backgrounds: An overview. *American Annals of the Deaf, 135*(2), 67–73.

Cook, W. C. (1930). A case of sickle cell anemia with associated subarachnoid hemorrhage. *Journal of Medicine, 11,* 541–543.

Crawford, M. R., Burch-Sims, G. P., Scott, D. M., & Turner, E. (1994). *Audiologic considerations in sickle cell disease.* Paper presented at the annual convention of the American Academy of Audiology, Richmond, VA.

Cummings, J. (1976). *The communication abilities of preschool children with sickle cell disease: A preliminary study.* Unpublished doctoral dissertation, Howard University, Washington, DC.

Delgado, G. (1981). International baseline on hearing-impaired children with non-native home languages. *American Annals of the Deaf, 126,* 118–121.

Delgado, G. (1984). *The Hispanic deaf: Issues and challenges for bilingual special education.* Washington, DC: Gallaudet Press.

Diamond, G. W., & Cohen, H. J. (1992). Developmental disabilities in children with HIV infection. In A. C. Crocker, H. J. Cohen, & T. Kastner (Eds.), *HIV infection and developmental disabilities: A resource for service providers.* Baltimore, MD: Paul H. Brookes.

Doyle, W. J. (1977). *A functiono-anatomic description of eustachian tube vector relations in four ethnic populations—an osteologic study.* Unpublished doctoral dissertation, University of Pittsburgh, Pittsburgh, PA.

Ellerbrock, T., Bush, T., Chamberland, M., & Oxtoby, M. (1991). Epidemiology of women with AIDS in the U.S., 1981–1990. *Journal of the National Medical Association, 256*(22), 2971–2975.

Fleming, P., Gwinn, M., & Oxtoby, M. (1992). Epidemiology of HIV infection. In R. Yogev & E. Connor (Eds.), *Management of HIV infection in infants and children* (pp. 7–22). St. Louis: Mosby-Yearbook.

Forman-Franco, B., Karayalcin, G., Mandel, D. D., & Abramson, A. L. (1982). The evaluation of auditory function in homozygous sickle cell disease. *Otolaryngology—Head and Neck Surgery, 89,* 850–856.

Friedman, E. M., Luban, N. L. C., Herer, G. R., & Williams, I. (1980). Sickle cell anemia and hearing. *Annals of Otology, Rhinology and Laryngology, 89,* 342–349.

Gerner de Garcia, B. (1990, March). *Multilingual education for Hispanic deaf children.* Paper presented at TESOL Convention, San Francisco, CA.

Gerner de Garcia, B. (1992). Diversity in deaf education: What we can learn from bilingual and ESL education. In D. S. Martin & R. T. Mobley (Eds.), *Proceedings of the first international symposium on teacher education in deafness* (pp. II-126–II-139). Washington, DC: Gallaudet Press.

Gerner de Garcia, B. (1993). Addressing the needs of Hispanic deaf children. In K. Christensen & G. Delgado (Eds.), *Multicultural issues in deafness* (pp. 69–90). White Plains, NY: Longman.

Gonzales, R. (1990). *Program to train Hispanic teachers to meet the cultural and educational needs of Hispanic hearing-impaired children in the United States.* Paper presented to 17th International Congress on Education of the Deaf, Rochester, NY.

Groce, N. E., & Zola, I. K. (1993). Multiculturalism, chronic illness, and disability. *Pediatrics, 91*(5), Suppl., 1048–1055.

Hanson, M. J., Lynch, E. W., & Wayman, K. I. (1990). Honoring the cultural diversity of families when gathering data. *Topics in Early Childhood Special Education, 10*(1), 112–131.

Jenkins, B. (1992). AIDS/HIV epidemics in the Black community. In R. L. Braithwaite & S. E. Taylor (Eds.), *Health issues in the Black community* (pp. 55–63). San Francisco: Josey-Bass Publishers.

Johnson, R., Liddell, S., & Erting, C. (1989). *Unlocking the curriculum: Principles for achieving access in deaf education.* Unpublished paper, Gallaudet Research Institute, Washington, DC.

Kampeier, R. H. (1936). Sickle cell anemia as a cause of cerebral vascular disease. *Archives of Neurology and Psychiatry, 36,* 1323–1329.

Lalwani, A., & Sooy, D. (1992). Manifestaciones otologicas y neuro-otologicas del SIDA. *Clinicas Otorrinolaringologicas de Norte America, 6,* 1239–1254.

Lane, M. (1984). Reaffirmations: Speaking out for children. A child's right to the valuing of diversity. *Young Children, 39*(6), 76.

Lynch, E. W. (1992). Developing cross-cultural competence. In E. W. Lynch & M. J. Hanson (Eds.), *Developing cross-cultural competence: A guide for working with young children and their families.* Baltimore, MD: Paul H. Brookes.

Madriz, J. J., & Herrera, G. (1995). Human immunodeficiency virus and acquired immune deficiency syndrome: AIDS-related hearing disorders. *Journal of the American Academy of Audiology, 6,* 358–364.

Orque, M., Block, B., & Monrroy, L. (1983). *Ethnic nursing care: A multicultural approach.* St. Louis: The C. V. Mosby Co.

Payan, R. (1989). Language assessment of the bilingual exceptional child. In L. Baca & H. Cervantes (Eds.), *The bilingual special education interface.* Columbus, OH: Charles E. Merrill.

Reis, P. W. (1986). Current estimates from the National Health Interview Survey, United States, 1984. *Vital and health statistics,* Series 10, No. 156. DHHS Pub. No. (PHS) 86-1584. National Center for Health Statistics, Public Health Service. Washington, DC: U.S. Government Printing Office.

Roseberry-McKibbin, C. (1995). *Multicultural students with special language needs: Practical strategies for assessment and intervention.* Oceanside, CA: Academic Communication Associates.

Rothenberg, R., Woefel, M., Stoneburner, R., Milberg, J., Parker, R., & Truman, B. (1987). Survival with the acquired immunodeficiency syndrome: Experience with 5833 cases in New York City. *New England Journal of Medicine, 317,* 1297–1302.

Schildroth, A. N., & Hotto, S. A. (1995). Race and ethnic background in the Annual Survey of Deaf and Hard of Hearing Children and Youth. *American Annals of the Deaf, 140*(2), 96–99.

Simmons de Garcia, J. (1988). *The linguistic and cultural diversity of deaf children: Implications for language and literacy development.* Unpublished qualifying paper, Harvard University, Cambridge, MA.

Simonds, R., & Rogers, M. (1992). Epidemiology of HIV infection in children and other populations. In A. C. Crocker, H. J. Cohen, & T. Kastner (Eds.), *HIV infection and developmental disabilities: A resource for service providers* (pp. 3–13). Baltimore, MD: Paul H. Brookes.

U.S. Bureau of the Census. (November 1992). *Population projections for states by age, sex, race, and Hispanic origin: 1992 to 2050.* Current Population Reports, P25-1092. Washington, DC: U.S. Government Printing Office.

U.S. Bureau of the Census. (February 1996). *Population projections for states by age, sex, race, and Hispanic origin: 1995 to 2050.* Current Population Reports, P25-1130. Washington, DC: U.S. Government Printing Office.

Waengler, H-H. B., & Bauman-Waengler, J. A. (1992). *Sickle cell anemia: Language performance in preschoolers.* Paper presented at the American Speech-Language-Hearing Association National Convention, San Antonio, TX.

Wayman, K. I., Lynch, E. W., & Hanson, M. J. (1990). Home-based early childhood services: Cultural sensitivity in a family systems approach. *Topics in Early Childhood Special Education, 10,* 65–66.

# 14

# AUGMENTATIVE/ALTERNATIVE COMMUNICATION AND ASSISTIVE TECHNOLOGY

## SHEILA J. BRIDGES and THOMAS E. MIDGETTE

Language is the vehicle by which culture is transmitted. It is, in fact, the essence of human existence and comes to shape our cultural self-identity. Within the realm of speech-language pathology, language (oral and non-oral) is identified as impaired or disordered when it deviates significantly from the recognized norms of the speaker's linguistic community or indigenous culture by drawing negative attention to itself, interfering with communication, and/or causing the individual to be maladjusted (Taylor, 1986). The interdependence of language and culture would imply that those factors contributing to impaired or disordered linguistic competence would further contribute to impaired cultural competence.

The challenge to speech-language pathologists who provide augmentative and alternative communication services to infants, toddlers, and their families is the responsibility of identifying an alternative (nonoral) mode of expression that adequately facilitates the transmission of culture. This mode of expression is often required to take an altered form, which, by nature of its definition (augmentative/alternative), deviates from the norm. In the absence of functional/traditional verbal expression, alternative modes of expression (aided and unaided) must be identified, developed, and applied within the infant's immediate linguistic family and larger language community. When the cultural background of the service provider differs from the culture of the family he or she is serving, this call for cultural sensitivity may be responded to with some trepidation and viewed as a challenge to the service provider's clinical competence.

To define augmentative and alternative communication within a cultural context demands a very broad perspective. Its actual application and integrated use in a diverse cultural context requires us to look beyond current documented AAC literature. It requires a transdisciplinary perspective that integrates family systems, counseling, sociolinguistics, and anthropology along with assistive/computer technology.

This chapter will examine AAC in early intervention across diverse cultural (racial and linguistic) groups from a transdisciplinary perspective. Beyond a theoretical view, practical application and critical use of alternative assessment and family-centered treatment models will be discussed.

## WHAT IS AUGMENTATIVE/ALTERNATIVE COMMUNICATION (AAC) AND ASSISTIVE TECHNOLOGY (AT)?

According to the American Speech-Language-Hearing Association,

> Augmentative and alternative communication is an area of clinical practice that attempts to compensate and facilitate, either temporarily or permanently, for the impairment and disability patterns of individuals with severe expressive communication and/or language comprehension disorders. AAC may be required for individuals demonstrating impairments in gestural, spoken, and/ or written modes of communication. (ASHA, 1991a, p. 8)

As an area of clinical practice, AAC services are addressed by a multidisciplinary or interdisciplinary team of professionals that includes, but is not limited to, a physical therapist, occupational therapist, speech-language pathologist, rehabilitation/vocational counselor, educator, psychologist, and rehabilitation technician/engineer. AAC intervention is multimodal, "utilizing the individual's full capabilities, including any residual speech or vocalizations, gestures, signs, and other aided communication" (ASHA, 1991b, p. 10). Other terms related to AAC include AAC system, symbols, aided and unaided, strategies and techniques (ASHA, 1991a, 1991b).

1. *An AAC system* is an integrated group of components that includes symbols, aids, strategies, and techniques used to enhance communi-

cation. Its augmentative function serves to augment or supplement gestural, spoken, and/or written communication abilities.

2. *Symbols* are visual, auditory, and/or tactile representations of conventional concepts ranging from gestures, picto-ideographs, printed text, and Braille, to spoken words. Symbols are representative in nature in that they are something that "stand for or represent something else."

3. *Aided symbols* are physical devices or objects that facilitate the transmission and/or reception of messages. Aided communication may take the form of a communication book, word board or chart, low or high technological dedicated communication device or computer. *Unaided symbols* require no external device for production and can range from facial expression, natural speech, and vocal and manual gestures to sign language. Table 14-1 provides examples of aided and unaided symbols and strategies.

## TABLE 14-1   Communication Symbols and Strategies

*Unaided Communication*
- Speech
- Vocalizations (intonation, inflection, volume, etc.)
- Facial expression
- Eye blink
- Body posture, position
- Natural sign languages (American Sign Language (ASL), British Sign Language, (BSL), etc.
- Educational sign systems (Seeing Essential English, Signing Exact English, Signed English, Linguistics of Visual English, Duffysigns, etc.)
- Gestural language codes (fingerspelling, Gestural Morse Code, Cued Speech)
- Other (natural gestures, pantomime, Amer-Ind gestural codes, etc.)

*Aided Communication Symbols*
- Tangible symbols
- Objects (real life, miniature)
- Representational symbol systems: photographs, pictures, drawings, graphic symbols (Blissymbols, Picsyms, PCS, Rebus, customized pictographs and ideographs)
- Abstract symbol systems (Logographs, Yerkish lexigrams, and Premack-type shapes, etc.)
- Symbolic language codes (traditional orthography, visual phonetic, phonemic symbols, Initial Teaching Alphabet [ITA], words, alphabetic clusters [WRITE 200], Braille, Morse code, NU-VUE-CUE, etc.)
- Synthetic speech and recorded/digitized speech

From: Beukelman & Mirenda, 1992; Blackstone, 1986; Musselwhite & St. Louis, 1988.

4. *Strategies* are the ways in which AAC aids, symbols, and/or techniques are utilized for the purpose of enhancing communication. Whether through formal training, self-teaching, or discovery, strategies determine the effectiveness and efficiency of an AAC system.
5. *Techniques* are the methods by which messages selected and transmitted. Techniques include direct selection, scanning, and encoding. These techniques are not mutually exclusive and often used in a complementary fashion. For example, direct selection (e.g., pointing manually by hand, via eye gaze, or with a pointing device such as a joystick, head pointer, mouth stick) may be used to encode a message. The symbols selected for encoding (alphanumeric, pictographs, Minspeak, Morse code, rebus symbols) are used in combination to communicate a single concept, message, or complete thought.
6. Similarly, a *scanning* (linear, row-column, etc.) *technique* may be used to encode a message as well, making selections using single or dual switch input.

Assistive technology includes AAC but also encompasses many other forms of technology. If you were to imagine any aspect of your life challenged by a sensory, motor, or cognitive disability, you would find an inexhaustible number of needs for which you could benefit from technological assistance, ranging from low tech, light tech, to high tech. Assistive technology provides aid for individuals with disabilities aid to increase their level of independence, productivity, and access to inclusive programs through computer access, auditory aids, educational and recreational access, environmental control, mobility, as well as electronic interfaces. Assistive technology areas include:

- Academic and vocational skills
- Augmentative communication
- Computer technology
- Daily living skills
- Engineering
- Mobility
- Seating and positioning
- Written communication (Church & Glennen, 1992)

There are a reported 32 million noninstitutionalized persons with chronic health disabilities (NIDRR, National Institute on Disability and Rehabilitation Research, as cited in Church & Glennen, 1992), and a significant number of individuals with acquired neurogenic disorders and traumatic injury that could benefit from assistive technology (AT) and equipment (Church & Glennen, 1992). Within this population are individuals with severe expressive and/or receptive language impairments that could benefit from augmentative or alternative modes of communication. Minorities with disabilities are significantly over represented in this population with a prevalence of disabilities 50 to 100 percent higher among minorities (Rehabilitation Act Amendment of 1992).

Technological advancements have contributed greatly to treatment alternatives for individuals with disabilities. Furthermore, state and federal policies have been crucial to contributing to the accessibility and advancement of technology for individuals with disabilities who could benefit from its application and use.

## Public Policy and Federal Law

A number of landmark cases and public laws have contributed to an increase in the quality and accessibility of services and support for children with disabilities and their families. The Individuals with Disabilities Education Act (IDEA) of 1990 (PL 100-476, formerly the Education for all Handicapped Children, PL 94-142, 1975) expanded the law to include early intervention services for children with special needs ages birth to 5 years and their families. In 1991, an amendment (PL 102-119) was passed making developmentally delayed 3- to 5-year-olds and all children eligible for receiving a publicly funded education or early intervention through special education and related services in the least restrictive environment. Thus, public schools could no longer disqualify students from educational services due to severe disabilities (Beukelman & Mirenda, 1992). Additional modifications included facilitation of the transition from early intervention programs to preschool programs and the use of Individual Family Service Plans (IFSPs) for preschool children with disabilities.

The Technology-Related Assistance for Individuals with Disabilities Act of 1989 (PL 100-407, Tech Act) provides financial incentives in the form of grants enabling states to make assistive technology services available to all persons regardless of age, disability, or location (Beukelman & Mirenda, 1992).

## IDENTIFYING THE DIVERSITY OF AAC SYSTEM USERS

### Culturally Diverse Populations

The growing diversity of families receiving early intervention AAC services reflects the demographic shift witnessed in the expansion of African American, Native American, Asian American, and Hispanic American populations in the United States. Diversity is further witnessed in the varying linguistic groups represented by these populations as well as in the diversity of young children with disabling conditions who could benefit from AAC.

The demographics shift anticipated for the twenty-first century suggests that racially diverse groups will increase to 45 million by the year 2000, 63 million in the year 2030, and 79 million in 2080. The shifting demographics are felt by large urban as well as small rural communities. States predicted to have an ethnically/racially diverse population exceeding 50 percent (and thus a majority) by the year 2020 include Washington DC, New Mexico, Hawaii, California, and Texas (Kuster, 1997).

In light of these demographic changes, AAC service providers in sparsely as well as heavily populated urban and rural communities will be required to meet the challenges of addressing the diverse needs of children and families whose cultural, life, and linguistic experiences vary greatly from the mainstream.

## Linguistically Diverse Populations

Linguistic diversity has been an inherent characteristic of racial, regional, and economically diverse English-speaking communities throughout U.S. history. The influx of non-English proficient (NEP) and limited English proficient (LEP) immigrants has served to expand the linguistic diversity of Americans by leaps and bounds within the past several decades. The major home languages of the current LEP students in U.S. schools include Spanish, Vietnamese, Cantonese, Cambodian, Hmong, Filipino, Korean, Lao, Armenian, Mandarin, Japanese, Farsi, Portuguese, Arabic, and many others (Cheng, 1996). The impact of the linguistic diversity of today's LEP student is most evident in California where over 100 languages are represented in California schools (Cheng, 1996). The 1990 Census reported 6 million foreign-born immigrants in California, reflecting a wide level of competencies in English proficiency (LEP, NEP, bilingual, etc.).

In spite of the diversification of American culture, there continue to be common threads that bind Americans of diverse cultural groups. The larger American society in which we live represents a macroculture in which we are all enculturated, while our families represent microcultures. Thus, cultural development includes elements of both (Hetzroni & Harris, 1996).

## Families with Children with Disabilities

Families with children with disabilities represent another microcultural group sharing similar behavior patterns, values, and common needs for interacting with their disabled children (Blackstone, 1993). Children with disabilities in turn are part of still another microcultural group. AAC users, like all children, first belong to their family, which provides them automatic membership in the family's cultural group. However, culturally and linguistically diverse children with severe communication impairment belong to another "minority" group, that of persons with disabilities (Blackstone, 1993).

Any infant or toddler at risk for speech-language delays as well as other developmental delays may be a potential candidate for AAC services. Most often these children are not identified as potential candidates for AAC until they reach preschool age. Such a delay may limit their opportunity to reap the benefits of early intervention while potentially placing them at further risk for increased delay. It is important to identify early those children who typically could benefit from augmentative and alternative modes of communication.

Table 14-2 provides a list of disabling conditions where AAC could potentially benefit. Candidates for AAC fall into wide ranges in age and in type and severity of disability, including those with congenital conditions, acquired disabilities, progressive neurological diseases, and temporary conditions (Beukelman & Mirenda, 1992; Blackstone, 1986). While this list is neither exhaustive nor predictive of the anticipated benefits AAC might contribute in the treatment of a specific disability, it does serve to alert the clinician to potential solutions in serving children with severe communication impairments.

## AAC AND CULTURALLY DIVERSE POPULATIONS

"**Culture** consists of all things that people have learned to do, believe, value, and enjoy in their history. It is the totality of ideals, beliefs, skills, tools, customs, and institutions into which each member of society is born" (Sue & Sue, 1990, p. 35).

### Cultural and Linguistic Considerations

Belonging to a particular culture may mean sharing common values and experiences of other group members; however, members within the group often differ as well. Individual differences should not be overlooked in the discussion of cultural generalizations.

There is an ever-present danger of overgeneralizing and stereotyping the values, characteristics, and experiences of culturally diverse groups. A discussion of the characteristics of any one group does not imply that these characteristics are evident in each individual member. A more efficient use of generalizations is to recognize their application and value

**TABLE 14-2    Disabling Conditions That Could Benefit from AAC and/or AT**

*Congenital Conditions*
Developmental apraxia
Specific language impairment (SLI)
Learning disability
Primary motor impairment
Severe intellectual disability
Autism
Visual, hearing, and dual sensory impairment
Developmental aphasia

*Acquired Conditions*
Traumatic brain injury
Cerebral vascular accident (stroke)
Spinal cord injury
Laryngectomy
Elective autism
Asphyxia
Glossectomy
Multiple sclerosis

*Progressive Neurological Conditions*
Multiple sclerosis (MS)
Multiple dystrophy (MD)
Parkinson disease
Huntington chorea
Acquired Immune Deficiency Syndrome (AIDS)
Amyotrophic lateral sclerosis (Lou Gehrig disease, ALS)
Alzheimer dementia

*Temporary Conditions*
Traumatic injury (emotional/physical trauma)
Invasive surgical intervention (intubation, tracheotomy, laryngectomy)
Guillian Barré syndrome (chronic condition)
Reyes syndrome (chronic condition)

From: Blackstone, 1986; Beukelman & Mirenda, 1992

in new situations by providing background, while acknowledging the need to verify, change, and redefine (Sue & Sue, 1990). On the other hand, the dangers of stereotypes, characterized as "rigid preconceptions" that are held about all members of a particular group without regard for individuality, puts one at risk for resisting change and redefinition in spite of evidence denying their validity. Recognizing that, stereotypes serve to distort conflicting data to make it conform to preconceived notions (Sue & Sue, 1990).

Culture is an intimate part of who we are. It pervades every part of our conscious and unconscious selves. While Table 14-3 provides an extensive list of the areas of our lives that culture pervades, it is not exhaustive. As service providers, the quality and effectiveness of our services are strongly influenced by our understanding and sensitivity to the communication style, language and dialect, family relationships and sex roles, acculturation, health care, beliefs, help-seeking behavior, and time orientation of the families we serve.

The following discussion is intended to contribute to the design and implementation of culturally sensitive services based on an understanding of the differences and similarities among the culturally and linguistically diverse children and families we serve. Particular attention is given to the cultural characteristics of Native American, African American, Asian Americans, and Hispanic American families.

## Native American Families

There is great diversity among Native Americans. Native Americans are a heterogeneous group comprised of approximately 530 tribes, 280 reservations, 209 Alaska Native Villages, and 200 distinct languages (G. Harris, 1993; Sue & Sue, 1990). Variations in customs, life experiences, and

**TABLE 14-3    Pervasive Influences of Culture**

- Family structure and orientation
- Important events in the life cycle
- Roles of individual members
- Rules of interpersonal interactions
- Rules for etiquette, decorum, and discipline
- Religious beliefs and spirituality
- Values and practices in health care
- Food preferences
- Generational status
- Holidays and celebrations
- Value and methods of education and learning
- Perception of work and play
- Perceptions of time and space
- Cultural history and traditions
- Value of music and other art forms
- Life expectations and aspirations
- Social mores
- Incidence and prevalence of disability
- Communication (semantic, syntactic, pragmatic, linguistic, etc.) patterns
- Perceptions of and attitudes toward impairments, illness, and disability

From: Blackstone, 1993; p. 1; Wallace, 1997.

family structure cover a wide range. However, certain generalizations can be appropriately made regarding Native American family orientation and value of sharing, cooperation, noninterference, time, and harmony with nature.

### Extended Family Orientation
In Native American traditional values, extended family is very important, and a high level of interrelationship is maintained between many relatives. Elders of the tribe are treated with respect and viewed as wise and knowledgeable.

### Sharing
Honor and respect are gained through sharing and giving rather than the practice of accumulating material goods, a respected practice by mainstream America.

### Cooperation
The family and group take precedent over any individual. This cooperative behavior may be viewed by mainstream Americans as lack of competitiveness with child peers in sports or academics; reticence to debate an issue, position, or point, or to stand in defense of oneself; or insincerity when harmonious agreement is verbalized but not played out by behavior.

### Noninterference
Less likely to "take charge," an asset by mainstream American standards, Native Americans more often assume a role of noninterference in others' behavior, a respect for other people's rights, and an avoidance of impulsive action.

### Time Orientation
With greater focus on and appreciation for the present, the future plays a role of less importance. Life is lived in the here and now and punctuality and planning are valued as less important and in some instances viewed negatively. Progress is made according to a rational order rather than confined by deadlines. This notion of time is contrary to mainstream society, which attributes achievement to the religious planning and implementation of goals.

### Harmony with Nature
Native Americans place value on nature and the acceptance of things as they are. This is contrary to mainstream American society, which values mastery and control of the environment (Sue & Sue, 1990).

A lack of awareness or sensitivity to the above Native American values can lead to erroneous interpretation, cross-cultural conflict, language barriers, bias assessment, and ineffective intervention resulting in early termination of services.

## African Americans

Representing the largest culturally diverse group in the United States, over 86 percent of African Americans reside in urban areas throughout the country. Current statistical data on the economic, health, and employment status of African Americans have provided a slanted look at the population by reflecting mostly individuals of lower socioeconomic status (Sue & Sue, 1990). The lack of representative data reflecting the diversity of African Americans has led to the perpetuation of stereotypes and overgeneralizations. However, the following data can provide insight to the status of African American families and their values.

### Extended Families
An extended family network continues to dominate most African American families. In spite of the ongoing concern for the rising number of matriarchal, female-headed households, extended African American families provide economic and emotional support. "Within the African American family there is an adaptability of family roles, strong kinship bonds, a strong work and achievement ethic, and strong religious orientation" (Sue & Sue, 1990, p. 211). Assertiveness and self-esteem are instilled in African American children by their families.

### Cultural Values
"African American values have been shaped by cultural factors, social class variables, and experiences with racism" (Sue & Sue, 1990, p. 215). These values include group-centered collaboration, interdependence, and sensitivity to interpersonal matters. A history of racism has contributed to mistrust and defensiveness in white-black relationships. Where black-black relationships tend to be playful, expressive, and open, white-black relationships tend to be more guarded, less verbal, and formal.

Understanding the above information should aid in early intervention with African American families.

## Asian Americans

Asian and Pacific Islanders are quite diverse groups representing over 60 separate ethnic and racial groups and subgroups (Cheng, Breakey, & Wallace, 1997). Asian American immigrants represent four major geographic regions: East Asia, representing people of Chinese, Japanese, and Korean descent as well as former residents of Hong Kong and Taiwan; Southeast Asia, including people once residents of Vietnam, Laos, Cambodia, Kampuchea, and Thailand; South Asia, including people of India, Pakistan, Bangladesh, Sri Lanka, Bhutan, and Nepal (Cheng et al., 1997; Shekar & Hegde, 1996); West Asia, includes Iraq, Afghanistan and Turkey and the Middle East include Iraq, Israel and Lebanon (Gall & Gall, 1993).

While Pacific Islanders are of Asian Pacific heritage, they too are quite diverse in their lifestyles, language, culture, religion, and child-rearing practices. Pacific Islanders include residents of the Polynesian, Micronesian, and Melanesian Pacific Archipelagos (Cheng et al., 1997).

The recent demographic shift in Asian American populations is attributed to the 1965 changes in the immigration laws. In 1985 over 282,000 Asians entered the United States. This number is expected to double by 2010. Currently, Chinese represent the largest subgroup, followed by Filipinos and Japanese. Within the next twenty years, it is predicted that the Filipinos will represent the largest group, followed by Chinese, Koreans, Vietnamese, Asian Indians, and Japanese (Cheng et al., 1997; Doerner, 1985). Demographic data provides evidence of the diversity that exists under the broad cultural heading of Asian Americans. "Although Asian immigrants and refugees form very diverse groups, there are certain areas of commonality" (Sue & Sue, 1990, p. 197). The following represent some of these traditional cultural values.

### Family Values

Within Asian culture the extended family is highly valued, and specified roles and hierarchical structure are respected. Family roles and relationships are viewed as interdependent (Tsui & Schultz, 1985).

### Relationships

Social roles are defined and structured with emphasis on appropriate social relationships, deference to authority, and emotional restraint. Relationships are expected to be harmonious.

### Mental Health Care

While health care is advanced in a number of Asian countries, mental health and psychotherapy are relatively foreign concepts. Consequently, there is an underutilization of these services because a negative stigma (e.g., equating psychological problems with insanity and attributing their cause to some failure of the family) has been associated with them. Recipients of these services were found to be less open about their problems with limited confidence in the effectiveness of the mental health professional As physical illness is more culturally accepted, psychological problems are most often manifested as physical complaints. In fact, it is a common belief that physical illnesses cause emotional disturbances and can be remedied by treating the physical symptoms. Alternatively, nature is held accountable for mental illness, holding cosmic forces or a shear lack of will power responsible for the disorder. When health care is sought, treatment is expected to be short and rapid and the "healer" is expected to assume an active role with solutions to the problem (Sue & Sue, 1990).

## Hispanic Americans

For the purpose of this chapter, the term Hispanic American will be used to encompass Spanish-speaking cultural groups, which consist of individuals living in the United States with ancestry from Mexico, Puerto Rico, Cuba, El Salvador, the Dominican Republic, and other Latin American countries (Sue & Sue, 1990). Terms denoting indigenous culture or country of origin are used and have been found more acceptable than others within Hispanic American communities. These terms include La Raza, Latino, Mexicano, Mexican American, Chicano, Spanish American, or more specifically Cuban, Argentinean, Costa Rican, Puerto Rican, and so on (Reyes & Peterson, 1997; Sue & Sue, 1990). The diversity of Hispanic subgroups is evident by the indigenous cultures they represent, encompassing African, Indian, Latin, Asian, and European ancestry.

While there are distinct differences between and within the different groups of Hispanic Americans, they share some common characteristics in family values, religious beliefs and practices, and lifestyles.

### Family Values

Traditional Hispanic families are hierarchical in structure, with special authority given to the elderly, the parents, and the males. Sex roles are clearly delineated, and fathers assume the role of primary authority figure. Children are required to be obedient and play a passive role when family decisions are made. Family members maintain a high level of support, which extends into adulthood as siblings support one another and children provide support to their parents.

For Hispanic families, interpersonal relationships among extended family members and friends are critical. Family relationships tend to be nurturing and cooperative rather than competitive among blood and nonblood family members. Unity, loyalty, and tradition are synonymous with family, as are respect and affection. Extended family members are a source of support and play a critical role in decision making. The interdependence that exists among many family members can be both a source of support as well as a source of stress.

### Religious Beliefs and Practices
The Catholic religion plays a central role in many Hispanic homes and communities. Religious beliefs and practices are a source of comfort in times of crisis. Prayer, particularly in Mass, is very important. Common religious views and beliefs strongly influence life practices. Most influential are the following views: (1) Sacrifice in this world is helpful to salvation; (2) being charitable to others is a virtue; and (3) one should endure wrongs done against him or her (Yamamoto & Acosta, 1982). These views have strong implications for receptivity to health care and rehabilitative services. For example, Hispanic patients and their families tend to take a passive rather than an assertive role in seeking services, because some problems are viewed as "meant to be" and not subject to change. Misfortunes are considered inevitable and Hispanic culture dictates a response of resignation.

### Lifestyle
Puerto Rican culture highly values "being" over "doing." Experiencing the family and placing family members as priorities take precedent over work and individual achievement. Prestige and status are accomplished by respect and cooperation in the family. Time and planning are less of a concern than enjoying the here and now.

Subgroups of Hispanic Americans exist among those who have achieved various degrees of acculturation. Large differences exist among these subgroups, which are reflected by language, physical characteristics, customs, and values. Acculturation may be influenced by any number of microcultures, resulting in bicultural characteristics.

## CURRENT ISSUES IN THE DELIVERY OF AAC SERVICES IN EARLY INTERVENTION

"**Culture** is what individuals need to know to be functional members of a community and to regulate interaction with other members of the community and with individuals from backgrounds different from their own" (Saville-Troike, 1989, p. 48).

To date a growing number of articles, papers, and manuscripts address the delivery of services to culturally and linguistically diverse populations. In addition to the literature emerging in speech-language pathology, contributions are being made by the disciplines of counseling, early intervention, and anthropology. Current service delivery issues regarding the provision of early intervention services to culturally diverse families in AAC include cross-cultural conflict, cross-cultural assessment, communication/language differences, and family involvement. Service delivery that is based on ethnographic study, non-biased assessment, cultural sensitivity, and family-centered models offers solutions to many of the above issues. Issues of cross-cultural conflict, cross-cultural assessment, and family-centered services will present challenges that are transdisciplinary in nature. The remaining section of this chapter addresses these issues from a transdisciplinary perspective, with appreciation for the vantage point brought by each discipline.

## Cross-Cultural Conflict

"The world view of the culturally different is ultimately linked to the historical and current experience of racism and oppression in the United States. A culturally different client is likely to approach services with a great deal of healthy suspicion as to the deliverer's conscious and unconscious motives in a cross-cultural context" (Sue & Sue, 1990, p. 5).

Cross-cultural conflict can create a barrier to learning (services) by the racial/ethnic child as well as to his or her parent's involvement in the delivery of services. Differences in language and culturally bound values (e.g., attitudes, beliefs, customs, and institutions) can create stresses for both the child and parent (Atkinson & Juntunen, 1994).

Cultural values theory or orientation is a fundamental concept that incorporates normative cognitive thoughts about the world, connotative inclination toward a specific course of action, and affective elements (Carter, 1991). People act out of their cultural norms, attitudes, thoughts, and beliefs from their existential reality. "Mismatches of cultural values may affect the delivery of health and educational services, the communication process, and interactional dynamics" (Carter, 1991, p. 165). Researchers (Midgette, 1988; Sue & Sue, 1990) contend that the reasons culturally diverse individuals underutilize and prematurely terminate services lie in culturally incongruent expectations about services. Services too often are antagonistic and in conflict with the world view and life experiences of the culturally different consumer (Midgette, 1988; Sue & Sue, 1990).

## Help-Seeking Behaviors

Tseng and McDermott (1975) warn that the client's orientation to the process of help-seeking and the "fit" between traditional treatment regimens and those implemented by providers may be critical to successful process and outcomes, particularly in a cross-cultural context. Clinical practices are most often carried out in a Western culture or European American model of service delivery, most often characterized as left-brain oriented, following a linear/logical/analytic/verbal model (Sue & Sue, 1990). This model serves to drive clinical training, program design, and intervention, as well as policy. Furthermore, traditional clinical models reflect the cultural experiences of the majority of service providers, many of whom represent mainstream society. Cross-cultural barriers imposed by this model can be ascribed to the following (Sue & Sue, 1990):

1. Culture-bound values
2. Class-bound values
3. Language variables

### Culture-bound Values
Entrenched in mainstream American health care practices, culture-bound values tend to be individual-centered and utilize a cause-effect approach to treatment. Based on the use of mainstream American norms, differences are often viewed as disorders, and cultural heritage is viewed as a handicapping condition. Treatment models are individual-centered (clinician-consumer), contrary to many cultures (Hispanic, Asian American, African American, and Native American) that traditionally value extended family, group, and community.

Another traditional clinical practice is the goal of eliciting self-disclosure through the intimate revelation of personal or social history (child case history, parent interview, etc.). Sharing personal and social histories may not be acceptable, because this information not only reveals personal history of the individual but also of the entire family. Further, mistrust may be a factor limiting self-disclosure, with some concern regarding the intent of the interviewer and how the information might be used. Gaining trust and sharing friendships are often prerequisites to self-disclosure (Sue & Sue, 1990).

### Class-bound Values
Clinical practices are often permeated by middle- and upper-middle-class values, adhering to restricted time schedules and utilizing unstructured approaches to problem solving and to seeking long-range goals and solutions (Sue & Sue, 1990). Consequently, the service provider may have difficulty relating to low-income and impoverished clients and their families who are challenged by unemployment, underemployment, little property ownership, lack of savings, and feelings of helplessness and dependency. Service providers may erroneously attribute these attitudes to cultural or individual traits. A conflict in expectations of services and roles by the consumer and service provider often lead to ineffective intervention and premature termination of services.

### Language Variable
The growing number of dialect, LEP, and NEP speaking groups greatly exceeds the number of service providers representing these groups. A lack of trained professionals competent in this area of service delivery

contributes further to the underrepresentation of culturally and linguistically diverse families in the delivery of AAC services (Cole, 1989). According to the most recent ASHA (1998) membership report, minority communication disorders specialists constitute 5.2 percent of the certified SLP/Aud clinicians. This percentage represents 1761 African Americans, 1477 Hispanics, 1004 Asian/Pacific Islanders, and 225 American Indian/Alaskan Natives. Language barriers serve to limit the extent of communication, interfere with relationship building, and contribute to failure in understanding cultural nuances (Sue & Sue, 1990). Sue and Sue (1990) state, "one of the major barriers to effective understanding is the common assumption that different cultural groups operate according to identical speech communication conventions" (pp. 63, 64).

A solution to these challenges to our current service delivery system demands the development of general principles of service delivery.

1. As providers we have an ethical, intellectual, and professional responsibility to provide clients with the most accurate, culturally appropriate, current, and effective practices to enhance their growth (Midgette & Meggert, 1991).
2. Multicultural competence involves learning about oneself as a prelude to understanding others. It is then that effective and meaningful cross-cultural interactions can take place.
3. Speech-language pathologists and other service providers should not assume universal *etic* (outsider's) applications of their concepts and goals to the exclusion of culture specific *emic* (participant's/insider's) views (Sue & Sue, 1990).

Culturally sensitive therapists must take into account the following factors to develop an *emic* view (Sue & Sue, 1990).

- Accept each ethnic minority reality
- Recognize conflicting value systems
- Understand the nature of biculturalism
- Respect ethnic differences in minority status
- Appreciate the roles of ethnicity and language
- Clarify the roles of ethnicity and social class

## Communication and Language Differences

Much of American society endorses a monolingual, standard English-speaking society, with little tolerance for those languages and dialects that stray from the "norm." The viewpoint expressed in the following quote by Hernandez (1996) echoes the intolerance reflected by the perspectives of many Americans regarding dialect and language differences.

The notion that Black English is a language and that Black kids are actually bilingual is ludicrous and patronizing. Ebonics is ungrammatical English. What students who speak Ebonics need to learn is that they are speaking substandard English and that substandard English brands them as uneducated. (Hernandez, 1996, p. A-21 in Reagan, 1997)

Approximately 35 million persons in the United States speak a language other than English at home, and 20 million of them are not fluent in English (Trueba, 1991). Census projections anticipate, within the next several decades, a dramatic increase in the number of language-minority children in the public schools as American society becomes more culturally and linguistically diverse (Baker, 1993; Corson, 1993).

Among language differences are differences in communication style. Hall (1976), an anthropologist, proposed the concept of high-low context cultures. Communication styles similarly reflect high-low context messages (Sue & Sue, 1990). High-context (HC) communication is less dependent on the verbal aspects of communication than on the nonverbal. Messages are further verified by shared group meaning. HC messages are interpreted based on the actual physical or situational context. Alternatively, low-context (LC) communication places greater emphasis on the explicit verbal code of the message. Cultural characteristics associated with this communication style are opportunism, individualism, and law and procedural orientation (Smith, 1981). HC and LC communication exist on opposing ends of the continuum.

Certain cultures have come to be identified with these styles. The United States is an LC culture as are Switzerland, Germany, and the Scandinavian countries. However, within American society, Asian Americans, African Americans, Hispanic Americans, and Native Americans, as well as other culturally diverse groups, emphasize HC messages (Sue & Sue, 1990). HC communication is slow to change and serves to unify members of its speaking community, unlike LC communication, which is not a unifying force but changes rapidly and easily. HC and LC orientations may lead to misunderstandings between their communicators as messages are subject to misinterpretation and contradiction.

HC communicators place greater value on the nonverbal nuances of proxemics, kinesics, paralinguistics, as well as pragmatic/contextual cues, while LC communicators place greater emphasis on the verbal message conveyed by phonetic, morphological, and semantic meaning. Tables 14-4 through 14-7 provide a summary of high-context communication patterns of African American, Hispanic Americans, Asian Americans, and Native Americans.

These subtle nuances in the communication patterns of culturally and linguistically diverse families may suggest that the task of providing

### TABLE 14-4 Communications Pattern of High-Context Communicators: Native American

Personal questions may be considered prying.

A bowed head is a sign of respect.

Repeating the same question is acceptable when doubting the truthfulness of the speaker.

Greater emphasis is placed on observing others' behavior than on what is said.

Speaking rate is more often slower and softer in intensity.

Response time is measured and slow.

Time and place are viewed as being permanent and settled.

Harmony is sought in relationships and criticism of others is avoided.

Communication style is low key and indirect.

Fewer interjections and less encouragement is communicated during conversation.

From: Cole, 1989; Joe & Malach, 1992; Lynch & Hanson, 1992; Sue & Sue, 1990.

### TABLE 14-5 Communications Pattern of High-Context Communicators: African American

Silence denotes refutation of accusation. Similarly, silence may be assumed in formal situations when interacting with an unfamiliar white speaker.

Communication style is more affective, emotional, and interpersonal.

Call and response patterns (a statement by the speaker is acknowledged or confirmed verbally by the listener) of interaction occur in general and within religious or church services.

Speech communicates affect and response time is quick.

Listeners display limited direct eye contact during conversation, denoting respect and attentiveness.

Touching another person's hair is considered offensive.

Intense (demonstrative, dynamic) emotions may be expressed publicly.

Narrative styles tend to be associational, such that single topics are not maintained but rather linked by the preceding statement.

Clear distinctions are made between aggressive verbal behavior, precipitous to fighting, versus arguing.

Personal inquiry by an unfamiliar person is considered offensive.

Turn taking during conversation is flexible, with tolerance for interruptions and assertiveness.

"Butting in" by outside parties during "private conversation" is not tolerated.

From: Cole, 1989; Lynch & Hanson, 1992; Sue & Sue, 1990; Willis, 1992.

**TABLE 14-6    Communications Pattern of High-Context Communicators: Hispanic American**

Reflecting a high sensitivity to interpersonal relations, nonverbal communication skills are typically used to assess interaction with others, particularly authority figures and others with status.

Hissing may be used as a way to get another person's attention.

Touching and close physical contact during conversation is often the norm.

Indirect eye contact during conversation is a sign of respect and attentiveness, while sustained direct eye contact suggests challenge to one's authority.

Gesturing with large arm movement when communicating is not considered exaggerated or too emotional.

Communication style is low-keyed and indirect.

Non-business-related discussion, greetings, and other pleasantries often precede business meetings and business-related discussions.

Mother–child interactions are primarily nonverbal.

From: Cole, 1989; Lynch & Hanson, 1992; Sue & Sue, 1990; Zuniga, 1992.

**TABLE 14-7    Communications Pattern of High-Context Communicators: Asian Americans**

Speakers tend to be soft-spoken and use silence to communicate agreement, politeness, and respect for the speaker.

Touching and hand-holding by members of the same sex is acceptable in public places, while public display of physical contact among individuals of the opposite sex is viewed as ridiculous and less acceptable.

Shaking the hand of a person of the opposite sex (male/female) is contrary to tradition.

Pragmatic rules regarding social distance, turn-taking, greetings, and politeness are dictated by the interactants' age, class, and marital status, and are strictly adhered to.

To slap another person on the back is not acceptable.

Communication style is low-keyed and indirect.

Beckoning another person with a finger is reserved for adults when beckoning children.

Humility is maintained in all instances.

From: Chan, 1992; Cole, 1989; Lynch & Hanson, 1992; Sue & Sue, 1990.

culturally competent AAC services to infants, toddlers, and their families is somewhat insurmountable. However, Blackstone (1993) provides the following guidelines for delivering AAC services to linguistically diverse children and their families.

1. Accommodate the primary language of the family.
2. Account for the language(s) of the child's communication partners (parents, siblings, etc.).
3. Assume a bilingual augmented communication system can be developed. Dialectal, bilingual, and limited English proficient children will need communication systems that enable them to code switch for home, school, and social use.
4. When possible, choose the child's native dialect.
5. Work closely with families, using a trained interpreter from the same cultural background as the family when needed.
6. Know that direct translations are not always possible and may change or distort meaning.
7. Identify how the family perceives the child's communication impairment and your role as AAC service provider.
8. Base vocabulary selection on the lexical, dialectal, and customary ways of interacting and verify by family members or other individuals of the same culture.
9. Know that commercially available symbols may distort or lack meaning for families that are ethnically, linguistically, or culturally different from the manufacturer. Customize symbols that are culturally relevant.
10. For bilingual and limited English proficient families, label symbols in both their primary and secondary languages.
11. In selecting a speech output communication device, select one that uses digitized speech or is capable of producing synthetic output in the family's language or dialect.
12. Remember that language (oral and non-oral) is culturally bound and must reflect the verbal and nonverbal rules for the child and family.
13. Always respect the culture of the family. Expand your knowledge by learning as much from the family and other available resources as you can and then incorporate it into your intervention.

While AAC infants and toddlers represent diverse cultural and linguistic groups, they share some common characteristics in how they communicate and use language. AAC children will rely on nonverbal forms of communication such as graphic symbols, print and signs, and other symbols outside of spoken words (Blackstone, 1993); communicate in short, simple, less varied linguistic productions; utilize techniques and strategies for enhancing message access and output; and depend on able-bodied communicative partners to co-construct messages.

Graphic symbols are a primary mode of aided expression used by early developing and preliterate AAC communicators. While there are over 35 commercially available symbols sets (Blackstone, 1993), there is limited research that culturally validates their selection and application with culturally and linguistically diverse infants and toddlers. Current practices of utilizing commercial symbol sets while modifying the text or label to reflect the language or dialect of the child loses sight of the linguistic, cognitive, and social value ascribed to graphic symbols. The early introduction of these symbols to young AAC users is important to the acquisition and transmission of communicative, linguistic, and social competence (Hetzroni & Harris, 1996). Harris and Hetzroni (in press) warn that "the choice and use of symbols may impact on the language of the user by imposing a lexical or syntactic organization that may differ from that used in the spoken language or dialect of the child's home."

Symbol selection must take into consideration the functionality or usefulness of the symbol as determined by its pragmatic application; the symbol's meaning as culturally determined; and the symbol's iconicity or clarity by which it resembles its referent (Harris & Hetzroni, in press). The application of these symbol sets must be effective in the social communicative context of the child's family, community, and school.

AAC children will use simple, shorter, and less varied linguistic productions (than their age-matched nondisabled peers) that do not necessarily reflect their linguistic competence (Blackstone, 1993). As members of two microcultures—family/community culture and community of disabled preschoolers—children with disabilities are required to establish linguistic competence that transcends both (family and disabled) cultures, mediating bicultural linguistic environments (Hetzroni & Harris, 1996). As AAC communicators rarely communicate with one another, linguistic competence must be acquired within the child's family/ cultural group.

AAC children will acquire strategies and techniques to enhance speed, coding, and speech output (Blackstone, 1993). Effective and efficient communication is culturally defined. For instance, rate enhancement may determine the efficiency of communication in a cultural context that is time-oriented, but be of less value in a cultural context where the present is valued as well as the importance of allotting time to reflect and to "just be." The technical skills required for a preschool child to operate and master an AAC system are culturally defined levels of access, transmission, and operational skill development (Hetzroni & Harris, 1996).

To operate an AAC device, the preschool AAC user acquires strategies that will differ from those of his or her family and community, yet these strategies (e.g., symbol selection, switch access, signaling, etc.) must meet cultural criteria for acceptability. These strategies are most often taught by the speech-language pathologist with the direct assistance and input of the child's family.

AAC children will depend on able-bodied communication partners to co-construct messages (Blackstone, 1993). Communication partners will have to assume an atypical role as active interactants and role models for the child communicator. Because as child AAC users have limited contact with other child AAC peers, their role models and interactants are most often able-bodied family members (parents, siblings, extended family members, and nondisabled child peers) who require training in system use and strategies. The child's family must assume an active role in decision making, assessment, and program implementation. Program success is dependent on family involvement. Family involvement must begin early in the intervention process, when initial groundwork is laid during the initial assessment.

## *Cross-cultural Assessment*

Taylor and Clark (1994) suggest the need for a "paradigm shift in the assessment of culturally and linguistically diverse children" (Kayser, 1996, p. 385). As language and culture are intertwined, the child's and family's culture must be acknowledged and respected in the assessment and intervention process. Cultural differences exist in family roles and relationships, childrearing practices, play and social relationships, language use, and communicative competence. Consequently, standardized measures based on mainstream norms are often culturally biased and invalid measures for culturally and linguistically diverse children with severe disabilities (Kayser, 1996; Stockman, 1996; Taylor & Clark, 1994). Proponents of this paradigm shift and advocates for culturally valid assessment propose the use of ethnographic interviewing (Blackstone, 1993; Westby, 1990).

Hymes (1962) first introduced the concept of ethnography of communication, describing it as an examination of cultural patterns of language and communication and the functions that they serve in everyday life. Westby (1990) advocates for its clinical application stating:

> to develop appropriate goals for children from diverse cultures, professionals must understand parents' beliefs and values regarding the family's and child's resources and needs; and they must adopt an ecological framework that considers children's

functioning within the broader aspects of their environment. Interviewing provides a means of obtaining the information necessary to develop culturally appropriate family-centered intervention goals. (Westby, 1990, p. 101)

An ethnographic approach requires the service provider to collect qualitative data through an initial interview and repeated observations and to participate in the cultural context of the child being served. Ethnographic assessment is dynamic and serves to tap the multifaceted, complex patterns of verbal and nonverbal interpersonal communication across social contexts (Blackstone, 1993). Procedures for obtaining descriptive documentation of communicative competence requires careful observation of the child and his or her interaction with family, along with family interviews (Blackstone, 1993; Westby, 1990).

As a descriptive measure of the communicative competence of the young AAC user, the ethnographic assessment must evaluate the communication functionality and adequacy of the child within his or her cultural framework. This requires assessing the child's functional communication and the communication of his or her interactants (Hetzroni & Harris, 1996). Both *emic* and *etic* perspectives are taken during assessment for cyclical data collection and analysis (Blackstone, 1993). For more information on ethnography, the reader is referred to the research of Westby (1990), Maxwell (1990), Blackstone (1993), and Spradley (1979).

Light (1989) discusses four interrelated culturally bound areas of communicative competence: linguistic, social, operational, and strategic competencies. As competencies are ever-evolving processes, assessment serves to establish the functionality and adequacy of these competencies in meeting the current demands of the child's social/interactive, family, community, and school needs.

### Communicative Competence

Communicative competencies are ever-evolving processes as the child acquires knowledge, judgment, and skills in the context of his or her cultural environment (Hetzroni & Harris, 1996).

### Linguistic Competence

Linguistic competence requires mastering two cultures, one's indigenous culture and the culture unique to those with a disability (Hetzroni & Harris, 1996). Areas of linguistic competence include semantics (vocabulary and symbol selection), syntax (word order, phrase structure), literacy (use, value, and purpose of written language), and discourse (rules for interrupting, turn-taking, initiating, etc.).

## Social Competence

Social competence or cross-cultural competence requires knowledge, judgment, and skills to understand and adequately function between one's own culture and across settings (Hetzroni & Harris, 1996). Rules for developing social and interpersonal relationships dictate the appropriateness of eye contact, social distance, physical contact, and silence.

## Operational Competence

Operational competency is comprised of those technical skills necessary for accessing, transmitting, and operating a communication device (Hetzroni & Harris, 1996). The selection and use of a communication device and other forms of assistive technology must take into account the social and cultural mores of the child's community and environment. Selection criteria must provide for the rejection or acceptance of high and low technology, mobility aids, speech output devices (synthetic versus digitized), and symbol use. These skills of access, transmission, and system use must be demonstrated within a level of acceptability within the child's family/cultural community.

## Strategic Competence

Strategic competence requires the use of particular systems of strategies of alternative and augmentative communication that vary from verbal communication systems common to the child's family and community (Hetzroni & Harris, 1996). In the absence of culturally matched role models with disabilities, questions must be posed regarding culturally acceptable modes of expression involving the use of symbols, gestures, cues, and so on.

Table 14-8 (O. Harris, 1993; Hetzroni & Harris, 1996) provides questions to assist in the assessment of the four interrelated culturally bound areas of communicative competence: linguistic, social, operational, and strategic competencies.

## Participatory Model of AAC Assessment

The participatory model for AAC assessment utilizes observations of the AAC child and his or her nondisabled peer(s) across settings (Beukelman & Mirenda, 1992) utilizing an activity/standards inventory. Daily activities that are important in the child's life across settings are outlined by the AAC team for observation. Similarly, observations of parallel activities are made and assessed of the nondisabled, age-, and culture-matched peer. Assessment of behaviors across settings allows for comparisons to be made between the nondisabled child and the child with disabilities. Comparing their level of performance, discrepancies are noted and examined

**TABLE 14-8    Guidelines for Cultural Assessment Intervention**

| | |
|---|---|
| *Linguistic Competency* | |
| Semantics | Are there lexical items particular to the culture, community, family, and/or peer group? What words are used with whom? |
| Syntax | What are the culture's syntax rules? Are there opportunities for code switching? |
| Literacy | Is written language prevalent? What is the level of literacy of peers and other interactants? |
| Discourse | What are the rules for social interaction, greeting, initiating, and terminating conversation? Is information repeated? Is turn taking encouraged? |
| Other | |
| | |
| *Social Competency* | |
| Eye Contact | When is eye contact used/avoided? |
| Nonverbal | Is touching appropriate? What is appropriate social distance? |
| Silence | When is silence expected? How long should silence be maintained? |
| Other | |
| | |
| *Operational Competence* | |
| Access | Are mobility aids accepted? Is increased independence desired by the client and family members? |
| Transmission | Is synthetic/digitized speech output accepted? Is silence expected? |
| Technology | Is technology (high/low) accepted? |
| System Use | Are symbols accepted? What types? |
| Other | |
| | |
| *Strategic Competency* | |
| Gestures | Are gestures accepted? What do they mean? |
| Cues | What cues are used to assist in communication? When are these cues used? |

From: O. Harris, 1993; Hetzroni & Harris, 1996.

to determine the presence of specific opportunity (interference outside of the AAC child) and access (capabilities of the AAC child's and/or AAC system) barriers.

Opportunity barriers include policy, practice, attitude, knowledge, and skill, while access barriers include current communication, environment, natural abilities, system utilization, capability, and operational requirements. The final goal of this process is to gather sufficient information for the child, child's family, AAC team members, and other professionals to establish intervention for the current and future communication needs (Beukelman & Mirenda, 1992).

Utilizing an ethnographic approach to AAC cross-cultural assessment of infants and toddlers of diverse cultural groups provides the clinician insight into the sociocultural and contextual aspects of emerging competencies in linguistic, social, operational, and strategic skill development.

Several principles of assessment and intervention for culturally and linguistically diverse AAC preschool children and their families are suggested by Hetzroni and Harris (1996). AAC service providers as well as all participants of the AAC team bring their own cultural experiences to the clinical process. However, communication and language are socially and culturally based and should occur as a collaborative process among the consumer, family, community, and service provider in spite of differences in cultural perspectives. Because the success of intervention is determined by the family's involvement, close communication between the family and AAC professional should occur through out the delivery of AAC services.

The *Scale to Assess World Views* (SAWV, Ibrahim & Kahn, 1987) is an instrument to assess and understand the client's/family's world view and cultural identity from a cognitive values perspective. Both the service provider's and the client's world view (e.g., ethnicity, culture, gender, age, life stage, socioeconomic status, education, religion, philosophy of life, beliefs, values, and assumptions) need to be clarified. Once clarified, the world views must be placed within a sociopolitical context (e.g., history of migration, acculturation level, languages spoken, and comfort with mainstream assumptions and value) (Ibrahim, 1991). Information gained from the SAWV can be instrumental in establishing appropriate intervention and goals that are culturally sensitive and culturally relevant.

Upon establishing the child's family cultural identity, the following areas should be considered via an ethnographic interview.

1. What are the perceptions of the child's/family's cultural group by society?
2. Is race a factor?
3. What is the sociopolitical history of the child's family group?
4. What language is spoken in the home (by parents, siblings, extended family members, etc.)?
5. What is the impact of gender from an ethnic/cultural and majority culture perspective?
6. What is the current neighborhood in which the child/family resides?
7. What religion(s) does the child/family subscribe to?
8. What is the family life/cycle history?

An awareness of and sensitivity to the child's family cultural identity is the first step to the delivery of culturally sensitive family-centered AAC services to culturally and linguistically diverse families.

## CULTURALLY SENSITIVE FAMILY-CENTERED EARLY INTERVENTION SERVICES IN AAC

"**Cultures** do not represent formulas or categories, nor do they prescribe service delivery methods" (Blackstone, 1993). Early intervention services cannot be relegated to generic strategies and techniques when serving specific culturally diverse families. The variations among and within groups are quite diverse. Culturally sensitive early intervention services must recognize diversity within groups, taking the following variables into consideration: (1) microcultures within macrocultures, (2) time of immigration, (3) past experiences, (4) socioeconomic status, (5) family unit, (6) ties to the community, and (7) level of acculturation.

These and other cultural issues must be considered prior to making recommendations for early intervention services and when prescribing AAC services (Ratcliffe, Cress, & Soto, 1997). It is the responsibility of the AAC early interventionist to address the needs of each family through collaborative efforts that serve to build on family strengths and empower family members. Furthermore, effectiveness of culturally sensitive early intervention services must be based on outcome measures that assess family satisfaction and need as well as provide qualitative and quantitative measures of the child's communicative skills.

### Principles of Family-Centered Services and Transcultural Caring

There is a wide acceptance of family-centered approaches to problem solving. However, there have been too few treatment theories and models that include the cultural values and family structures of ethnic families. The following principles of family-centered services (Blackstone, 1993) should be considered in the delivery of early intervention services to culturally and linguistically diverse families.

1. Culture influences each family's life cycle, structure, and relationships.
2. Each family member's roles, values, and perceptions are influenced by the family member with a disability. The level of influence is determined by the disabled family member's level of adaptation.

3. Each family's personal reactions to disability impacts the family's reaction to intervention (e.g., trust, knowledge, ambivalence, fear, resistance).
4. In spite of the diversity of the AAC community, diverse groups share some characteristics while exhibiting divergence in others.
5. Family-centered early intervention services in AAC require an ethnographic approach incorporating both *emic* (participant's/insider's) and *etic* (outsider's) perspectives.

Researchers (Leininger, 1987; Mizio & Delaney, 1981; Tseng & McDermott, 1975) have called for transcultural learning modes of helping culturally diverse families. Transcultural caring of culturally diverse families means the deliberate and creative use of cultural care knowledge and skills to assist families in attaining their well-being and living productively (Leininger, 1987).

Acknowledging the multiple sources of stress that impact families' lives is important to effective transcultural caring. The stress of day-to-day living, life changes, birth, death, financial problems, moving, divorce, illness, and having a child with a disability are all challenges to family structure and stability (Blackstone, 1993). Service delivery systems can be another source of stress, particularly if they are not collaborative and lack sensitivity/attentiveness to these compounding stressors. In addition to the limited research to date examining family-centered services in AAC, we can build from research in family systems theory, family-centered planning, and team process techniques. Few studies to date address family-centered early intervention in AAC. The following studies serve to illustrate the impact of family-centered services on the success of AAC service delivery to culturally diverse families.

One particular study by Smith-Lewis (1993) examined the home/school interaction of culturally diverse students receiving AAC services. The study participants were three African American, two Latino, two Italian, and three Anglo-American families. The participants in the study were middle and high school students who had received AAC services for three to four years. Three of the students were using electronic communication devices, while the remaining used sign language or low-tech devices.

An interview of both parents and teachers in this study found that the two groups used quite different descriptors in their discussion of the children's performance. Where school personnel described the children using medical and diagnostic terms, families gave psychosocial descriptions of their children, their dislikes and likes, and certain personality traits. Review of home videotapes of the children's interactions revealed a surprising level of communicative competence in the absence of home and community use of the prescribed AAC system.

Differences were also noted in the degree of input and consequently the level of acceptance parents had in the selection of their child's AAC system. Anglo-American families proved to be the only families who expressed an interest in technology; however, none of the participating families felt they had agreed on the AAC system prescribed for their children. In one instance where sign language was attempted in one Latino home, it was reported that the use of American Sign Language (ASL) served to further separate the child from her family, who spoke primarily Spanish.

This study serves to illustrate what has been reported in other case studies and ethnographic studies (Meyers & Blancher, 1987; Sims, 1997): Recommendations for AAC systems were made with little or no parent input. In such instances, AAC systems often go unused and unsupported by families. Family members have a critical impact on the success of AAC practices.

The limited knowledge base in the area of family-centered services in AAC has caught the attention of the International Society for Augmentative and Alternative Communication (ISAAC). A research agenda (Blackstone, 1994) for examining the impact of AAC on family systems across the life span was proposed to address the following questions:

1. What do families do for and with AAC users and their AAC devices?
2. What are families willing to do?
3. How do families adapt to professionals?
4. What are major issues that families face across the life span?
5. How do families' perceptions of professionals affect outcome?
6. What are appropriate outcome measures: parent's perception of support, observation, questionnaires, rating scales, interviews, etc.?

An ethnographic approach in investigating family satisfaction and need provides some insight to answering these and other questions pertaining to family-centered services. Bridges and Pottschmidt (1996) investigated parent satisfaction and needs in early intervention in AAC across culturally diverse families using an ethnographic approach. Six families (three African American, three European American) in North Carolina were interviewed using an ethnographic interview instrument designed and validated by the investigators. Results of the study revealed that parents felt that AAC systems were important to meeting their children's communication needs in most family and social situations. The areas identified as important for the application of an AAC system included home/family activities, personal needs, play, and recreation, classroom participation, community participation, studying/learning, and religious activities and celebrations.

Further, parents ascribed a high level of performance to their child's participation in the following activities: expression of daily needs, answering questions, expressing feelings, understanding directions, establishing relationships with children of the same culture, interacting with role models of the same culture, and participating in cultural activities/celebrations.

When asked, "What good experiences (e.g., things you liked best, were helpful, etc.) have you had in receiving AAC services?" and "What bad experiences (e.g., frustrations, anxieties, disappointments, etc.) have you had in receiving AAC services?", parents' reports revealed repeated themes of teaching/learning, capabilities, collaboration, struggle, responsiveness, time, finances, and implementation across good and bad experiences.

Bridges and Pottschmidt (1996) summarized their findings by stating that it is critical that service delivery models serve to empower families by:

1. Being responsive and sensitive to family values, needs, and priorities.
2. Recognizing families' time constraints and coordinating services accordingly.
3. Demonstrating to families within their homes and cultural/family context functional ways of integrating the use of AAC systems in their day-to-day routines.
4. Identifying and responding to family stressors with appropriate supports and resources.
5. Collaborating with other professionals and family members (parents, siblings, and extended family members) in developing an appropriate AAC system and treatment approach.
6. Teaching and aiding parents in learning ways to assist their children in communicating in a variety of settings across a variety of activities.

The application of these findings can be best illustrated in the following case study of "S" (Bridges & Pottschmidt, 1996; Jarvis, 1997) a 4-year-old African American child, henceforth referred to as Michael. This case study illustrates the application of an ethnographic model to service delivery and family empowerment in early intervention AAC services.

## A Case Study

Michael is a 4-year-old African American child with a diagnosis of spastic quadriplegic cerebral palsy. Motor limitations restrict his ability to pick up, grasp, and manipulate objects, as well as his ability to reach and point. Michael is nonambulatory but recently received an adapted wheelchair with postural supports. The older son of Tracie and Albert, Michael has a younger brother, Derrick. At 18 months of age, Derrick was recently diagnosed with developmental delays and evaluated for speech and language therapy. Michael attends an inclusive day program with disabled and nondisabled peers where he receives occupational, physical, and speech therapy services. Classroom activities include circle time, snack, lunch, and free time (play).

At the time of our initial contact, Michael had previously been evaluated at the Children's Hospital for an augmentative communication system. A Mac Powerbook with switch access (Buddy Buttons), synthetic voice output, and software support (Board-maker, Mayer-Johnson Co.; Speaking Dynamically, Mayer-Johnson, Co., etc.) were recommended. The goal of our initial contact was to identify family need and satisfaction with AAC services to date and to establish an AAC early intervention program that would serve to meet Michael's needs now and support his needs for the future. Such a program requires establishing the family's level of satisfaction and need using an ethnographic approach, establishing Michael's current level of communication, and identifying the discrepancies that exist between his communication ability and that of his nondisabled peer (within an appropriate cultural context).

### An Ethnographic Approach
An ethnographic interview was conducted with Michael's mom, using the *Family Satisfaction and Needs Interview* (Bridges & Pottschmidt, 1996). Tracie reported that an important need for her was to have a team of professionals assist her in making her home more adaptable for Michael and to advise her as to what to do and where to go. She felt she could benefit from support from other African American families with children with disabilities and gain greater knowledge and access to resources. Financial support was needed to assist with the purchasing of special equipment for Michael and for seeking respite services.

For Michael's communication needs, Tracie reported that she would like her son to be able to make choices and to play with his brother and independently play with his toys. She believed it was most important that Michael be able to express his daily needs, share personal information and ideas, ask and answer questions, and read and write stories. Other activities reported to be very important were expressing feelings, playing with other children and adults, establishing relationships with children of the same culture, interacting with role models of like culture and participating in cultural activities and celebrations. She also added that attending church was an important family activity, such that she wanted Michael to be able to participate in Sunday School and church service (lead and sing along with the church congregation, greet the minister and other parishioners, etc.) and answer questions posed during Sunday School.

## Formal and Informal Assessment

The *Nonspeech Test* (Huer, 1988), an assessment instrument for children with varying levels of disability, was administered via family interviews, observation, and elicitation to establish receptive and expressive levels of communication. Michael received receptive and expressive age equivalent scores of 23 to 26 months.

The participation model (Beukelman & Mirenda, 1992) was used to assess Michael's communication needs and skills, to identify barriers, and to establish treatment approaches. Peer observations at home and school revealed that Michael enjoyed looking at *Barney* videotapes, but was unable to participate in the singalong with his classmates. Limited participation was evident during circle time as well, as Michael responded vocally when his name was called and smiled during singalong and when questions were asked about days of the week, colors, and numbers. Participation was further limited when Michael's physical therapy overlapped with circle time.

At snack time Michael was able to communicate his snack preferences by smiling/frowning and responding yes/no to choice-making questions. Free play provided the children with several play options, including activities with toys, the computer, and the sand table. During lunch, Michael was placed at a table separate from his classmates. Food options were not made available to him, although he could indicate yes/no when he wanted more or less of any one item. Similar observations were noted at home where Michael was observed engaging in play, eating at meal time, and interacting with his parents and his brother.

Children with disabilities are often at risk for delayed social, cognitive, and linguistic abilities as a result of lack of opportunity to engage in those experiences (play, life experiences, social interaction, exploration, interaction, etc.) that are critical to their development. Consequently, a treatment model that serves to identify and remove or overcome those barriers is essential to the initiation of any treatment approach that purports to be practical and effective.

Numerous barriers were evident when Michael's performance was compared to that of a nondisabled African American classmate as well as that of his younger brother. Discrepancies were particularly evident when barriers to access were a factor. Overcoming accessibility barriers required modifying Michael's positioning by placing him in a supported position on the floor to play with his peers; making switch-activated toys available for him to have play options during free time; providing switch access to the classroom computer for increased learning opportunities; providing voice output for expanding opportunities for choice making and participating in group (classroom, church, community) and one-on-one activities; and providing opportunities for engaging in interactive play with his peers, family members, and role models. Overcoming these barriers required prioritizing and establishing goals.

Communication goals were established by Michael's interdisciplinary team and his parents. IFSP goals were as follows:

Michael will play with a toy independently.

Michael will interact with his peers during free play and structured activities.

Michael will indicate his preferences given two choices.

Michael will answer questions using a multimodal AAC system.

Several switches were identified for Michael's trial use. These included a puff and sip switch that Michael used in the classroom for activating the desktop computer to access computer games and preliteracy/talking book software programs. This further provided him a wealth of other learning options available through computer access. A wobble switch was used on a trial basis for activating battery-operated adapted toys that Michael could access while supported on the floor and playing with the other children. Similarly, both switches were available for his use once he began using his laptop Powerbook computer.

Providing Michael with opportunities to engage in play served to encourage his growth in a variety of areas: social skills, language skills (content, form, function), functional age and culturally appropriate communication style, and an active role in initiating and maintaining interaction. Through play, children learn the properties of objects and the relationship between them. They learn interaction with peers and adults and gain opportunities to directly control their environment and make choices. Furthermore, participation in reading and story telling activities is important for the development of early literacy skills.

Recommendations were made for recording simple choice-making messages and interactive phrases on loop tapes and talking switches that allowed the use of prerecorded voice and other recorded messages. The voice of another child matched for age, gender, and voice type (e.g., an

African American peer who was a friend of Michael's) was used to record interactive messages, and familiar classroom and Bible songs for Michael to "sing along."

Michael's mother met with the assistive technology specialist to develop an initial vocabulary of symbols and phrases for Michael to use as well as family pictures and photos to scan into his computer. Much of this vocabulary was for home and community use. Inservice training was provided to Michael's mother for symbol selection and programming and storing vocabulary. Tracie was put in touch with the Parent to Parent Family Support Network, which provides family support services. Currently, an updated directory is being completed of early intervention services highlighting programs with specialized services for culturally and linguistically diverse families. In addition, Michael's family was placed in touch with several loan programs and assistive technology lending libraries in the area.

### Concluding Remarks

Michael's communication needs and abilities will continue to change as he continues to develop and grow. He will continue to benefit from a multimodal communication system and assistive devices to support his multiple needs and abilities. The assessment and intervention model illustrated in this case study emphasizes the need for disciplines to provide a partnership with one another as well as families in a way that is sensitive to their needs and serves to empower them. Assessment and intervention is a dynamic and ongoing process. An ethnographic approach in the delivery of early intervention AAC family-centered services to culturally and linguistically diverse families is key to designing intervention that is culturally sensitive and relevant to the families that we serve.

## STUDY QUESTIONS AND ACTIVITIES

1. What are some disabling conditions where AAC could potentially be of benefit to clients?
2. What are some reasons culturally diverse individuals underutilize and prematurely terminate health and educational services?
3. Discuss three general principles that may be a solution to some of the current challenges to providing culturally appropriate service delivery.
4. List six factors that culturally sensitive therapists must take into account to develop an *emic* view.
5. Discuss Blackstone's (1993) guidelines for delivering AAC services to linguistically diverse children and their families.

# REFERENCES

American Speech-Language-Hearing Association. (1991a). Report: Augmentative and alternative communication. *Asha, 33*(Suppl. 5), 8.

American Speech-Language-Hearing Association. (1991b). Augmentative and alternative communication. *Asha, 33*(Suppl. 5), 9–12.

American Speech-Language-Hearing Association. (1993). *1993 Omnibus survey results.* Rockville, MD: Author.

American Speech-Language-Hearing Association. (1998). *Summary membership and affiliation counts by race/ethnicity for the period January 1–June 30, 1997.* Rockville, MD: Author.

Atkinson, D. R., & Juntunen, C. L. (1994). School counselors and school psychologists as school-home-community liaisons in ethnically diverse schools. In P. Pedersen & J. C. Carey (Eds.), *Multicultural counseling in schools.* (p. 103–120). Boston: Allyn & Bacon.

Baker, C. (1993). *Foundations of bilingual education and bilingualism.* Clevedon, Avon, England: Multilingual Matters.

Beukelman, D., & Mirenda, P. (1992). *Augmentative and alternative communication: Management of severe communication disorders in children and adults.* Baltimore: Paul H. Brookes.

Blackstone, S. (1986). *Augmentative communication: An introduction.* Rockville, MD: ASHA.

Blackstone, S. (1993). *Augmentative Communication News, 6*(2).

Blackstone, S. (1994). *Augmentative Communication News, 7*(6).

Bridges, S. & Pottschmidt, M. (1996). *Early intervention in AAC: A survey of parent satisfaction.* Presented at the American Speech-Language-Hearing Association Annual Convention, Seattle, WA.

Carter, R. T. (1991). Cultural values: A review of empirical research and implications for counseling. *Journal of Counseling and Development, 70,* 164–173.

Chan, S. (1992). Families with Asian American roots. In E. Lynch & M. Hanson (Eds.), *Developing cross-cultural competence.* (p. 181–257). Baltimore, MD: Paul Brookes.

Cheng, L. (1996). Enhancing communication: Toward optimal language learning for limited English proficient students. *Language, Speech and Hearing in Schools, 27,* 347–354.

Cheng, L., Breakey, L., & Wallace, G. (1997). Asian Americans: Culture, communication, and clinical management. In G. Wallace (Ed.), *Multicultural neurogenics* (p. 227–242). San Antonio: Communication Skill Builders.

Church, G., & Glennen, S. (1992). *The handbook of assistive technology.* San Diego, CA: Singular Publishing.

Cole, L. (1989). E pluribus pluribus: Multicultural imperative for the 1990s and beyond. *Asha, 31*(9) 65–70.

Corson, D. (1993). *Language, minority education and gender.* Clevedon, Avon, England: Multilingual Matters.

Doerner, W. (1985, July 8). Asians: To America with skills. *Time,* pp. 42–44.

Gall, S. B., & Gall, T. L. (1993). *Statistical record of Asian Americans*. Washington, DC: Gale Research.

Hall, E. T. (1976). *Beyond culture*. New York: Anchor Press.

Harris, G. (1993). American Indian cultures: A lesson in diversity. In D. Battle (Ed.), *Communication disorders in multicultural populations* (pp. 79–113). Boston: Andover Medical Publishers.

Harris, O. (1993). Role of cultural elements in communication behaviors. *Augmentative Communication News, 6*(2), 5.

Harris, O., & Hetzroni, O. (in press). Cultural issues in symbol selection for AAC users. *ECHO*.

Hernandez, R. (1996, December 26). Never mind teaching Ebonics: Teach proper English. *The Hartford Courant*, p. A-21.

Hetzroni, O., & Harris, O. (1996). Cultural aspects in the development of AAC users. *AAC: Augmentative and Alternative Communication, 12*(1), 52–58.

Huer, M. (1988). *The nonspeech test*. Wauconda, IL: Don Johnston, Inc.

Hymes, D. (1962). The ethnography of speaking. In T. Gladwin & W. C. Stortevant (Eds.), *Anthropology and human behavior* (pp. 13–53). Washington, DC: Anthropological Society of Washington.

Ibrahim, F. A. (1991). Contribution of cultural world view to generic counseling and development. *Journal of Counseling and Development, 70*, 13–19.

Ibrahim, F. A., & Kahn, H. (1987). Assessment of world views. *Psychological Reports, 60*, 163–176.

Jarvis, M. (1997). *Development of a family-centered AAC system for multicultural populations: A treatment model*. Unpublished master's project, North Carolina Central University, Durham, NC.

Joe, J., & Malach, R. (1992). Families with Native American roots. In E. Lynch & M. Hanson (Eds.), *Developing cross-cultural competence* (pp. 89–119). Baltimore: Paul Brookes.

Kayser, H. (1996). Cultural/linguistic variation in the United States and its implications for assessment and intervention in speech-language pathology: An epilogue. *Language, Speech, and Hearing Services in Schools, 27*, 385–387.

Kuster, J. (1997). Multicultural/diversity internet resources. *Asha, 39*(2), 46.

Leininger, M. M. (1987). Transcultural caring: A different way to help people. In P. Pedersen (Ed.), *Handbook of cross-cultural counseling and therapy* (pp. 107–115). New York: Praeger Publishing.

Light, J. (1989). Toward a definition of communication competence for individuals using augmentative and alternative communication systems. *Augmentative and Alternative Communication, 5*, 137–144.

Lynch, E., & Hanson, M. (Eds.). (1992). *Developing cross-cultural competence*. Baltimore: Paul Brookes.

Maxwell, M. (1990). The authenticity of ethnographic research. *Journal of Childhood Communication Disorders, 13*(1), 1–12.

Meyers, C. B., & Blancher, J. (1987). Parents' perceptions of schooling for severely handicapped children: Home and family variables. *Exceptional Children, 53*(5), 441–449.

Midgette, T. E. (1988). *Effects of a structured program about psychotherapy on low-income psychiatric inpatients.* Unpublished doctoral dissertation, Michigan State University, East Lansing, MI.

Midgette, T., & Meggert, S. S. (1991). Multicultural counseling instruction: A challenge to faculties in the 21st century. *Journal of Counseling and Development, 70,* 136–141.

Mizio, E., & Delaney, A. (Eds.). (1981). *Training for service delivery to minority clients.* New York: Family Service Association.

Musselwhite, C., & St. Louis, K. (1988). *Communication programming for persons with severe handicaps: Vocal and augmentative strategies.* Boston: College-Hill Publications.

Ratcliffe, A., Cress, C., & Soto, G. (1997). Communication isn't just talking: What's new in AAC. *Asha, 39*(2), 30–36.

Reagan, T. (May–June 1997). The case for applied linguistics in teacher education. *Journal of Teacher Education, 48*(3), 185–196.

Reyes, B. A., & Peterson, C. (1997). Hispanic Americans: Culture, communication, and clinical management. In G. Wallace (Ed.), *Multicultural neurogenics* (pp. 165–191). San Antonio: Communication Skill Builders.

Saville-Troike, M. (1989). Anthropological considerations in the study of communication. In O. Taylor (Ed.), *Nature of communication disorders in culturally and linguistically diverse populations* (pp. 47–72). Austin, TX: Pro-Ed.

Shekar, C., & Hegde, M. N. (1996). Cultural and linguistic diversity among Asian Indians: A case of Indian English. *Topics in Language Disorders, 16*(4), 54–64.

Sims, M. (1997). *Survey of parental satisfaction and need for family centered augmentative alternative communication services.* Unpublished master's project, North Carolina Central University, Durham, NC.

Smith, E. J. (1981). Cultural and historical perspectives in counseling blacks. In D. W. Sue (Ed.), *Counseling the culturally different: Theory and practice.* New York: John Wiley.

Smith-Lewis, J. (1993). Culturally diverse nonspeakers: Home/school interactions. *Augmentative Communication News, 6*(2), 6.

Spradley, J. (1979). *The ethnographic interview.* New York: Holt, Rinehart and Winston.

Stockman, I. (1996). The promises and pitfalls of language sample analysis as an assessment tool for linguistic minority children. *Language, Speech, and Hearing Services in Schools, 27,* 355–366.

Sue, D. W., & Sue, D. (1990). *Counseling the culturally different: Theory and practice* (2nd ed.). New York: Wiley & Sons.

Taylor, O. (1986). *Nature of communication disorders in culturally and linguistically diverse populations.* Austin, TX: Pro-Ed.

Taylor, O., & Clark, M. (1994). Culture and communication disorders: A theoretical framework. *Seminars in Speech and Language, 15*(2), 103–114.

Trueba, H. (1991). The role of culture on bilingual instruction: Linking linguistic and cognitive development to cultural knowledge. In O. Garcia (Ed.), *Bilingual education: Focusschrift in honor of Joshua A. Fishman on the occasion of his 65th birthday* (Vol. 1, pp. 43–55). Amsterdam: John Benjamins.

Tseng, W., & McDermott, J. (1975). Psychotherapy: Historical roots, universal elements and cultural variations. *American Journal of Psychiatry, 132,* 378–384.

Tsui, P., & Schultz, G. (1985). Failure of rapport: When psychotherapeutic engagement fails in the treatment of Asian clients. *American Journal of Orthopsychiatry, 55,* 561–569.

Wallace, G. (1997). *Multicultural neurogenics.* San Antonio: Communication Skill Builders.

Westby, C. (1990). Ethnographic interviewing: Asking the right questions to the right people in the right way. *Journal of Childhood Communication Disorders, 12*(1), 101–111.

Willis, W. (1992). Families with African American roots. In E. Lynch & M. Hanson (Eds.), *Developing cross-cultural competence* (pp. 121–150). Baltimore: Paul Brookes.

Yamamoto, J., & Acosta, R. X. (1982). Treatment of Asian-American and Hispanic-Americans: Similarities and differences. *Journal of the Academy of Psychoanalysis, 10,* 585–607.

Zuniga, M. (1992). Families with Latino roots. In E. Lynch & M. Hanson (Eds.), *Developing cross-cultural competence* (pp. 151–179). Baltimore: Paul Brookes.

# INDEX